D0210312

Health Care Reform
& the Law in Canada

Meeting the Challenge

Health Care Reform
& the Law in Canada

Meeting the Challenge

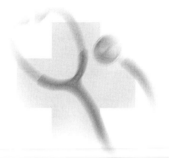

Timothy
A. CAULFIELD
Barbara   *editors*
VON TIGERSTROM

Published by
The University of Alberta Press
Ring House 2
Edmonton, Alberta T6G 2E1

This volume copyright © 2002 The University of Alberta Press
All rights reserved.

National Library of Canada Cataloguing in Publication Data
Main entry under title:
Health care reform and the law

Includes bibliographical references.
ISBN 0-88864-366-7

1. Health care reform--Canada. 2. Medical laws and
legislation--Canada. I.Von Tigerstrom, Barbara, 1969- II.
Caulfield, Timothy A., 1963-
KE3404.Z85H42 2001   344.71'04   C2001-910941-5
KF3605.A75H42 2001

No part of this publication may be produced, stored in a retrieval system, or
transmitted in any form or by any means—electronic, photocopying, recording, or
otherwise—without the prior permission of the copyright owner.

The University of Alberta Press acknowledges the financial support of the
Government of Canada through the Book Publishing Industry Development
Program for its publishing activities. The Press also gratefully acknowledges the
support received for its program from the Canada Council for the Arts.

 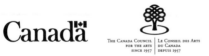

Printed and bound in Canada by Hignell Book Printing Ltd., Winnipeg, Manitoba.
∞ Printed on acid-free paper.
Copyedited by Carol Berger.
Proofreading by Tara Taylor.
Book design by Gregory Brown.

CONTENTS

CONTRIBUTORS

PETER CARVER is assistant professor, Faculty of Law and Faculty of Rehabilitation Medicine, University of Alberta.

TIMOTHY A. CAULFIELD is Canada Research Chair in Health Law and Policy; associate professor, Faculty of Law and Faculty of Medicine and Dentistry; Research Director, Health Law Institute, University of Alberta, and a Population Health Investigator, Alberta Health Foundation for Medical Research.

SUJIT CHOUDHRY is assistant professor, Faculty of Law and Joint Centre for Bioethics, University of Toronto. An earlier version of this talk was presented at the Canadian Association of Law Teachers Annual Congress in May 2000. This paper is the first part of a larger project tentatively entitled "Recasting Social Canada: A Reconsideration of Federal Jurisdiction over Social Policy," and was previously published in *Osgoode Hall Law Journal* 38:1, July 2000.

COLLEEN M. FLOOD is assistant professor, Faculty of Law, University of Toronto.

E. RICHARD GOLD is BCE Chair in E-Commerce, Faculty of Law, McGill University; senior fellow, Einstein Institute for Science, Health and the Courts; and research associate, Health Law Institute, University of Alberta. The opinions expressed in this chapter are those of the author and do not necessarily represent those of the Einstein Institute for Science, Health and the Courts or of the Health Law Institute.

MOE M. LITMAN is professor of law and chair of the Health Law Institute, Faculty of Law, University of Alberta. The research for this article was funded by a grant from the University's Small Faculties Research Fund.

BARBARA VON TIGERSTROM was the project coordinator for the Health Law Institute in 1999–2000 and led the Institute's health reform project in its first year. She is currently working towards her Ph.D. in the Faculty of Law at the University of Cambridge.

BRENT WINDWICK is executive director of the Health Law Institute, University of Alberta, and a partner with the firm of Field Atkinson Perraton in Edmonton, Alberta.

PREFACE

The question of health care reform has emerged as one of Canada's "hot button" issues, preoccupying not only our politicians but the medical community and the public it serves. Surveys consistently show that Canadians view health care to be *the* critical social issue, over even the economy and education. It is no surprise, then, that the issues and implications of health care reform are keeping a broad array of academic disciplines very busy. Economics, ethics, political science, sociology and health administration are but a few of the disciplines that are engaged in the health care debate.

Of course, legal scholars have also contributed to this area. In fact, it is hard to imagine a facet of health care reform that doesn't have some type of legal ramification. Cost-containment initiatives trigger unique malpractice dilemmas. Policies to allow the further privatization of our health care system raise questions about the application and adequacy of the Canada Health Act. New health care initiatives, such as a home care program, may require novel legal structures. The law is also closely tied to the making of broader health care policies. Whether it is the constitution, case law, legislation or regulatory policy, law can represent both the practical application of health policy and a reaction to it. It sets the framework within which policy decisions are made, establishes the legal duties and obligations of health professionals and ascribes rights and remedies to the users of Canada's health care system. The language of the law has come to permeate much of contemporary policy and ethical discourse, providing both a vocabulary and a public forum—courts and legislatures—for health policy debates.

In the summer of 1999 the Health Law Institute at the University of Alberta received funding from the Alberta Law Foundation for an education and research project on the legal aspects of health care reform. Given the dynamic nature of the province's health care reform, such an initiative seemed both essential and timely. This ongoing initiative has resulted in a series of public lectures, the publication of articles on various health reform topics in academic journals and the popular press, and the compilation of a bibliography of materials on legal issues in health reform. The bibliography has already been used by many individuals and organizations and is included in this book to provide those interested in reading further with a guide to some of the literature on this topic. Finally, this collection of essays was conceived as a way of engaging Canadian legal academics in the project and advancing the literature on a broad range of subjects relating to health reform and the law.

Although not intended to be a comprehensive overview of the relevant issues, this collection does provide a sense of the breadth of legal topics. The collection includes papers on everything from topics not usually associated with health law, such as international trade, to the more conventional, such as the Canada Health Act and malpractice. The papers also highlight how legal scholarship analyzes not only how the law is responding to challenges in health reform but how it ought to. For example, the chapters on fiduciary and malpractice law seek to describe how the current jurisprudence might respond to the current health reform environment. The chapters on international trade and human rights law suggest how the law in these areas establishes some limits and a framework for analyzing proposed reforms. The chapter on mental health law shows how the law can be used both to construct and to critically assess reforms in health care. Legal institutions, specifically supervisory institutions, are the central concern of the chapter on the Canada Health Act and Bill 11.

It has been a pleasure working with all of the contributors to this collection. We thank them not only for contributing their excellent written work, but also for participating more broadly in the exchange of ideas about law and health reform that we sought to encourage as part of our project. We would also like to thank Nina Hawkins, Vanessa Cosco and Bonnie Bokenfohr for their invaluable assistance with the project and this collection and, of course, the Alberta Law Foundation for its continued and generous support of the Health Law Institute.

I

MALPRACTICE IN THE AGE OF HEALTH CARE REFORM

TIMOTHY A. CAULFIELD

O ver the past ten years it has been difficult to pick up a newspaper without finding some reference to the perceived failures of the Canadian health care system. "Doctor Blames 'Needless Death' on Health Cuts,"[1] "Hospital Apologizes to Parents After Baby Born on Road,"[2] "Overcrowding Blamed for Deaths,"[3] "Emergency Backlog Led to Patient's Death"[4]—the examples of headlines underscoring the turmoil in the health care sector seem endless. And, indeed, few would disagree that the health care system has been under tremendous pressure. There have been massive cuts in provincial and federal health care budgets, a broad array of new technologies has been introduced, health delivery systems have been restructured and private for-profit alternatives expanded. And all at a time when the population is aging and becoming more demanding of the health care system. Providing health care in this environment is an increasingly difficult and complex challenge.

This chapter investigates how Canadian malpractice law may respond to the dramatic changes that are occurring in the health care system. In particular, I explore how cost restraint pressures, both formal and informal, and the growing availability of private options may impact physicians' obligations and liability exposure. In many respects, the application of existing malpractice law in the context of health care reform and cost-containment pressures adds confusion to an already chaotic situation. Indeed, malpractice law generates unique dilemmas for both physicians and patients. For physicians, the law creates unusual and onerous disclosure obligations and places them in precarious conflicts of duty. From the perspective of the patient, malpractice law has the positive effect of reinforcing the health care provider's obligation to do that which is in the patient's best interest. However, in some situations the application of existing tort principles, such as the modified objective test used in informed consent cases, may actually magnify the inequities inherent in a two-tiered system.

An examination of malpractice law in this context also highlights the disconnect between the operation of tort principles and more broadly based engines of social change, such as the political process.[5] Simply put, whether one favours privatization or is an advocate of the public system, tort law is not the best tool for effectuating health care reform. Malpractice lawsuits are determined on a case-by-case basis. They focus on the rights and legal duties of individual physicians and patients. And while the principles of tort law obviously have social utility, such as the compensation of patients who are injured by negligence, the rights and duties of patients and physicians are rarely subordinated to the needs of the broader health care system. For example, the current malpractice jurisprudence, rightly or not, encourages physicians to ignore cost-constraint policies while, at the same time, obligating physicians to disclose information about private health care options. Although many citizens may turn to malpractice law when they believe health care reform has resulted in an injustice,[6] the resolution of such lawsuits will be based more on the relevant malpractice jurisprudence than on the social policies that inform health care reform initiatives. This chapter seeks to shed some light on how such cases may actually play out.

The chapter begins with a brief discussion of the general policy and ethical issues associated with health care reform. While many of these issues are not strictly legal in nature, it is important to ground the chapter in the context of the current health care environment. This section is followed by an examination of a selection of private law issues associated with health reform initiatives. Much of the chapter focuses on the issues associated with the informed consent obligations of physicians. Given the relevance of disclosure obligations to waiting lists and the growing for-profit health care industry, two hot topics in the health care debate, emphasizing the informed consent issues seemed a logical approach. The paper ends with a brief review of several other issues relevant to malpractice law in this context, including a discussion of the standard of care and the legal liability of third-party decisionmakers.

The Current Context

If asked, it seems certain that health care providers would view the increasing need to "do more with less" as one of the most pervasive themes of this era of health reform and cost-containment. As long ago as 1994, a study found that

70 percent of the Canadian physicians surveyed thought that government cuts have hurt the quality of care.[7] Since then, more cuts have occurred. Whether the result of an explicit policy or a reaction to an implicit need, institutions have had to provide care in a climate of significantly reduced resources.[8] It is only recently that there has been a re-injection of government funds into the health care system.[9] Though increased federal and provincial funding will undoubtedly relieve some of the financial pressures experienced by health ministries and regional health authorities, the need to contain health expenditures will not diminish. A variety of pressures seem likely to continue to push up health care costs: new technologies, the aging of society and increased private investment are but a few examples. The philosophy of cost-containment is here to stay. And because physicians continue to control a large portion of the health care budget—through the direct utilization of resources, referrals and admitting privileges—cost-containment strategies have been (and will continue to be) relevant to the clinical decisions made by physicians.[10]

As a result, a number of commentators have noted that this era of health care reform challenges the very nature of the duties owed by the physician to the patient.[11] From the Hippocratic oath to recent professional codes of ethics, the physician's responsibility has historically focussed on the individual patient. While the reality of a busy practice and the financial incentives inherent in a fee-for-service system have always put pressure on this perceived ethical ideal, "a physician's dedication to serving the needs of his or her patients has remained the 'immutable bedrock of medical ethics.'"[12] To a large degree, a physician's legal obligations have mirrored this ethical standard. A physician's fiduciary obligations, discussed below and in another chapter of this book, stand as the best example of the degree to which Canadian law expects physicians to place the interests of their patients above all else.[13] There are also a few recent negligence cases which suggest that the legal standard of care should not be compromised by cost-containment pressures.[14] Even asking (let alone requiring) physicians to consider the broader financial and policy implications of their clinical decisions requires a shift in the focus of the physician's traditional legal and ethical duties. As noted by Marc Rodwin, "[Health reform] trends and views encourage the idea that rather than strive to promote only the welfare of individual patients, doctors and medical organizations must also act in the interest of the population they serve."[15]

Cost-containment strategies can take a variety of forms, from simply restricting access to a particular service, to informal policies which pressure physicians to "do less," to highly structured, explicit strategies designed to encourage physicians to provide less expensive care. The growth of managed care initiatives throughout the United States is perhaps the most obvious example of the latter. While the term "managed care" is used to describe a wide variety of health care delivery systems,[16] it can generally be said to apply to the "controlled" delivery of health care services in a way that promotes efficiency and cost effectiveness.[17] Such programs often "place the primary physician as gatekeeper with an eye toward controlling utilization everywhere in the system."[18] From the perspective of this chapter, one of the key features of managed care programs is that they may provide incentives to actually provide less or a particular type of care.[19] Due to the structure of these delivery systems (which often include mechanisms such as capitation),[20] health care providers may make more if they do less or if they provide a certain type of care. Such arrangements have obvious ethical and policy implications.[21]

In Canada, the spirit of financial and resource management—which is at the heart of managed care programs—has been embraced by numerous ministries, regional health authorities and health care institutions.[22] For example, it has been argued that the decrease in the average length of stay in some Ontario hospitals can be attributed, at least in part, to the financial incentives built into policies such as "case costing."[23] Other examples include the various global caps placed on the provincial budgets for physician fee-for-service expenditures[24] and fee-adjustment mechanisms such as "holdback" and "payback" which allow a reconciliation between the provincial government and the province's physicians at the end of the fiscal year.[25]

Though more formal allocation and incentive mechanisms affecting physicians may emerge, the most common form of cost-containment pressure remains the informal, often unspoken, institutional policies and allocation decisions.[26] Despite the fact that this is not a empirically documented phenomenon,[27] it seems reasonable to conclude that health care institutions throughout Canada are increasingly asking frontline workers to make tough allocation decisions.[28]

The bottom line is that at some level most cost-containment mechanisms control costs by trying to control physician practice or, at least, by instituting policies that will impact physician practice.[29] And, while such policies may make a great deal of sense from the perspective of distributive justice, they have the potential to severely compromise the classic physician/patient relationship—largely because they require or encourage physicians to integrate the needs of others into their clinical decision-making process.[30] The private law principles relevant to health care—be they in relation to consent, the standard of care or fiduciary law—are built on the obligations which flow from the health care provider/patient relationship; these are legal duties owed by one individual to another.[31] As shown in the following section, the law has already had some difficulty injecting the notions of "third-party needs" into this historically exclusive relationship.

Specific Legal Issues

A number of jurisdictions throughout the world have struggled with the legal issues and conflicts which seem endemic to health reform and cost-containment in health care. In the United States and Britain there is a good deal of case law and legislation which flows directly from the pressure which cost-containment places on the physician/patient relationship.[32] A number of jurisdictions have gone so far as to pass legislation which either prohibits financial incentives to physicians aimed at cost-containment or requires the disclosure of the nature of such incentives.[33] Indeed, the concerns about the impact of incentive mechanisms may be addressed by the US Congress.[34] There have also been a number of US and British cases, some of which will be reviewed below, that are relevant in this context.[35]

There have only been a handful of Canadian decisions which directly address the private law issues which have arisen as a result of health reform initiatives. Despite this dearth of specific jurisprudence, there are a number of legal trends and emerging principles which are highly relevant in this context. In this section I will discuss how health reform in Canada might impact the physician's disclosure obligations. This includes a discussion of general informed consent law, the policy arguments for and against an expanded disclosure obligation and how this obligation might manifest itself in relation to the practical issue of waiting lists. Second, by way of example, I briefly explore another liability issue—the use of a "cost-containment" excuse as a defence to malpractice claim.

A. Informed Consent

Susan Wolf recently characterized the twentieth century as "the century of informed consent."[36] Though it may seem a grand statement, it is clearly not far from the truth. With each passing decade, common law courts have given health care providers increasingly onerous disclosure obligations. This is particularly so in Canada. Since the seminal Supreme Court of Canada case of *Reibl* v. *Hughes*,[37] informed consent jurisprudence has consistently expanded the duty of physicians to provide patients with "material information" concerning proposed treatment. "Material information" is defined in terms of what a reasonable person in the patient's position would want to know. Failure to provide this information constitutes negligence on the part of the physician.[38]

The duty is firmly based on the ethical principle of autonomy. Ours is a society with a deep reverence of the right of individual choice. It has been suggested that other principles, such as the communitarian ethical approach,[39] are gaining prominence, but there is little evidence that autonomy has lost any ground. Indeed, the increasing consumerization of Canadian culture,[40] and health care in particular, has arguably intensified the sway of autonomy. Patients are now consumers. In this context, the process of informed consent has emerged as the practical manifestation of the theoretical ideal of patient autonomy and as a necessary tool for the increasingly information-hungry "patient consumer."[41]

This deference to the notion of autonomy is found throughout Canadian jurisprudence. For example, in the case of *Malette* v. *Shulman*, the Ontario Court of Appeal upheld the importance of the consent process noting that "[i]ndividual free choice and self-determination are themselves fundamental constituents of life."[42] Likewise, in *Ciarlarliello* v. *Schacter*, the Supreme Court of Canada declared that "the concept of individual autonomy is fundamental to the common law and is the basis for the requirement that disclosure be made to a patient."[43]

It is this close link to autonomy which seems certain to keep pushing back the bounds of the disclosure obligation. As noted by Bernard Dickens, "The respect for personal autonomy shown in modern health law makes it likely that courts will continue to broaden the scope of required disclosure."[44] Over the years, Canadian courts have had many opportunities to interpret the physician's duty of disclosure, and generally this has resulted in the predicted expansion of the duty. There have been remote risks of an adverse event deemed material[45] and an emphasis on the need to inform the patient of a broad range of material information, including a consideration of nonmedical information and the existence of any alternative treatments or procedures.[46]

Disclosure Obligations and Health Reform

How might this onerous obligation play out in the context of health care reform? How might reduced resources, cost-containment mechanisms and expanding private sector involvement in health care delivery impact the physician's duty of informed consent? First, there is a strong argument that a physician will need to disclose information about the existence of any mechanisms, implicit or explicit, which may influence the physician to use less (or even different) health care resources than would otherwise be suggested.[47] That is, a physician must tell a patient of a hospital or regional health authority policy to use, for example, fewer diagnostic imaging services. This would be particularly so if the policy was associated with some type of an incentive mechanism (e.g., a financial incentive to provide less care). While this information is not the medical risk data traditionally associated with the consent process, the informed-consent process has never been focussed solely on medical considerations.[48] Surely factors that may impact the physician's autonomy and ability to deliver care could also be considered material. Indeed, as noted by Wolf, "[I]t is hard to imagine information more material."[49] This is information that a reasonable person in the patient's position would want to know. And, as care becomes more closely tied to economic consideration, the relevance and materiality of this information will increase.

In the US, managed care strategies, such as utilization review and capitation mechanisms, are more common and explicit. As such, the informed consent controversy has already led to a great deal of academic debate, case law and even legislation compelling disclosure of cost-containment mechanisms and incentives to provide less care.[50] As noted by Miller and Sage, in the US "[r]equirements to disclose financial incentives have been enacted in many states and are included in recent reforms to Medicare and Medicaid."[51] Given the aggressive and often profit-oriented approach of many US managed care organizations, the requirement for a comprehensive disclosure of factors influencing physician practice is clearly essential. It has been argued that "failure to provide detailed information about these practices to consumers confirms their already vulnerable position and induces further erosion of the physician-patient relationship."[52] It is important to note that these disclosure requirements are part of a broader US trend toward a much more transparent system which includes the disclosure of information on everything from hospital outcomes to physicians' practice profiles (e.g., the education of a physician and the number of successful lawsuits that have been brought against him or her).[53] So, in the US, a country which has historically had a less patient-centred approach to the informed-consent process, as compared to Canada, the legal and political winds clearly point toward an inclusive disclosure policy.

Can the same arguments for the disclosure of health policy and cost-containment information be used in Canada? Unlike US citizens, Canadians cannot use the information to select between different medical care organizations (MCOs). Moreover, there are, as yet, few explicit and well-defined cost-containment mechanisms which are aimed at curtailing physicians' ability to utilize health care resources. As noted above, Canadian physicians are, in general, under more amorphous cost-containment pressure.

Despite these differences between the US and Canada, there are policy and legal justifications for disclosure in the Canadian situation. First, this information "can empower consumers" and "encourage dialogue among consumers, physicians [and] local regulators."[54] Even information about a policy to use fewer CT scans, for example, can enable patients to consider "whether it is worthwhile pressuring decision-makers to change the policy in question."[55] Second, though patients cannot select between different health management organizations (HMOs) they can choose between different providers. A patient may wish to find a physician who is not under the same constraints or who does not, for example, have a long a waiting list. As noted by Lewis, *et al.*, "[A] patient may languish on a particular physician's waiting list for a long time without ever knowing that another physician could provide the needed service much sooner."[56] This, in turn, may encourage physicians to be more efficient in their management of resources (i.e., the management of waiting lists). Third, and most importantly, to withhold information that is potentially relevant to the provision of a health care service is to adopt a paternalistic approach which would be in stark contrast to the current philosophical and legal trend. Since the case of *Reibl* v. *Hughes* the standard of disclosure has been viewed through the lens of the patient. If it is something that a reasonable person in the patient's position would want to know, it should be disclosed.[57]

A related issue is whether a physician is under a legal duty to inform patients of alternative treatments or procedures which are not available (for example, at the hospital where the physician practises) because of cost-containment policies or resource shortages. Does the patient have the right to be informed by the physician that these alternatives may be available elsewhere? As was stated by the Alberta Court of Appeal in a 1998 case, "A patient should be advised of a known treatment which others in the same specialty consider superior, even if the doctor does not agree. It is the kind of information a patient fairly could expect to receive."[58] This line of case law can be used to support the idea that physicians have a duty to disclose information to patients about the existence of private options that may be available both within and without a given jurisdiction if it can be conceived as something that a reasonable person in the patient's position would want to know. For example, private options which are not substantially different, faster or more convenient may not have to be disclosed. However, if a private option is available that would allow access to a procedure that would provide treatment in a manner that would lower the risks to the patient or speed access to a medically necessary service, that private option should probably be disclosed. Again, this is something that a reasonable person in the patient's position would want to know.[59] As suggested by Professor Dickens:[60]

> If patients have the means to obtain indicated care in another hospital, town, province or country, physicians may be obliged to inform them, because the option may be material to patients' choice between accepting the lesser care or seeking superior care elsewhere. Physicians who do not know whether patients have such means should ask them.

Policy Arguments Against Disclosure

There are, of course, a number of policy arguments which suggest that the disclosure of private options may not always be such a good idea. First, for those who are not enthusiastic about the introduction of more private for-profit options, giving patients information about queue-jumping alternatives could be viewed as a process that will do little more than promote the proliferation of private facilities. From the perspective of patients, hearing about private options from a physician in a clinical setting could help to legitimize a decision to access a private service (for example, a patient might think, "If my physician believes it is a reasonable alternative, perhaps I should give it a try"). Second, providing this information may also be against some physicians' ideological stance on private medicine. That is, they may feel uncomfortable "advertising" for private alternatives. Third, some patients may not have the financial resources to access the private tier and, as such, one could argue that it would be cruel to "tantalize" these patients with information about faster, or more elaborate, private services.

Though these arguments may seem quite persuasive, they do not mediate the physician's legal disclosure duties. Withholding information for the good of the patient, a concept known as therapeutic privilege,[61] is a legal doctrine that is rarely used in Canadian law. It is a practice that has been overwhelmed by the dominance of autonomy and, as such, can only be applied in rare circumstances (e.g., situations of severe emotional distress).[62] It seems doubtful a court would characterize the possibility that a patient with a low income may become upset about the inability to purchase private options as a justification for the exercise of therapeutic privilege. On the contrary, the physician should not presume to know how the patient would react or use such information (e.g., perhaps the patient would borrow the needed money). Likewise, personal concern about the social consequences of providing information will likely do little to limit the physician's disclosure duties. As with other value laden issues, such as abortion, physicians must be careful not to allow personal views to interfere with their legal and ethical obligations. Regardless of a physician's personal convictions, enough information should be provided to allow patients to make informed treatment decisions.[63] Those physicians who truly want to distance themselves from the growth of the private for-profit health care industry could explain their positions regarding private options to their patients.

The Causation Dilemma

Up to this point I have been arguing that Canadian informed-consent jurisprudence supports the idea that physicians have an obligation to disclose a variety of issues associated with health care reform and cost constraints. Though there seems little doubt that recent Canadian jurisprudence has created very onerous disclosure obligations, this does not mean that a patient could easily succeed in a claim against a physician who failed to provide relevant health reform information. There are many challenges that stand in the way of patients seeking to bring informed-consent lawsuits. Canadian plaintiffs face a very difficult "causation hurdle." A plaintiff must be able to demonstrate that "but for" the negligent nondisclosure, the treatment would have been declined.[64] Historically, patients have not been very successful at meeting this legal test.[65]

In other words, a plaintiff/patient would need to show that if all of the appropriate information had been disclosed, he/she would have made a different decision about the treatment. If a patient is injured by a cost-containment mechanism or a resource shortage (e.g., he/she reacted to a cheaper contrast medium or was injured on a waiting list) and was not informed of a private option, the causation hurdle may be relatively easy to pass. The patient would be claiming that "but for" the nondisclosure he/she would have purchased the private option and would not have been injured. However, for many of the possible lawsuits in this context, the causation hurdle creates some interesting legal dilemmas. For example, what if there is no option other than what is provided in the public system? If the physician failed to disclose information about cost-containment pressures (e.g., a policy to do fewer CT scans) and the patient could not use this information to access a different provider or a private option, it is difficult to see how a patient could satisfy the causation test. This is because the negligent nondisclosure would not, or so it is argued, have a significant impact on the patient's actual treatment decision.

More interesting, however, is the situation where a patient cannot afford or does not have access to private options. In such circumstances it will also be difficult for the patient to argue that "but for" the nondisclosure, he/she would not have been injured. Would a court investigate the personal characteristics of the patient/plaintiff, including the patient's financial situation, to determine if a "reasonable person in the patient's position" would have opted for the private alternative? Though it remains a point of legal controversy,[66] there are many examples of cases where the courts have seemingly used very personal characteristics to determine this causation issue. For example, in *Mickle* v. *Salvation Army Grace Hospital* the plaintiff parents alleged that a negligently performed ultrasound resulted in the birth of a child with congenital hemihypoplasia ichthyosis erythroderma (CHILD Syndrome) and limb deficiencies.[67] The court held that because the child's disabilities were not severe, a reasonable woman in Mickle's position would not select abortion. Likewise, in the Supreme Court of Canada decision in *Arndt* v. *Smith* the court concluded that despite a negligent nondisclosure by the defendant physician of the risks associated with having chicken pox during pregnancy, the characteristics of the plaintiff/mother were such that she would not have terminated the pregnancy even if given the option.[68] Given this case law, it seems entirely possible that a Canadian court could use the fact that a patient/plaintiff has a low income to conclude that the plaintiff cannot satisfy the causation test—that is, that a reasonable person in the patient's position would not have opted for the private alternative.[69]

If Canadian courts were to apply the causation test in such a manner it would lead to the ridiculous situation where wealthy Canadians could recover damages for nondisclosure while lower income Canadians would have more difficulty, thus compounding the inequities of a two-tiered system. Unfortunately, such is the state of informed-consent case law. From the perspective of this chapter, this causation problem stands as an example of how tort principles can amplify, rather than mitigate, many of the concerns associated with health care reform initiatives. Those with money will have access to a broader range of services, will be entitled to hear about those private options as part of the informed-consent process,[70] and will be more likely than lower income Canadians to recover damages when the disclosure process is inadequate.

Consent, Conflicts of Interest and the Physician's Fiduciary Duty

Because the principles which underlie fiduciary law flow from the unique nature of the physician/patient relationship, fiduciary obligations are also particularly relevant in the context of cost-containment initiatives and resource allocation policies.[71] In Canada, fiduciary law requires health care providers to "act with utmost good faith and loyalty"[72] in their dealings with patients. Indeed, fiduciary law arguably compels physicians to do that which is in the patient's best interest, even at the expense of the physician's interest or that of any other person or entity.[73]

One of the effects of characterizing the doctor-patient relationship as fiduciary is that it likely expands the doctor's duty of disclosure.[74] In particular, fiduciary law compels physicians to disclose potential conflicts of interest including, arguably, pressures to withhold treatment for the purposes of cost-containment.

There have been a number of relevant US and Canadian legal cases that address both specific health care reform conflicts and, more generally, the nature of the physician/patient relationship.[75] One of the most famous American decisions is *Moore* v. *Regents of the University of California*.[76] While Mr. Moore was receiving treatment for hairy-cell leukemia, his doctor discovered that Moore had unique cells which had the potential to be of both research and commercial value. Mr. Moore alleged that, without his knowledge or consent, his physician subsequently took cells from his spleen to develop a profitable cell line. Mr. Moore sued for damages and the defendant applied to the court to have the action summarily dismissed. The court held that Mr. Moore had a good cause of action and that his physician had a fiduciary duty to "disclose personal interests unrelated to the patient's health, whether research or economic, that may affect his medical judgement."[77] In the US, this disclosure obligation has also been held to apply to institutions that provide health care services. For example, in the decision of *Shea* v. *Esensten*, the court held that an MCO violated its fiduciary duty to disclose all material facts because it failed to disclose the existence of incentive structures that limited care.[78]

Though there have been no Canadian fiduciary cases which deal specifically with cost-containment issues, there are cases which support the principle that fiduciary law requires doctors to inform their patients of any financial or other conflict of interest which they may have in treating the patient.[79] This issue has not yet been considered by the courts, but it may well be that fiduciary obligations extend to disclosure of this type of information.

The Waiting List Example

There is a sound legal and policy case favouring the disclosure of a broad amount of information on cost-restraint policies and private treatment options. Both consent and fiduciary law seem to support some degree of disclosure in this context. How might these legal principles play out in the setting of today's health care system? In this section I examine the practical example of waiting lists.

Over the past few years much has been made of the waiting list problem in Canada. Rightly or not, waiting lists have emerged as a tangible symbol of the perceived failures of the current health care system. In reality, the cause and dynamics of waiting lists are complex and ill-defined.[80] Nevertheless, those favouring a strong public health care system use waiting lists as an argument for more government funding of specific services such as MRIs.[81] And many of those who support more private involvement in the health care system see waiting lists as an opportunity and justification for the introduction of more private options.[82]

Liability issues have also been associated with waiting lists. What if a patient dies or becomes injured while waiting for treatment? What if a patient could have received a quicker diagnosis at a private facility? Issues such as this have, in fact, led some hospitals and regional health authorities to the conclusion that they have a legal duty to inform patients of the risks of waiting for the public service and that private or out of jurisdiction (i.e., the US) alternatives may exist.[83] The Calgary Regional Health Authority recently recommended that physicians send a letter to patients that both explains some general concerns and risks associated with waiting lists and provides information about private options.[84] Likewise, in January 2000 it was reported that a number of hospitals in Toronto asked patients to sign waivers "spelling out the dangers of long waiting lists for care."[85] It was suggested that the "waiver would establish, in writing, that the patient was fully aware of the health risk of joining a lengthy queue."[86] Is such action justified? How might a waiting list lawsuit unfold?

Recently, there was a well-publicized story of an Edmonton, Alberta man who was having persistent headaches.[87] Because he would have to wait five months to access a publicly funded MRI, he decided to pay $1,000 for a private MRI. This privately financed test, which he received almost immediately, revealed that he had a rapidly growing brain tumour. A week later he had surgery to have the tumour removed. But what if this man did not know about the private option and his physician failed to inform him of this possible alternative? Could he successfully sue his physician for nondisclosure of material information? If, in fact, he was unaware of his private options, had the financial resources available to purchase a private test and was injured by the delay between the public and private alternatives, it seems entirely possible that a successful lawsuit could be mounted. The patient would be arguing that "but for" the nondisclosure of the private alternatives and the risks associated with being on a waiting list he would not have been injured. Though it would undoubtedly be controversial, such a claim is well within the bounds of current tort theory.[88]

But even if this man's physician did have a legal obligation to disclose the risks and alternatives associated with waiting lists (and I believe he probably did), a number of interesting practical issues remain. For example, what would the physician tell her patient? What are the actual risks associated with waiting for a public service? In fact, it is only now beginning to be understood what risks can reasonably be associated with being on a waiting list.[89] The gap in knowledge in this area will undoubtedly be alleviated as more data emerges from various waiting list research initiatives.[90] At the current time, however, physicians will largely be speculating on the health risks of waiting and the benefits of purchasing quicker services. This uncertainty regarding the magnitude of the risks will also create some ambiguity regarding what the courts will characterize as material risk information worthy of disclosure. In addition, most physicians and patients probably know little about the dynamics associated with waiting lists or, for that matter, cost-containment in general.[91] If it is accepted that physicians must disclose information about health care policies and resource shortages that may affect patient care, physicians will undoubtedly need to learn more about this area.[92]

Examining a physician's disclosure obligations in the context of waiting lists also highlights how the informed-consent process can help patients become more informed participants in health policy debates. Though the informed-consent process is not the best nor the only place for a dialogue about health reform pressures and the mechanics of waiting lists, a brief discussion of why a given service is unavailable may provide a patient with important, previously unknown, information. While this disclosure obligation could be seen as a mechanism that will only encourage the growth of a two-tiered system, that doesn't necessarily have to be the outcome. Indeed, just because a patient utilizes a private option does not necessarily mean that he or she is "pro-privatization." On the contrary, the need to access a private facility may spur a patient to speak out in support of the public system. This point is nicely illustrated by a recent letter to the *Edmonton Journal*. Due to a long waiting list for what she perceived to be a needed MRI, the author of the letter struggled with the possibility of accessing a private option. "I agonized for five days about whether or not to accept [an anonymous donation of money for a private MRI] because of my belief in, and commitment to, the principles of the Canada Health Act and our public health care system."[93] The author concludes thus: "I challenge Premier Klein to begin seriously to care for the health needs of the people he is mandated to serve by ensuring equal and timely access to all necessary healthcare services including diagnostic tests."

B. Standard of Care and the "Cost-Containment" Defence

Health reform initiatives will have an impact on much more than just physicians' disclosure duties. They will, for example, create many other liability pressures. In this section I will briefly look at one interesting aspect of this area—the use of cost-containment strategies and resource shortages as an "excuse" or defence to a malpractice action.

"ER Crisis May Bring Rash of Suits"[94] was the prognosis of one recent headline. Given the strain that the system has been under, the suggestion that there may be more lawsuits is hardly a courageous prediction. As resources are stretched further, it may become difficult for physicians and health care institutions to provide services that meet previously established standards of care or, at least, that satisfy the expectations of the public. As noted by a nurse involved in an Ontario incident where resource shortages caused a baby to be born on a roadside, "We are not always going to be able to provide the service people expect at all times."[95] Likewise, as noted above, physicians are necessarily implicated in most resource allocation schemes. If an institution is going to try to save dollars by doing fewer diagnostic services, for instance, it is the physicians who must select who will not get tested.[96]

It is easy to envisage how these factors may be relevant to future negligence actions. If an injured plaintiff/patient did not receive an expected test or subsequently discovers that a usually used procedure was withheld for purposes of fiscal restraint, this fact will undoubtedly form part of the lawsuit. From the perspective of this chapter the question is whether a physician could use the existence of health reform initiatives or cost-containment mechanisms as an excuse for the provision of substandard care. In other words, could a physician successfully argue, "Yes, I usually provide that test, but we have been asked to try and conserve costs and, therefore, I shouldn't be held liable for the decision not to provide the service"?[97]

In general, a doctor is required to exercise the same degree of skill and care which could reasonably be expected of a practitioner of the same experience and standing. The Supreme Court of Canada has characterized the principle as follows:[98]

> Every medical practitioner must bring to his task a reasonable degree of skill and knowledge and must exercise a reasonable degree of care. He is bound to exercise that degree of care and skill which could reasonably be expected of a normal, prudent practitioner of the same experience and standing, and if he holds himself out as a specialist, a higher degree of skill is required of him than of one who does not profess to be so qualified by special training and ability.

In assessing whether a doctor has met the appropriate standard of care, a court will place particular importance on evidence of accepted practice. As a general rule, save in exceptional circumstances, a doctor who is shown to have acted in accordance with the generally accepted practice will be found to have met the appropriate standard of care and will not be found negligent.[99] Conversely, if a doctor is shown to have departed from the accepted practice this will provide very strong evidence (though not necessarily determinative in itself) that the doctor was negligent.

Given this approach, could a physician use the existence of a cost-containment initiative as an excuse for substandard care? Is the desire to save money an acceptable reason to depart from an accepted clinical practice? The leading Canadian case on this issue is *Law Estate* v. *Simice*,[100] in which a widow sued several physicians as a result of the death of her husband due to a ruptured aneurysm. In defence, one of the excuses forwarded for not providing a CT scan in a timely manner was that there were constraints imposed by the provincial insurance scheme on the use of such diagnostic tools. The court did not accept this "economic defence" and went on to conclude that:[101]

> [I]f it comes to a choice between a physician's responsibility to his or her individual patient and his or her responsibility to the medicare system overall, the former must take precedence in a case such as this. The severity of the harm that may occur to the patient who is permitted to go undiagnosed is far greater than the financial harm that will occur to the medicare system if one more CT scan procedure only shows the patient is not suffering from a serious medical condition.

One of the few other Canadian decisions directly on point is the Newfoundland decision of *McLean* v. *Carr*.[102] In this case the court was again faced with an allegation that a CT scan was improperly withheld. While the court again rejected an economic defence, the court implicitly suggested that, at a minimum, the use of an economic defence must be accompanied by cogent evidence of cost-effectiveness:[103]

> In the present case everyone agrees a CT scan on admission would decrease the risk of death resulting from a developing epidermal hematoma. The question is one of the cost-effectiveness of precautions which could have been taken. It was allegedly too costly in 1987 to do a CT scan on all head-injured patients. I was not, however, provided with any evidence to establish that the cost would be prohibitive to scan, not all, but just patients whose skulls had considerable force applied and who had a resulting skull fracture.

There have also been a number of US decisions that are relevant to this issue. For example, in the now well-known American malpractice case of *Wickline* v. *State of California*, the court concluded: "While we recognize, realistically, that cost-consciousness has become a permanent feature of the health care system, it is essential that cost limitation programs not be permitted to corrupt medical judgement."[104]

Practically, there are not enough recent cases to make a safe prediction on how a court would react to a plea of economic pressure. Indeed, despite projections of a huge number of resource allocation related lawsuits,[105] very few relevant cases have actually been reported. That said, the thrust of existing and related jurisprudence clearly points to a rejection of the defence. Courts seem hesitant to allow goals of economic restraint to interfere with the obligations that physicians owe to individual patients.[106] If one considers the strength of a physician's fiduciary duties under Canadian law—a duty of utmost good faith and loyalty—an erosion of the physician's focus on the patient's best interest seems all the more unlikely.

To be clear, I am not referring to a circumstance where there is an actual scarcity of a given resource (e.g., a lack of advanced diagnostic technologies in rural settings or the unavailability of needed specialists). Canadian courts have always been sympathetic to the plight of physicians and hospitals struggling to do their best with inadequate resources. As noted by Picard and Robertson, "[I]n determining the applicable standard of care a Court will take into account the facilities and equipment available to the doctor. If some are unavailable because of scarcity of resources, this will have an impact on what can reasonably be expected of the doctor in these circumstances."[107] However, as highlighted by *Law Estate* v. *Simice*, if a physician makes a conscious decision not to provide an available resource for the purpose of saving the broader system money, courts seem likely to be much less sympathetic. A defence of "trying to save the system money" will not stand as an excuse for substandard care.

In this context then, malpractice law encourages physicians to place the interests of patients over the goals of economic restraint. From the perspective of patients this may seem a comforting conclusion. However, from the perspective of physicians, such liability pressure will add to an already confusing situation. Indeed, one could argue that if Canadian courts completely ignore the fiscal realities faced by today's health care providers, they will place an unfair and unrealistic burden on physicians. In addition, a rejection of the economic defence has the potential to frustrate cost-containment initiatives, thereby making potentially useful health reform policies more difficult to implement. But, as was noted in the informed consent section, malpractice law generally operates independent of broader health policy agendas. Physicians who place the goals of a macro-allocation policy over the needs of their patients do so at their peril.

Conclusion

Two broad themes emerge from the law in this area. First, health care providers seem to be in an almost inescapable conflict of duty that creates novel liability dilemmas. In the eyes of the law, the physician's primary duties remain focussed on the patient. Because health reform programs often ask (or force) physicians to curtail costs for the good of other members of society, however, this patient-focussed ethic is strained to the point of becoming a liability issue. Physicians may understandably be frustrated and confused by the current situation. They are asked to participate in global reform but also held personally liable for negligent acts that result from that participation. Rightly or not, Canadian malpractice jurisprudence does not seem well placed to accommodate this increasingly stark conflict. On the contrary, health care reform initiatives and the growth of private treatment options have created unique malpractice issues.

Second, the obligations placed on physicians by existing malpractice jurisprudence do not fit nicely into any particular health policy agenda. Because malpractice law continues to reinforce the paramount issue of a physician's duty to her patients, it does little to facilitate the introduction of broader cost-containment initiatives. Because malpractice law has created tremendously demanding disclosure obligations, physicians are required to provide patients with information about private alternatives—a practice that will arguably help the growth of for-profit medicine. And, because Canadian courts have continued to retain the troublesome "causation hurdle" used in informed-consent cases, wealthy patients may have the most success pursuing lawsuits against physicians who negligently withhold information about private options. This will only compound the inequities inherent in a two-tiered system.

The common law will always lag behind broader social change. It is, to a large degree, a reactive mechanism. Before a specific issue can be addressed it must be brought before the courts by an individual seeking compensation. To date, there have been surprisingly few Canadian malpractice cases that are a direct result of health care reform initiatives. There is, however, a rich body of tort law jurisprudence which allows some conclusions to be drawn about the legal duties of physicians in this age of health care reform. Respect for patient autonomy and an emphasis on the physician's duty to the patient seem likely to remain the two dominant considerations. Though future cases may erode these fundamental tenets of Canadian health law, such a move would constitute a radical shift in the direction of malpractice jurisprudence. Radical shifts are an uncommon phenomenon in the world of tort law—a world where incremental and subtle change is the more common approach. In many ways, legal academics are in the business of making predictions. I predict tough times for Canadian physicians as they struggle to balance their well-established duties toward their patients against the broader demands of our ever-changing health care system.

NOTES

A portion of this paper builds on T. Caulfield and G. Robertson, "Cost Containment Mechanisms in Health Care: A Review of Private Law Issues" (1999) 27 *Manitoba Law Journal* 1.

1   C. Rusnell, *The Edmonton Journal* (5 September 1997) B3.
2   P. Fayerman, "Hospital Apologizes to Parents After Baby Born on Road," *The National Post* (26 September 2000) A4.
3   R. Brennan, *The Edmonton Journal* (5 February 1998) A8. The story's subheading states: "Hospital patients at risk as wait for treatment grows, nurses say."
4   R. Walker, "Emergency Backlog Led to Patient's Death," *The Edmonton Journal* (18 November 2000) A7.
5   See R. Epstein, "The Social Consequences of Common-Law Rules" in S. Levmore, *Foundations of Tort Law* (Oxford University Press, 1994).
6   See N. Wyatt, "Grieving Brother Threatens Lawsuit over Sister's Death," *The Edmonton Journal* (5 February 1998) A8.
7   *Medical Post*, 1994 Physician Survey at 55. There is evidence that the public feels the same way. See R. Mackie, "Most Ontarians Believe Health Care Deteriorating," *The Globe and Mail* (17 January 2000) A2, where it is reported that 71 percent of Ontarians believe that "health care is currently in a crisis."
8   See P. Armstrong and H. Armstrong, *Wasting Away: The Undermining of Canadian Health Care* (Toronto: Oxford University Press, 1996); D. Angus, *et al.*, *Sustainable*

Health Care for Canada: Synthesis Report (Queen's-University Ottawa Economic Project, 1995); M. Brown, "Changes in Alberta's Medicare Financing Arrangements: Features and Problems," in M. Stingl and D. Wilson, eds., *Efficiency v. Equality: Health Reform in Canada* (Halifax: Fernwood Publishing Co., 1996) at 148; M. Brown, "Rationing Health Care in Canada" (1993) 2 *Annals Health L.* 101.

9   A. Geddes, "$54 M pumped into health care," *The Edmonton Journal* (19 May 2000) A1.

10   Indeed, the *Medical Post* survey found that 72.4 percent of physicians thought government intervention had the potential to seriously impact the way they practised.

11   S. Shortell, *et al.*, "Physicians as Double agents" (1998) 280 *J.A.M.A.* 1102; E.H. Morreim, *Balancing Act: The New Medical Ethics of Medicine's New Economics* (Washington D.C.: Georgetown University Press, 1995); J. Lairson, "Re-examining the Physician's Duty of Care in Response to Medicare's Prospective Payment System" (1998) 2 *Washington L. Rev.* 791.

12   Shortall, *ibid.* at 1102.

13   See Section, *infra*, entitled "Consent, Conflicts of Interest and the Physician's Fiduciary Duty."

14   *Law Estate, infra* note 97.

15   M. Rodwin, "Strain in the Fiduciary Metaphors: Divided Physician Loyalties and Obligations in a Changing Health Care System" (1995) 11 *Am. J.L. & Med.* 241 at 254. See also R. Perkel, "Ethics and Managed Care" (1996) 80 *Med. Clin. North Am.* 263 at 266; C. Perry, "Conflicts of Interest and the Physician's Duty to Inform" (1994) 96 *Am. J. Med.* 375: "[T]he economic benefits and hazards of today's practice of medicine provide sundry and frequently subtle opportunities for fiduciary conflicts of interest"; Policy Perspective, "For Our Patients, Not for Profit" (1997) 278 *J.A.M.A.* 1733 at 1733: "Patent financial incentives that reward overcare or undercare weaken patient-physician and patient-nurse bonds and should be prohibited. Similarly, business arrangements that allow corporations and employers to control the care of patients should be proscribed."

16   See K. Christensen, "Ethically Important Distinctions Among Managed Care Organizations" (1995) 23 *J.L. Med. & Ethics* 223, for a review of the key differences between various managed care organizations.

17   Managed care initiatives have been criticized on numerous levels. One of the more interesting observations is that they may, in fact, encourage patients to exaggerate their problems in order to gain access to health care resources. See A. Barsky and J. Borus, "Somatization and Medicalization in the Era of Managed Care" (1996) 274 *J.A.M.A.* 1931.

18   Perkel, *supra* at 15. See also "Managed Care: What to Expect as Medicare-HMO Enrollment Grows" (1996) 51 *Geriatrics* 35.

19   Christensen, *supra* note 16 at 225.

20   For a brief general discussion of capitation, see C. Donaldson and K. Gerard, *Economics of Health Care Financing: The Visible Hand* (London: MacMillan Press, 1992) at 110–12.

21   See E. Emanuel and N. Neveloff Dubler, "Preserving the Physician-Patient Relationship in the Era of Managed Care" (1995) 273 *J.A.M.A.* 323; B. Culliton, "Managed Care and Conflict of Interest" (1996) 2 *Nature Med.* 489 at 489: "To the extent that the switch to managed care in the name of sound economy is ...

undermining patients' legitimate need to be able to trust that their physicians are first and foremost on their side."

22 See F. Caruth, "Redirecting Incentives in the British Columbia Health Care System: Creating a Consequence" in R. Deber and G. Thompson, eds., *Restructuring Canada's Health Services System: How Do We Get There From Here?* (Toronto: University of Toronto Press, 1992).

23 M. Waldman, "Conflicts of Interest, Physicians and Physiotherapy" (1996) 154 *C.M.A.J.* 1737 at 1737. This author argues that "case costing" drove down the "length of stay for a patient with a fractured hip ... from fifty-six days in 1992 to 24.2 days in 1995." Case costing is a funding mechanism which allots a fixed amount of money for a given diagnosis regardless of time spent in the hospital. Therefore, it is in the best interests of physicians and the institution to turn over beds quickly, as this will allow more patients to be treated thus generating more income for providers and saving money for the institution.

24 J. Hurley and R. Card, "Global Physician Budgets as Common-Property Resources: Some Implications for Physicians and Medical Associations" (1996) 154 *C.M.A.J.* 1161 at 1162. For example, in 1996 it was reported that some provinces have caps on individual physician incomes (e.g., Ontario's upper range is $454,000 for all physicians, Newfoundland's is $350,000 for general practitioners and $450,000 for specialists). Other provinces use a formula to determine the income cap. Nova Scotia, for instance, sets the threshold at "1.8 standard deviations above the mean for the group."

25 See *ibid.* for a review of each province's global cap policy as of 1995. With holdback, a portion of a percentage of payments is held back during the year and then paid out after the reconciliation. In a payback scheme any excess expenditures are repaid at year's end. These devices are broad-based incentives which aim to subtly compel physicians to consider the financial implications of their individual clinical decisions. For an example of a specific agreement see Alberta Medical Association and Alberta Health, *Letter of Understanding Between the Minister of Health of the Government of Alberta and the President of the Alberta Medical Association* (1 April 1995–March 1998) at 1. This agreement, which was designed to help to secure the funding envelope for Alberta physicians until spring of 1998, states that the "parties believe that change can best be brought about by the introduction of incentives at the provider level." The letter states: "Savings achieved under $50 million will be shared one-third AMA and two-thirds government. Savings achieved in excess of $50 million will be shared equal proportions of one-half AMA and one-half regions."

26 J. Williams and E. Beresford, "Physicians, Ethics and the Allocation of Health Care Resources" (1991) 24 *Annals R.C.P.S.C.* 305 at 309.

27 There are many explicit institutional policies concerning the use of various procedures and pharmaceuticals (e.g., contrast media). See D. Roy, B. Dickens and M. McGregor, "The Choice of Contrast Media: Medical, Ethical and Legal Considerations" (1992) 147 *C.M.A.J.* 1321.

28 *On the Front Lines: Hard Choices: Resource Allocation at the Caregiver Level,* Provincial Health Ethics Network Annual General Meeting and Workshop, Red Deer, Alberta, 28 May 1997. See also D. Roy, J. Williams and B. Dickens, *Bioethics in Canada* (Scarborough: Prentice Hall Canada, 1994) at 351–3, for a brief discussion of the physician's role in the allocation of resources.

29 J. Martin and L. Bjerknes, "The Legal and Ethical Implications of Gag Clauses in Physician Contracts" (1996) 22 *Am. J.L. & Med.* 433 at 438.

30 See Emanuel and Neveloff Dubler, *supra* at 21: "The physician patient relationship is the cornerstone for achieving, maintaining, and improving health. The structure of financing and regulation should be designed to foster and support an ideal relationship between the physician and the patient." Of course, physicians have always been influenced by nonmedical factors. See G.R. Langley, *et al.*, "Effects of Non-medical Factors on Family Physicians' Decisions About Referral for Consultation" (1992) 147 *C.M.A.J.* 659; M. Chren, "Physicians' Behaviour and Their Interactions With Drug Companies" (1994) 271 *J.A.M.A.* 684.

31 See J. Lomas and A. Harmony in Public and Self-Regulation" in R. Evans, M. Barer and T. Marmur, eds., *Why are Some People Healthy and Others Not?* (New York: Aldine De Gruyter, 1994) at 256, where the authors' note that the system of professional regulation is similarly focussed on the relationship of physician/ patient:

> The self-regulation process in medicine has focussed on the individual practitioner-patient encounter, a framework that both discourages re- sources consideration in making judgements of "good care" and makes it difficult to ascertain overall impacts on population health.

32 For a review of key cases in Britain, see M. Blake, "Battling the Budget: Judicial Review of National Health Resources" (1996) 6 *Dispatches* 1.

33 See M.R. Anderlik, "Efforts to Regulate Physician Financial Incentives" (1998) Perspective in Health Law, online at http://www.law.uh.edu/ healthlawperspectives/Managed/990120Efforts.html (accessed on 30 November 2000), where it is noted that "[a]t least 20 states have legislation or administrative regulations that prohibit certain kinds of incentives, and at least 16 states require disclosure of incentive to enrollees under at least some circumstances." For instance, an Idaho statute requires that no "MCO shall offer a provider any incentive plan that includes a specific payment made to a provider as an inducement to deny, reduce, or delay specific medically necessary, and appropriate services...." *Ibid.*

34 E.D. Burrus, "Managed Care Will Receive an Overhaul with the 106th Congress" (1998), online at http://www.law.uh.edu/healthlawperspectives/ (accessed on 30 November 2000).

35 See L. Sederer, "Judicial and Legislative Responses to Cost Containment" (1992) 149 *Am. J. Psychiatry* 1157.

36 S. Wolf, "Toward a Systemic Theory of Informed Consent in Managed Care" (1999) 35 *Houston L. Rev.* 1631 at 1631.

37 *Reibl* v. *Hughes* (1980), 114 D.L.R. (3rd) 1 (S.C.C.).

38 See *Reibl* v. *Hughes* (1980) 114 D.L.R. (3rd) 1 (S.C.C.) and, generally, E.I. Picard and G.B. Robertson, *Legal Liability of Doctors and Hospitals in Canada* (Scarborough, Ont.: Carswell, 1996).

39 See S. Hellsten, "Biotechnology, genetic information and community: from individual rights to social duties?" in A. Thompson and R. Chadwick, eds., *Genetic Information: Acquisition, Access, and Control* (New York: Kluwer Academic/Plenum Publishing, 1999) at 297–308.

40 B. Barber, *Jihad vs. McWorld* (New York: Times Books, 1995); R. Porter, *The Greatest Benefit to Mankind: A Medical History of Humanity* (New York: Norton and Company, 1997).

41 See Wolf, *supra* note 36 at 1641, who argues that "the core problem that bioethics has addressed is how to make patient autonomy a reality in the clinic, an ideal achieved in large part through the requirement of informed consent."

42 *Malette* v. *Shulman,* (1990), 72 O.R. (2d) 417 (Ont C.A.).

43 *Ciarlariello* v. *Schacter*, [1993] 2 S.C.R. 119. See also *B.(R)* v. *Children's Aid Society of Metropolitan Toronto* [1995] 1 S.C.R. 315.

44 B.M. Dickens, "Informed Consent" in J. Downie and T. Caulfield, *Canadian Health Law and Policy* (Toronto: Butterworths, 1999) at 131.

45 For examples of risks held to be material, see *Meyer Estate* v. *Rogers* (1991), 78 D.L.R. (4th) 307 (Ont. Gen. Div.) (a 1-in-100,000 risk of a fatal reaction to a contrast media dye); *Arndt* v. *Smith,* [1997] 2 S.C.R. 539 (0.23-per-cent chance of a fetal anomaly); *Leung* v. *Campbell* (1995), 24 C.C.L.T. (2d) 63 (Ont. Gen. Div.) (1-in-300,000 risk of suffering paralysis as a result of spinal manipulation by a chiropractor).

46 See Picard and Robertson, *supra* 38 at 129–31.

47 T. Caulfield and D. Ginn, "The High Price of Full Disclosure: Informed Consent and Cost Containment in Health Care" (1994) 22 *Man. L.J.* 328. See also F. Miller, "Denial of Health Care and Informed Consent in English and American Law" (1992) 18 *Amer. J.L. & Med.* 37; R.C. Fraser and K.M. Avery, "What You Don't Know Can Hurt You" (1994) 3 *Health L. Rev.* 3; Picard and Robertson, *supra* note 38 at 131–2.

48 Even in the case of *Reibl* v. *Hughes,* the risk that the carotid artery surgery might jeopardize the plaintiff's pension plan was held to be a factor that should have been considered in the informed-consent process. *Reibl, supra* note 37.

49 Wolf, *supra* note 36 at 1661.

50 See generally V. Khanna, H. Silverman and J. Schwartz, "Disclosure of Operating Practices by Managed Care Organizations to Consumers of Health Care: Obligations of Informed Consent" (1998) 9 *J. Clin. Ethics* 291; T. Miller and W. Sage, "Disclosing Physician Financial Incentives" (1999) 281 *J.A.M.A.* 1424; Wolf, *ibid.*, at footnote 97 for a list of state laws.

51 Miller, *ibid.* at 1424.

52 Khanna, *supra* note 50 at 292.

53 See A. Twerski and N. Cohen, "The Second Revolution in Informed Consent: Comparing Physicians to Each Other" (1999) 94 *Northwestern U.L. Rev.* 1; E. Kluge, "Informed Consent in a Different Key: Physicians' Practice Profiles and the Patient's Right to Know" (2000) 160 *C.M.A.J.* 1321. It is interesting to note that Kluge's hypothesis is that Canadian informed-consent law might reasonably lead to the conclusion that practice profiles should also be available. "If the practice profiles of physicians reflect their proficiency as practitioners, does the logic of *Reibl* v. *Hughes* not support the disclosure of such information?" *Ibid.* at 1322.

54 Khanna, *supra* note 50 at 292.

55 Caulfield and Ginn, *supra* note 47 at 339.

56 Lewis, *infra* note 80 at 1299.

57 Though there seems to be some agreement that physicians must disclose information about conflicts of interest and private options (both discussed more fully below), it should be noted that not all legal commentators are convinced that physicians have a legal obligation to disclose information about health reform policies. For example, Dickens has suggested that the disclosure required by *Reibl* "may be only of risks of available treatments, not of risks of potentially helpful treatments that are unavailable" (Dickens, *supra* note 44 at 133. For an alternate view see Picard and Robertson, *supra* note 38). However, policies that are keeping a more beneficial treatment from a patient are relevant to the risks associated with the treatment the patient is being offered and, as such, should be disclosed. Moreover, if a physician has a duty to disclose alternate procedures, why those treatments are not being offered ought to be explained.

58 *Seney v. Crooks* [1998] A.J. No. 1060 (QL) (C.A.).

59 Must a physician disclose information about the availability of services available throughout the world? Probably not. The test is what would a reasonable person in the patient's position want to know. Information about private options within reasonable access of the patient is probably sufficient. However, this obligation may vary between patients. If a physician knows that a particular patient has interest in a wide range of private options, more should probably be disclosed. Likewise, if specific questions are asked, they should be answered in a comprehensive fashion.

60 Dickens, *supra* note 44 at 133.

61 In *Reibl v. Hughes, supra* note 37 at 13, Laskin noted: "[I]t may be the case that a particular patient may, because of emotional factors, be unable to cope with facts relevant to recommended surgery or treatment and the doctor may, in such a case, be justified in withholding or generalizing information as to which he would otherwise be required to be more specific."

62 See *Meyer Estate v. Rogers* (1991), 78 D.L.R. (4th) 307 (Ont. Gen. Div.), where a physician intentionally withheld information about the risks associated with contrast media. The court stated that the "therapeutic privilege" exception to the doctor's duty of disclosure should not be part of Canadian law because it has the potential to erode the requirement of informed consent. Likewise, in *McInerney v. MacDonald*, [1992] 2 S.C.R. 138, where the court held, in the context of a patient's right of access to medical records, that the doctrine should only be resorted to in extreme circumstances. See also, Picard and Robertson, *supra* note 38 at 147–9; Dickens, *supra* note 44 at 137–40.

63 College of Physicians and Surgeons of Alberta, Policy on Termination of Pregnancy, June 2000, online at http://www.cpsa.ab.ca/policyguidelines/term_preg.html (accessed on 30 November 2000).

64 See *Arndt v. Smith* (1997), 148 D.L.R. (4th) 48 (S.C.C.); E. Nelson and T. Caulfield, "You Can't Get There From Here: A Case Comment on *Arndt v. Smith*" (1998) 32 *U.B.C.L. Rev.* 353; J. Katz, "Informed Consent—A Fairy Tale? Law's Vision" (1977–78) 39 *University of Pittsburgh L. Rev.* 137; G.B. Robertson, "Informed Consent Ten Years Later: The Impact of Reibl v. Hughes" (1991) 70 *Can. Bar Rev.* 423; E.I. Picard and G.B. Robertson, *Legal Liability of Doctors and Hospitals in Canada* (Toronto: Carswell, 1996) 157–69; P.H. Osborne, "Causation and the Emerging Canadian Doctrine of Informed Consent to Medical Treatment" 1985), 33 *C.C.L.T.* 131; M. Crow, "Confusion over Causation: A Journey through *Arndt v. Smith*" (1998) 7 *Health L. Rev.* 3.

65 In a survey of 117 informed-consent cases between 1981 and 1991 it was found that 82 percent were unsuccessful. In forty-five of the 117 cases the physician was found to be negligent (e.g., had not disclosed enough information) but in 56 percent of these cases causation was not established. See Robertson, *ibid.*

66 See, generally, *supra* note 64.

67 *Mickle v. Salvation Army Grace Hospital Windsor Ontario* [1998] O.J. No. 4683 (Ont. Crt. Justice).

68 *Arndt, supra* note 64.

69 A plaintiff could argue that he/she would have taken out a loan or borrowed money from relatives in order to purchase the needed test. But this is the classic "hindsight is 20/20" suggestion that led the Supreme Court to refrain from adopting a subjective causation test. The SCC noted that all plaintiffs/patients will say that a different treatment option would have been selected (if not, then why would they sue?). As a result, the SCC has maintained the much-criticized "modified objective" test. In applying the "modified objective" test set out in *Reibl*, and affirmed in *Arndt*, a court must decide what a reasonable person in the patient's situation would likely do. See *Reibl* and *Arndt, supra.*

70 The fact that the informed-consent process must be tailored to the particular patient's individual interests and characteristics is another example of how the law may differentiate between patients with financial resources and those without. As noted by Dickens, "The physician must learn enough about the patient to know reasonably what information is material to the patient." *Supra* note 44 at 124. Does this mean that a physician must disclose more information to wealthy patients? Dickens goes onto suggest that this may well be the case. "If patients have no means to avail themselves of options, however, it is not obvious that physicians are legally bound to tantalize them by disclosing choices beyond their reach." *Ibid.* at 133.

71 Rodwin, *supra* note 15 at 241; B. Dickens, "Medical Records—Patient's Right to Receive Copies—Physician's Fiduciary Duty of Disclosure: *McInerney* v. *MacDonald*" (1994) 73 *Can. Bar. Rev.* 234.

72 *McInerney* v. *MacDonald* (1992) 93 D.L.R. (4th) 415 (S.C.C.) at 423. See also *Norberg* v. *Wynrib* (1992) 92 D.L.R. (4th) 449 (S.C.C.); *Henderson* v. *Johnston* (1956) 5 D.L.R. (2d) 524 (Ont. High Ct.); *Cox* v. *College of Optometrists of Ontario* (1988) 65 O.R. 461 (Ont. High Ct.).

73 See, generally, J. Erlen and M. Mellors, "Managed Care and the Nurse's Ethical Obligations to Patients" (1995) 14 *Ortho. Nurs.* 42 at 43, where the authors note that the nurses' "fiduciary relationship is grounded in the ethical principles of respect for persons and beneficence ... Patients expect that nurses will act in accord with their interests and that nurses will not abandon them whenever they need help." See also, C. McDaniel, "Ethics and Mental Health Service Delivery Under Managed Care" (1996) 17 *Issues in Mental Health Nurs.* 11; F. Chervenak, L. McCullough and R. Chez, "Responding to the Ethical Challenges Posed by the Business Tools of Managed Care in the Practice of Obstetrics and Gynaecology" (1996) 175 *Am. J. Obs. Gyn.* 523 at 523–4.

74 Kluge, *supra* note 53 at 1322: "Physicians operate within a fiduciary relationship with their patients. ... [This] means that physicians and patients should come together in an atmosphere of openness and mutual trust. It may reasonably be asked whether such trust is possible when significant information is withheld by either side."

75 For a review of conflict of interest case law and legislation see Dickens, *supra* note 44.

76 *Moore* v. *Regents of the University of California*, 793 P.2d 479 (Cal. 1990).

77 *Ibid.* at 485. See also, E. Picard and G. Robertson, *supra* at 133.

78 107 F. 3d 625 (8th Cir. 1997). See Moe Litman's chapter elsewhere in this collection. See also L. Gostin, "Managed Care, Conflicts of Interest, and Quality" (2000) 30 *Hastings Center Rep.* 27.

79 *Henderson* v. *Johnston* (1956), 5 D.L.R. (2d) 524 at 534 (Ont. H.C.), aff'd (1958), 11 D.L.R. (2d) 19 (C.A.), aff'd (1959), 19 D.L.R. (2d) 201 (S.C.C.).

80 S. Lewis, *et al.*, "Ending waiting-list mismanagement: principles and practice" (2000) 162 *C.M.A.J.* 1297.

81 See B. Gilmour, "$1M to Shorten Waits for MRIs," *The Edmonton Journal* (27 July 2000); H. Smith, "Medical Need, Not Size of Wallet, Should Determine Priority for MRI," *The Edmonton Journal* (10 June 2000).

82 See L. Priest, "MRI Clinics Put Medicare to Test," *The Globe and Mail* (21 August 2000) A2.

83 See S. Lightstone, "Waiting-list Worries Cause Calgary MDs to Prepare Letter for Patients" (1999) 161 *Can. Med. Assoc. J.* 183.

84 A copy of a draft letter from the Calgary Regional Medical Staff Association is on file with the author.

85 "Treatment Wait May Harm Health, Cancer Centre Warns," The Canadian Press, ~~(9 January 2000) *Edmonton Journal* A9.~~

86 *Ibid.*

87 B. Gilmore, "$1,000 to Catch Deadly Cancer," *Edmonton Journal* (26 July 2000) A1; Opinion, "Scan Reveals Dangers in Medicare" *The Edmonton Journal* (27 July 2000).

88 As part of a recent article on the risks associated with waiting lists, *The Globe and Mail* told the story of a man who had waited eight months and lost three months work before getting a publicly funded MRI. The patient commented: "I suffered for eight months waiting for the test. If I knew ... the surgery would be this great, I would have paid the $850 [for the private MRI]." D. Walton, "Waiting for the Diagnosis is a High Price to Pay," *The Globe and Mail* (15 November 2000) A9.

89 See C. Naylor, *et al.*, "Benchmarking the Vital Risk of Waiting for Coronary Artery Bypass Surgery" (2000) 162 *C.M.A.J.* 775; D. Hadorn, "What Can Comparisons of Mortality Rates Tell Us About Waiting Lists?" (2000) 162 *C.M.A.J.* 794; S. Lewis, *et al.*, "Ending Waiting-List Mismanagement: Principles and Practice" (2000)162 *C.M.A.J.* 1297; A. McIlroy, "Doctors' lists may be inflated, study suggests," *The Edmonton Journal* (2 September 1998) A4.

90 See Western Canada Waiting List Project, *From Chaos to Order: Making Sense of Waiting Lists in Canada: An Interim Progress Report, September 2000* (WCWLP: University of Alberta, 2000) for a discussion of a multi-disciplinary project designed solely for the study of waiting lists.

91 This is particularly so given that many patients probably have little understanding of health reform initiatives. In the US it was found that only 27 percent of the public knew what "managed care" meant. Khanna, *supra* note 50 at 291.

92 The physician has a legal responsibility to take steps to ensure that the patient has understood the disclosed information. As noted in the Supreme Court of Canada

decision of *Ciarlarliello* v. *Schacter*, "[I]t is appropriate that the burden should be placed on the doctor to show that the patient comprehended the explanation and instructions given." *Ciarlarliello* v. *Schacter* [1993] 2 S.C.R. 119 at 140. See also, *Adan* v. *Davis* [1998] O.J. No. 3030 (QL) (Gen. Div.).

93 V. Elton-Eerkes, "Letter: Why Didn't Gov't Use Available MRI Machine?" (24 May 2000) *The Edmonton Journal.*

94 L. Priest, "ER Crisis May Bring Rash of Suits" (17 January 2000) *The Globe and Mail* A1.

95 Fayerman, *supra* note 2 at A4.

96 See T. Stoltzfus Jost, "Health Care Rationing in the Courts: A Comparative Study" (1998) 21 *Hastings Int'l. and Comparative L. Rev.* 639 at 640–1.

97 I have discussed this issue in more detail elsewhere. See, for example, T. Caulfield, "Health Care Reform: Can Tort Law Meet the Challenge?" (1994) 32 *Alta. Law Rev.* 685. See also, J. Irvine, "The Physician's Duty in the Age of Cost Containment" (1994) 22 *Man. L.J.* 345; Irvine, "Case Comment: Law Estate v. Simice" (1994) 21 C.C.L.T. (2d) 259; Picard and Robertson, *supra* note 38 at 207–10.

98 *Crits* v. *Sylvester* (1956), 1 D.L.R. 502 at 508 (Ont. C.A.), *aff'd* [1956] S.C.R. 991. See also Picard and Robertson, *supra* note 38 at 132–4.

99 *ter Neuzen* v. *Korn*, [1995] 10 W.W.R. 1 (S.C.C.).

100 (1994), 21 C.C.L.T. (2d) 228 (B.C.S.C.), *aff'd* [1996] 4 W.W.R. 672 (C.A.).

101 *Ibid.* at 240.

102 *McLean* v. *Carr* (1994), 363 APR 271 (Nfld. TD).

103 *Ibid.* at 289.

104 *Wickline* v. *State of California*, 228 Cal. Rptr 661 (Cal. App. 2 Dist. 1986) at 672.

105 See Fayerman, *supra* note 2.

106 For a discussion of the US situation, see M. Frankel, "Medical Malpractice Law and Health Care Cost Containment: Lessons for the Reformers from the Clash of Cultures" (1994) 103 *Yale L.J.* 1297; Morreim, *supra* note 11.

107 Picard and Robertson, *supra* note 38 at 207. For an example case, see *Bateman* v. *Doirin* (1993), 18 CCLT 1 (NBCA).

2

Bill 11, the Canada Health Act and the Social Union

The Need for Institutions

Sujit Choudhry

M edicare has been a source of ongoing controversy between provincial governments, which separately administer the ten provincial health insurance schemes that constitute the Canadian health care system, and the federal government, which provides financial support to the provinces in exchange for compliance with the national standards spelled out in the Canada Health Act (CHA).[1] Indeed, in the spring of 2000, two events thrust Medicare back onto the front pages and into the centre of the public policy agenda. The first event was the passage of the federal budget.[2] Prompted by growing public concern regarding waiting lists and over-crowded emergency rooms, the federal government announced a one-time supplement to federal transfer payments to the provinces in the amount of $2.5 billion. Instead of welcoming the new federal monies, however, the provinces were outraged, claiming that the federal initiative was grossly insufficient to deal with the fiscal crisis that has allegedly engulfed Medicare. Far from deflecting provincial criticism, the federal budget had exactly the opposite effect, precipitating a new round of federal–provincial negotiations that may yield a new set of principles for Medicare. The second event was the passage of Bill 11.[3] Bill 11 will permit the operation of private, for-profit clinics in Alberta. These clinics will be able to offer services covered by the provincial health insurance plan.

They will also be able to offer "enhanced" medical services on a fee-for-service basis. These may differ from insured services only in that they are of higher quality, or provided more quickly. In addition to generating massive

Table 1: History of the mandatory enforcement mechanism of the Canada Health Act (in 1,000s of dollars)

Fiscal year	Reason for deduction	Nfld.	PEI.	NS	NB	Que.	Ont.
1984–85	User charges	0	0	0	3,015	7,893	0
	Extra-billing	0	0	0	63	0	39,996
1985–86	User charges	0	0	0	3,222	6,139	0
	Extra-billing	0	0	0	84	0	53,328
1986–87	User charges	0	0	0	296	0	0
	Extra-billing	0	0	0	206	0	13,3322
1987–88[1]	User charges	0	0	0	0	0	0
	Extra-billing	0	0	0	0	0	0
1988–89[2]	User charges	0	0	0	0	0	0
	Extra-billing	0	0	0	0	0	0
1989–90	User charges	0	0	0	0	0	0
	Extra-billing	0	0	0	0	0	0
1990–91	User charges	0	0	0	0	0	0
	Extra-billing	0	0	0	0	0	0
1991–92	User charges	0	0	0	0	0	0
	Extra-billing	0	0	0	0	0	0
1992–93	User charges	0	0	0	0	0	0
	Extra-billing	0	0	0	0	0	0
1993–94	User charges	0	0	0	0	0	0
	Extra-billing	0	0	0	0	0	0
1994–95[3]	User charges	0	0	0	0	0	0
	Extra-billing	0	0	0	0	0	0
1995–96	User charges	46	0	32	0	0	0
	Extra-billing	0	0	0	0	0	0
1996–97	User charges	96	0	72	0	0	0
	Extra-billing	0	0	0	0	0	0
1997–98	User charges	128	0	57	0	0	0
	Extra-billing	0	0	0	0	0	0
1998–99	User charges	53	0	38.9	0	0	0
	Extra-billing	0	0	0	0	0	0
Gross	User charges	323	0	199.9	6,533	14,032	0
Total	Extra-billing	0	0	0	353	0	106,656
Net total	User charges	323	0	199.9	0	0	0
	Extra-billing	0	0	0	0	0	0

1. "Running net total" refers to the sum of withheld federal transfer payments of net returned monies.

2. In the preface to the *Canada Health Act Annual Report 1987–88*, federal Minister of National Health and Welfare Jake Epp wrote:
The year 1987–88 has been a landmark in the Canadian health care system. As provided for under the Canada Health Act, by April 1, 1987, all provinces and territories had taken steps to comply with the extra-billing and user charges provisions of the Act. This report therefore differs slightly from its previous editions. It no longer contains a table of deductions made from the federal transfer payments, and it has been amended to show that all provinces that received deductions in their payments have been granted full refunds during the year (see Health Canada, *Canada Health Act Annual Report 1987–88* (Ottawa: Supply & Services Canada, 1988) at 3).

Man.	Sask.	AB	BC	Yuk.	NWT	Annual total	Running net total[1]
0	0	1,827	22,797	0	0	35,532	35,532
810	1,451	8,109	0	0	0	50,429	50,429
0	0	2,640	30,620	0	0	42,621	78,153
460	656	9,216	0	0	0	63,744	114,173
0	0	1,362	31,332	0	0	32,990	111,143
0	0	5,878	0	0	0	19,416	133,589
0	0	0	0	0	0	0	0
0	0	0	0	0	0	0	0
0	0	0	0	0	0	0	0
0	0	0	0	0	0	0	0
0	0	0	0	0	0	0	0
0	0	0	0	0	0	0	0
0	0	0	0	0	0	0	0
0	0	0	0	0	0	0	0
0	0	0	0	0	0	0	0
0	0	0	83	0	0	83	83
0	0	0	0	0	0	0	0
0	0	0	1,223	0	0	1,223	1,306
0	0	0	0	0	0	0	0
0	0	0	676	0	0	676	1,982
269	0	2,319	0	0	0	2,666	2,666
0	0	0	43	0	0	43	2,025
588	0	1,266	0	0	0	2,022	4,688
0	0	0	0	0	0	0	2,025
587	0	0	0	0	0	772	5,460
0	0	0	0	0	0	0	2,025
612	0	0	0	0	0	703.9	6,163.9
0	0	0	0	0	0	0	2,025
2,056	0	9,414	84,749	0	0	117,306.9	
1,270	2,107	23,203	2,025	0	0	135,614	
2,056	0	3,585	0	0	0	6163.9	
0	0	0	2,025	0	0	2,025	

3. The CHA annual reports between 1987–88 and 1992–93 inclusive make no reference to any deductions in federal transfer payments to the provinces. However, the *Canada Health Act Annual Report 1994–95* contains three tables of deductions, one for each of the following fiscal years: 1992–93, 1993–94, 1994–95 (see Health Canada, *Canada Health Act Annual Report 1994–95* (Ottawa: Supply and Services Canada, 1995)).

4. The *Canada Health Act Annual Report 1994–95* contains the following explanation: Subsection 20(5) of the Act provided an incentive for the early elimination of these charges. A province that ended extra-billing or user charges within three years of the coming into force of the Act, that is, before April 1, 1987, was entitled to have the total amount of deductions refunded. All provinces in which direct charges existed did, in fact, establish or revise laws, regulations or practices to comply with the extra-billing and user charges conditions by the established deadline. Consequently, prior withheld funds were paid to the provinces as required under the Act. Any deductions made beginning April 1, 1987 were not to be refunded (see *ibid.* at 14)

public opposition within Alberta, Bill 11 has sparked a war of words between the Alberta government and Ottawa regarding Alberta's compliance with the CHA.

These two events provide a useful occasion to reflect on the current state of Medicare. What is particularly striking is that the public debate spawned by each event has been dominated by financial considerations. There are three interrelated issues here. First, there is the question of the level of funding for Medicare. Are current levels of funding adequate? If not, what level of funding would be required to ensure that the system fulfills its objectives of providing comprehensive and accessible medical care to all Canadians? Second, there is the question of the source of funding. Assuming that more monies are required, where are they to come from? If the sources of funding are to be strictly public, should these new monies come from the federal or provincial governments? If nonpublic sources are an option, what kinds of sources should be considered? Should we encourage private investment, particularly with respect to large capital expenditures? Or should we re-open the question of whether patients should pay directly for the medical services that they receive? Third, there is the question of distribution or allocation. Once we have identified the level and sources of funding, according to what principles or criteria should we distribute medical goods and services?[4]

Financial issues have dominated the discourse of all political actors on all sides of the debate over the future of Medicare. And to be sure, funding is of fundamental importance, particularly if the federal government proposes to create national homecare and pharmacare systems. But my concern is that the fixation on funding has occurred at the expense of an examination of the place of supervisory institutions in the health care system. Supervisory institutions are of central importance to the future of Medicare, no matter what scenario unfolds, because any future system will include some national standards. To be effective, these standards must be interpreted, applied and enforced by institutions of some kind.

Because I approach Medicare as a student of federalism, institutions hold a particular interest for me. The basic question of federalism is who governs or, more specifically, which set of institutions, federal or provincial, has jurisdiction to regulate a certain area of socio-economic activity. An analogous question—which institutions should govern Medicare?—is central to the debate over the future of health care in this country. However, it is a question that has been largely ignored by politicians on all sides of the debate, the media and even academic commentators. This omission is problematic and short-sighted because institutions are central to the durability of Medicare. Simply put, without institutions to enforce them, national standards for Medicare are merely political platitudes. In this article I focus on two specific institutional questions: the federal enforcement of the existing national standards of the CHA, and the pressing need for dispute-settlement machinery under the Social Union Framework (SUF) signed by Ottawa and nine provinces in 1999.[5]

Federal Enforcement of the Canada Health Act

A Legal Primer on the Canada Health Act

Let me begin with a legal primer on the CHA.[6] The political rhetoric surrounding the CHA appears to suggest that it imposes legally binding obligations on provincial governments that receive federal monies for Medicare. Since jurisdiction over health care is thought to go to the provinces under the division of powers, the CHA has accordingly been portrayed by some as a massive incursion by the federal government into provincial jurisdiction.[7] The legal situation, however, is sharply at odds with this picture. The CHA does not purport to legally bind provincial governments. Rather, it binds the federal government by defining the conditions that must be met for federal payments to the provinces to be legal. The interesting feature of the CHA is that the legality of federal payments is conditioned upon provincial compliance with the conditions spelled out therein. The CHA also contains enforcement mechanisms that are triggered in cases of provincial noncompliance, which I discuss in detail below.

Why is the CHA framed in this way? There is a complicated constitutional story here. The starting point is a pair of decisions made by the Supreme Court of Canada and the Privy Council in 1938, which held that jurisdiction over unemployment insurance rests with the provinces.[8] Although rather specific in focus, the judgements also contain broader language that suggests that publicly operated insurance schemes which seek to safeguard persons against the risk of illness or poverty lie outside federal jurisdiction.[9] As a consequence, the conventional wisdom is that direct federal regulation of social policy, including health insurance, is unconstitutional.[10] It would be unconstitutional, for example, for the federal government to operate a national health insurance scheme.[11] However, these decisions also stated that it would be entirely constitutional for the federal government to spend monies in areas of provincial jurisdiction by making transfer payments to provinces, and by attaching conditions to those funds.[12] The rather obvious concern raised by these holdings is that conditional grants to the provinces allow the federal government to indirectly regulate social policy through the use of financial incentives, an end they are constitutionally precluded from achieving directly through legislative or "coercive" means. As well, as Andrew Petter has argued, this distinction finds little support in the text of the Constitution Act, 1867,[13] which allocates jurisdiction not on the basis of policy instruments, but rather on the basis of subject matter, a point relied on by the Supreme Court itself in the context of jurisdiction to implement international treaties and Crown immunity.[14] Petter has also argued that, in addition to resting on a weak doctrinal foundation, the federal spending power runs counter to important constitutional values, for example, because it allows national majorities to determine policy in areas of provincial jurisdiction, and because it weakens the lines of political accountability by divorcing jurisdiction over policy areas from control over policy outcomes.[15] By and large, the courts have been unsympathetic to these criticisms, responding to them by drawing fairly questionable distinctions between legislative activity on the one hand and spending on the other, and ignoring altogether the arguable tension between spending power and important constitutional values.[16] And as it turns out, conditional grants have been an extremely effective policy instrument. The end result is that spending power has allowed the federal government to play a central role in the development of the postwar welfare state in Canada (now dubbed "the Social Union"), although it lacks jurisdiction over social policy.[17]

The Enforcement of the CHA: The Ideal

With this brief introduction in mind, let us turn to the dispute over Bill 11.[18] Aside from the massive public opposition to Bill 11 within Alberta, one of the notable features of the dispute has been the active role of the federal government. On 16 November 1999, Alberta announced its intention to allow for-profit clinics to offer insured medical services; a short time thereafter, Allan Rock expressed concern in a letter to his provincial counterpart, Halvar Jonson, that such a course of action might run afoul of the CHA.[19] Federal expressions of concern turned into public criticism once the text of Bill 11 was tabled on 2 March 2000. A few days later, in a remarkable spectacle, Rock gave a public address at the University of Calgary's Faculty of Medicine, arguing that Bill 11 would do nothing to reduce costs, cut waiting lists or to improve the quality of care.[20] Federal criticism of Bill 11 peaked in a letter Rock sent to Jonson on 7 April 2000. In that letter Rock requested amendments to Bill 11, *inter alia*, prohibiting overnight stays in for-profit clinics and the sale of enhanced services in combination with the provision of insured services, and by so doing, implied that Bill 11 (before it was amended) might not comply with the CHA.[21] On 11 May 2000, however, Rock effectively conceded, in a speech to the House of Commons, that Bill 11 on its face did not violate the CHA.[22] I will return to the question of Bill 11's compliance with the CHA below.

The impression created by the energetic and aggressive federal stance toward Bill 11 is that bureaucrats in the Canada Health Act Division of Health Canada are actively monitoring the provincial health care systems, and constantly assessing them for compliance with the national standards spelled out in the CHA. Moreover, Rock's very personal, and very public, involvement in the issue suggests that the federal government is willing to take the provinces to task for noncompliance with the CHA and to bear the political consequences of doing so. In fact, the available evidence points in exactly the opposite direction. There is a yawning gap between the rhetoric surrounding Bill 11 and the reality of the federal government's enforcement of the CHA. The truth is that the federal government is largely unaware of the degree of provincial compliance with the CHA, and, in suspected cases of provincial noncompliance, has followed the traditional norms of intergovernmental relations in Canada, shrouding its interactions with provincial governments in secrecy.

To provide a framework for critical analysis, let us consider what the CHA contemplates in terms of the enforcement of the conditions laid out therein. It is fairly clear that the CHA envisages a scheme approximating the image created by the rhetoric surrounding Bill 11, whereby the federal government monitors provincial compliance with the terms of the CHA and, in cases of noncompliance, moves to ensure provincial compliance. This conclusion follows from the terms of the CHA itself. The CHA spells out a public enforcement machinery, centred on the federal government or, more accurately, two enforcement tracks for two different sets of conditions. For the conditions of universality, comprehensiveness, accessibility, nonprofit public administration and portability, the CHA provides that provinces "must" satisfy these criteria in order to qualify for federal transfers.[23] However, the CHA provides that for breaches of these conditions, the federal cabinet "may" withhold funds from the offending province after mandatory consultation with the province.[24] The cabinet need not withhold these funds; its power to do so is discretionary. By contrast, for the CHA's bans on extra-billing and user charges, the CHA provides for mandatory deductions in an amount equal to the amount of those charges.[25] Another feature of the CHA's enforcement machinery which is frequently overlooked is the requirement that the minister of health submit an annual report to Parliament respecting the administration and operation of the CHA that documents the extent of provincial compliance with national standards. The direct role of Parliament in monitoring compliance with the CHA illustrates the special importance of Medicare.[26]

What would the ideal system of federal enforcement look like? Surprisingly, aside from the provisions I mentioned above, the CHA hardly speaks to this crucial issue. However, if we proceed from first principles, a very general picture emerges. An effective enforcement scheme would require that an institution be vested with responsibility for assessing provincial compliance with the standards laid down by the CHA. This institution could be a government department (like the Canada Health Act Division of Health Canada), or an arms-length agency; to date, the federal government has opted for the former approach. What would this institution do? A large part of its work would be devoted to gathering information about provincial health insurance plans. It could gather information in one of two ways. First, it could receive reports from provincial governments that document, in detail, their compliance with the CHA. Second, it could gather information through a complaints procedure, whereby aggrieved individuals or public interest organizations could bring alleged breaches of the CHA to the attention of federal authorities, which could then launch an investigation.

What kind of information would this institution gather? For some standards, all that would be required would be an examination of the relevant provincial statutes and regulations. Universality and portability fall into this category. However, other standards raise complex questions of fact that would require the federal enforcement agency to gather information regarding the actual operation of provincial health plans. Consider accessibility. For provincial plans to satisfy this criterion, they must "provide for insured health services on uniform terms and conditions and on a basis that does not impede or preclude, either directly or indirectly, whether by charges made to insured persons or otherwise, reasonable access to those services by insured persons."[27] The definition of accessibility clearly contemplates both financial and nonfinancial barriers to access. Some financial barriers, such as extra-billing and user fees, are specifically prohibited by the CHA. Nonfinancial barriers would probably include the lack of resources to meet the demand for medical services, manifested in the form of waiting lists, as well as geographic disparities in the availability of medical treatments. Presumably, relevant information would include patient-to-bed ratios, physician-to-patient ratios, specialist-to-patient ratios, and the length of waiting lists, among a host of other data.[28] Finally, the federal enforcement agency would need to be staffed with experts who could interpret this data. Moreover, either provinces would be obliged to provide this sort of information to the federal enforcement agency, or the agency would require both the resources and the legal authority to gather this data itself.

The Enforcement of the Canada Health Act: The Reality

The reality on the ground differs markedly from this sketchy and idealized picture. In order to get a sense of the nature and extent of federal enforcement, I have relied on four sources of evidence: the track record of the CHA's enforcement machinery, as contained in the annual reports submitted by the minister of health to Parliament; reports of the auditor general on the administration of the CHA; records of proceedings of the House of Commons in Hansard; and media reports regarding alleged violations of the CHA.

Let me begin with two facts. The first is that, despite the explicit bans on user charges and extra-billing—which are remarkably specific in a statute otherwise marked by its use of open-ended language—provinces continue to violate these conditions of federal funding (see Table 1 below). Since these conditions are subject to the mandatory enforcement mechanism, the federal government is legally obliged to make deductions in federal transfer payments, and it appears that the federal government complies with the CHA. The latest year for which information is available is the 1998–99 financial year (1 April 1998 to 31 March 1999), during which the federal government withheld $703,950 from Newfoundland, Nova Scotia and Manitoba.[29] This figure is comparable to the mandatory deduction in 1997–98 of $772,000. By contrast, in 1995–96 and 1996–97, the mandatory deductions were much higher, totalling $2,666,000 and $2,022,000 respectively. The difference can be accounted for in part by large penalties imposed on Alberta ($2,319,000 in 1995–96, $1,266,000 in 1996–97) due to the operation of the Gimbel Eye Clinic, which I discuss below. Overall, the federal government has withheld a gross total of $252,920,950 from provincial governments that permitted extra-billing and user charges. Of these monies, however, 96.8 percent ($244,732,000) was returned to provincial governments pursuant to section 20(5) of the CHA, which provides that if, in the opinion of the minister, extra-billing and user charges had been eliminated in a province by 1 April 1987, the total amount deducted in respect of extra-billing or user charges before that date would be refunded. Of the remaining funds ($8,188,950), 43.7 percent ($3,585,000) was withheld from Alberta.

In stark contrast, the discretionary enforcement mechanism, which attaches itself to the important conditions of universality, comprehensiveness and accessibility, has never been used. Juxtaposed against the active use of the mandatory deductions scheme, a casual observer could reasonably conclude that the federal government is actively monitoring provincial compliance with the terms of the CHA, and has come to the conclusion that provincial plans meet those national standards. Alternatively, one could conclude that instances of noncompliance have been resolved without the need for financial penalties. Indeed, Health Canada consistently makes these sorts of claims in the annual CHA reports.[30]

However, the reports of the Auditor General tell a radically different story. The Auditor General has examined the enforcement of the CHA on three occasions, in 1987, 1990 and 1999. I focus on the last report because it is by far the most detailed, and because it repeats many of the concerns advanced in the first two. The Auditor General indicated in 1999 that there had been numerous instances of noncompliance in the last five years. Six cases were resolved without the use of financial penalties; the report did not provide any details. However, the Auditor General noted that there were other cases of

Table 2: ~~Alleged violations of the~~ Canada Health Act's prohibition of extra-billing and user fees and federal responses

Date	Alleged violation	National standard
27/06/84	Ontario refuses to ban extra-billing.	Extra-billing
06/07/84		Extra-billing
19/07/84		Extra-billing, user fees
14/07/86		Extra-billing
09/02/88	Women in BC are forced to pay for their own abortions even if a fetus is severely deformed, as BC covers only those abortions where the mother's life is in danger. NDP health critic Marion Dewar asks the federal government to penalize BC.	Extra-billing
10/12/90	Jim Karpoff (Surrey North, NDP) asks the Minister of Health to comment on Quebec's plan to levy "deterrence" or user fees on patients ($5 for each "non-essential" emergency room visit).	Extra-billing
17/12/90	Rey Pagtakhan (Winnipeg North, Lib.) revisits the $5 user fee.	Extra-billing
20/03/91	Jim Karpoff once again raises the $5 user fee issue, following comments by the Quebec minister of health that the fees would proceed.	Extra-billing
16/09/91	Following passage of Bill 120 on 28 August 1991, Jim Karpoff notes the federal government's inaction in regards to Quebec's user fees.	Extra-billing
19/09/91	Karpoff calls on the minister of health to "inform Quebec that he will proceed immediately under the Canada Health Act to penalize Quebec for Bill 120, which imposes user fees in emergency wards. He should also inform the premier of the province of BC, who has been advocating user fees, that he will not accept user fees in that province."	Extra-billing
19/05/94		Extra-billing
20/09/94	Hon. Audrey McLaughlin (Yukon, NDP) asks the Prime Minister to raise the issue of "the private clinics which clearly contravene the Canada Health Act" with Alberta's premier, with whom he was meeting that day.	Extra-billing
28/11/94	McLaughlin revisits the same issue.	Extra-billing
29/11/94	Various user fees are charged by private clinics— prostate surgery in Toronto and Windsor, kidney stone treatment in Ontario, express executive checkups in Montreal, abortions in most provinces, among other procedures.	User fees

Violating province	Public federal response
Ontario	Ottawa is reportedly set to impose penalties of approximately $50 million.
All	Federal government announces that medicare penalties will begin on 19 July.
Ontario, BC, Alberta, NB, Saskatchewan, Manitoba, Quebec	Penalties of $9.5 million per month go into effect against 7 provinces. The penalties to be repaid if the provinces get rid of extra charges by 1 April 1987.
Ontario	Transfer payments withheld since 1984 returned to Ontario after the province bans extra-billing.
BC	Federal health minister Jake Epp says he lacks the power to decide that abortions are "medically necessary" under the CHA.
Quebec	Hon. Perrin Beatty responds that he asked his officials to contact the Quebec government "to seek information with regard to the proposals" and says he will "ensure that the principles underlying the Canada Health Act are fully respected."
Quebec	Perrin Beatty responds that he had not yet received a reply from Quebec.
Quebec	Perrin Beatty says the minister "indicated that he believes that what he is doing can be done within the confines of the Canada Health Act. The ball is in Quebec's court to demonstrate that it can be done."
Quebec	No action.
Quebec	No explicit federal follow-up.
BC	BC fined almost $2 million for extra-billing.
Alberta	Right Hon. Jean Chretien responds, *inter alia*, "I hope that Mr. Klein will respect the laws of Canada."
Alberta	Mary Clancy (parliamentary secretary to minister of citizenship and immigration, Lib.) notes that all health ministers, with the exception of Alberta, agreed at a September 1994 conference to regulate private clinics.
Ontario, Quebec	

Date	Alleged violation	National standard
07/01/95	Reports resurface of direct billing practices by private clinics such as the Gimbel Eye Centre in Calgary.	User fees
07/11/95	Alberta fails to ban user fees by the 15 October deadline.	
18/11/95	Newfoundland women pay facility fees to get abortions at the province's only private abortion clinic in St. John's; women in Halifax pay an average of $400 for abortions at a private clinic; five small surgery clinics in Manitoba charge fees for, *inter alia*, eye cataract operations, disposable equipment used in operations; and knee operations on patients who want to bypass the surgery waiting list at local hospitals.	Extra-billing
30/09/97	Manitoba, Newfoundland, Nova Scotia continue to pay penalties for allowing private clinics to charge extra fees.	
06/09/96	Gimbel Eye Centres still charges out-of-province patients "facility" fees two months after Alberta agreed to end extra-billing.	Extra-billing
02/11/96	Gimbel patients pay a new kind of fee for "enhanced services," but the clinic says these services are not "medically necessary."	Extra-billing
31/05/96		
05/10/97	Alberta allows HRG (Health Resource Group) to open its first private hospital in Calgary's former Grace Hospital. It says no "medically necessary" procedures will be done. HRG charges a facility fee and bills medicare for procedures.	Extra-billing
16/12/99	Trillium Health Centres (Mississauga, Toronto) charges patients up to $300 extra, in cash, to jump the MRI queue.	Extra-billing
23/03/00	A Montreal clinic charges hundreds of dollars an hour for the use of operating rooms so that patients can jump the queue for minor surgeries. The clinic's owner says the province knows about its practices.	Extra-billing
04/04/00	Alexa McDonough asks Allan Rock about an Albertan who needed an MRI, was told that there was a nine-month waiting list, but if she paid $600 she could be seen the next day.	Extra-billing
10/05/00	Bill 11 is passed by the Alberta legislature.	Extra-billing, accessibility

This table covers the period from 17 April 1984, when Royal assent was given to the Canada Health Act, to the present. Whereas alleged violations are often described by critics or the media as engaging a particular principle of the CHA, the listed national standard has been reformulated wherever necessary to reflect my own understanding of the relevant CHA condition.

Violating province	Public federal response
All	Federal government gives provinces until 15 October to comply with CHA's ban on user fees or face transfer payment reductions.
Alberta	Marleau imposes $420,000 per month penalty on Alberta.
Manitoba, Newfoundland, Nova Scotia	Marleau penalizes Newfoundland and Nova Scotia $20,000 per month, and cuts Manitoba's transfer payments by $49,000 per month.
	Health Canada says the federal government cannot do more.
Alberta	No action.
	No federal follow-up.
Alberta	Joseph Volpe (parliamentary secretary to minister of health, Lib.) announces that an agreement to end, by 1 July, facility fee billing of patients for insured services in private clinics was reached between Alberta and the Minister of Health.
Alberta	No action.
Ontario	No federal follow-up.
Quebec	Both the Quebec's health insurance board and Health Canada launch investigations.
Alberta	Allan Rock says he is investigating the incident and took the matter up with Alberta's health minister when they met on 31 March 2000 in Markham, Ont.
Alberta	The following day, Allan Rock tells the House of Commons: "We are therefore serving notice today that we will monitor closely what may happen on the ground in private for-profit facilities permitted under Bill 11 to ensure that queue jumping and other accessibility issues do not arise."

noncompliance that had not been resolved. A number of provinces (which the Auditor General did not name) contravened the portability condition, which requires that medical services received outside of a province (including outside of the country) by insured persons temporarily absent from that province be reimbursed at the same rate as inside the province. The portability condition was apparently violated by five provinces with respect to treatment received outside of Canada; in addition, one province violated the condition with respect to treatment received in other provinces. The Auditor General also stated, without providing any detail, that "[o]ther examples of suspected noncompliance with the comprehensiveness and accessibility criteria have been the subject of considerable discussion between the federal government and the provinces and territories."[31] These disputes remained unresolved.

The most charitable interpretation of the Auditor General's findings to this point of the report is that the federal government has been aware of the extent of provincial noncompliance, has been able to resolve some but not all disputes through negotiation, and has been reluctant to use the powerful financial levers available to it to secure better compliance. However, the report then went on to state that the federal government was largely unaware of the true extent of provincial noncompliance, because it lacked the required information. The root of the problem was the federal government's approach to information gathering. Rather than taking an active approach to gathering relevant information from the provinces—which, as I argued above, follows from the logic of the CHA—the report stated that Health Canada "has taken a passive stance."[32] The provinces voluntarily submit annual reports which are reproduced or summarized in the annual CHA reports. But, as a perusal of the annual CHA reports reveals, the provincial reports are rather general in nature, and lack the specific data that would be necessary to assess compliance with criteria like accessibility and comprehensiveness. It appears that regulations that would have required more extensive provincial reporting were drafted in 1984, when the CHA was adopted, but faced stiff provincial opposition and were therefore never promulgated.[33]

Other sources of information are restricted to "regional staff reports, correspondence and complaints from the public, newspaper clippings and other media reports."[34] The report did note that the federal government monitored changes to provincial laws and regulations but, as I argued above, some of the funding criteria require information about the actual operation of health care systems.

Worryingly, these are not new criticisms. In his first report on the enforcement of the CHA in 1987, the Auditor General stated that the actual operation of provincial plans was not being monitored by Health Canada. It recommended that steps be taken to do so.[35] In his 1990 report, the Auditor General noted that this recommendation had not been adopted.[36] The Auditor

General made a similar recommendation in his 1999 report. In response, Health Canada agreed to assess the adequacy of its current information-gathering system and to determine how it can be improved.[37] Allan Rock recently announced that the federal government would allocate an additional $4 million to the existing annual budget of $1.5 million to monitor and assess provincial compliance.[38] These monies will go toward increased staff and developing better methods of tracking information. The details of these arrangements, however, have yet to be announced.

The general lack of federal enforcement of the CHA is also evident from media reports and Hansard, although this source of information is far from comprehensive. Between 17 April 1984 (when the CHA came into force) and May 2000, there were numerous alleged violations of the CHA. Of these, several involved alleged violations of the prohibitions on user fees and extra-billing (see Table 2 below). In most cases, the federal government did respond to the alleged violation through discussions with the relevant provincial government, and/or the imposition of a cash penalty. The most prominent example here is the dispute surrounding the Gimbel Eye Clinic in Calgary. The eye clinic is a privately owned facility which specializes in laser surgery. From 1989 onward, the provincial health insurance plan covered the cost of these laser treatments. However, the clinics charged patients a "facility fee" which was not covered by the provincial health insurance plan. In a letter to provincial and territorial ministers of health (dated 6 January 1995), then Minister of Health Diane Marleau took the position, for the purposes of the CHA, that the Gimbel clinic was a "hospital" and that the facility fee therefore amounted to a kind of user charge for medically necessary services covered by the provincial health insurance plan, which is clearly prohibited under the Act.[39] The letter imposed a deadline of 15 October 1995 for provincial compliance. Alberta did not meet this deadline and, as a result, the federal government imposed a penalty of $420,000 per month in November 1995. Soon thereafter, the federal government imposed penalties on Manitoba, Newfoundland and Nova Scotia. Alberta later, in July 1996, complied.

However, the aggressive and public stance of the federal government with respect to the Gimbel Eye Clinic stands in stark contrast to the relatively timid federal response to a Quebec proposal in December 1990 that patients visiting emergency rooms be charged a $5 user fee. In response to questions in the House of Commons at that time, then Minister of Health Perrin Beatty "indicated that he believes that what he is doing can be done within the confines of the Canada Health Act."[40] However, he did not provide any details. The federal government made no further public statements on the matter. The provincial proposal was eventually withdrawn. It is not clear whether the proposal was withdrawn in response to federal pressure; at the very least, the federal government made no announcement to this effect in the House of Commons.

With respect to the funding conditions subject to the discretionary enforcement mechanism (see Table 3 below), however, the facts tell a different story. As I have mentioned, federal funds have never been withheld under this mechanism. However, since the CHA came into force, there have been several alleged violations of these funding criteria. Most of these appear to have generated no federal response in public. They are certainly not mentioned in any of the CHA reports. Indeed, this is even so for alleged violations of the portability condition, which is not subject to the difficulties of interpretation that bedevil comprehensiveness and accessibility. To be fair, the Auditor General's report does suggest that Health Canada is aware of the various breaches of the portability criterion; however, if this is true, the fact remains that these violations are ongoing. There have been complaints against several provinces regarding the rates of reimbursement for out-of-country treatment that are lower than that provided for treatment within the province. In two provinces (British Columbia and Ontario), the question ended up before the courts; Canada declined to intervene in one case, *Collett* v. *Ontario (A.G.)*,[41] and in the other, *Brown* v. *British Columbia (A.G.)*,[42] conceded that the provincial health plan appeared to contravene the CHA, but asked the court to dismiss the action so that the matter could be resolved through intergovernmental negotiation. In addition, Quebec does not provide reimbursement for treatment received in provinces other than Ontario.[43] The federal government has taken no public position here as well.

A large number of complaints have turned on waiting lists and whether the threat they pose to health contravene the accessibility criterion. The issue has been raised in the House of Commons on several occasions.[44] In not one case did the federal government publicly promise to look into the matter, even though these complaints related to important services. On three occasions, for example, Members of Parliament alleged that women lacked access to abortion services, widely recognized by health professionals as being a crucial component of women's reproductive health. Other complaints related to waiting times for breast cancer treatment, hip replacements and cataract surgery. Similarly, there have been a handful of complaints regarding alleged violations of the comprehensiveness and universality criteria. Likewise, these generated no federal response in public.

What has been the response of political actors, the media and academic commentators to the lack of federal enforcement? To a large extent, this issue has been ignored. By comparison, other issues in health policy, particularly declining federal support for health care, have received an enormous amount of attention. The portions of the Auditor General's report in 1987 that dealt with the CHA prompted one question in the House of Commons;[45] the same portions of the 1990 report did not prompt a single question. However, the

1999 report did prompt three questions, although the report was not made into an issue by members of the opposition.[46] The media coverage has been equally scant.[47] Moreover, of the published articles on the CHA in the legal and medical literature, only two refer to the report of the Auditor General, or the issue of nonenforcement generally.[48]

In my view, the federal government's nonenforcement of the CHA, along with the failure of political actors and the academic community to highlight the federal government's abdication of its responsibilities, is a national embarrassment. In this connection, it is worth highlighting a remarkable statement in the Auditor General's 1999 report: "Parliament cannot readily determine the extent to which each province and territory has satisfied the five criteria [i.e., universality, comprehensiveness, accessibility, portability and nonprofit public administration] and the two conditions [i.e., the bans on extra-billing and user fees] of the Act."[49] This criticism was offered in connection with the content of the annual CHA reports presented to Parliament by the Minister of Health. The auditor general's concern (expressed also in 1987 and 1990) was that the reports are fundamentally flawed because they fail to indicate the degree of provincial compliance. This view, however, put together with the Auditor General's finding that Health Canada really has no idea of the degree of provincial compliance with the CHA, suggests that the CHA is potentially being violated with impunity and that this fact is being kept from Parliament. Although politely worded, the overall message contained in the Auditor General's report is damning.

Why the lacklustre federal performance? There would appear to be two reasons why the federal government has failed to aggressively enforce the national conditions spelled out in the CHA. The first is a lack of institutional capacity. Information gathering of the kind that is required to gauge provincial compliance with the conditions of accessibility and comprehensiveness, in particular, requires a serious commitment of human and capital resources. As I mentioned earlier, an expert staff, including persons with training in health services research, is a must.

However, it would a mistake to reduce the federal government's neglect of the CHA to a lack of resources. The more fundamental problem is a lack of political will. The Auditor General's report made an oblique yet revealing reference to this problem when it stated that the enforcement of the CHA had been tempered by national unity concerns.[50] What the report was referring to was a long history of tense federal-provincial relations surrounding the federal spending power. Particular exercises of the federal spending power have long been regarded as federal impositions by provincial governments (although only one province, Quebec, has ever challenged the constitutionality of federal government expenditures in areas of provincial jurisdiction).[51] The dynamic of fiscal federalism has also been profoundly affected by the dramatic decline in federal transfer payments, a point I discuss below with respect to the SUF. But I can state the basic point here: the legitimacy of the federal enforcement of national standards has been diminished along with its financial involvement.[52] The failure to exercise its discretionary enforcement power accordingly reflects a loss of legitimacy and political capital on the part of the federal government.

To be fair, Bill 11 may mark a dramatic turning point in the federal government's stance toward the CHA. The federal government has responded energetically from the start. As well, insofar as the federal government has passed judgement on the compatibility of Bill 11 with the CHA, and has made that judgement public, the federal government's actions are radical and new.[53] But again, it is important to note that the Canadian Union of Public Employees (CUPE) had released its own legal opinion on the compatibility of Bill 11 with the CHA.[54] Had the federal government not made its view public, it would have lost face. On balance it is fair to say that the experience surrounding Bill 11 is exceptional, not representative. The federal government has a long way to go.

The Future

What is the relevance of the federal government's nonenforcement of the CHA for the future? My sense is that national standards are here to stay and may in fact become more, not less, important, in the years to come. As I have argued before, Canadians take Medicare to be constitutive of social citizenship, and are unlikely to accept a scenario in which that component of Canadian identity is abolished. If the federal government creates national homecare and pharmacare programs, for example, federal financial support will probably come with conditions attached. If federal financial support for existing programs is increased, the standards in the CHA will remain and, indeed, might be supplemented by standards regarding waiting lists, as Allan Rock has suggested.[55] If federal financial support remains at current levels or declines, the standards in the CHA may be replaced by joint federal-provincial standards, as is provided by the CHST, or even interprovincial standards, as was contemplated by Tom Courchene's ACCESS proposals.[56] If private financing becomes a more prominent feature of the system, standards to ensure reasonable access will be absolutely critical. And any scenario which involves national standards by necessity has an institutional component.

A second point is the importance of accountability.[57] Accountability for performance is an idea that has historically been identified with the private sector. In the 1990s, however, it attracted support in public policy circles. As Colleen Flood has argued, enhanced accountability is a crucial component of any strategy to maintain public confidence in Medicare, which is the key to ensuring the survival of the public system. Accountability, at the very least, includes informing citizens of provincial compliance with benchmarks for performance. Typically, these benchmarks have been framed in terms of indicators that measure the quality of care. The Canadian innovation is to frame performance benchmarks in terms of distributive justice which, as I have argued elsewhere, is the best way to understand the national standards of comprehensiveness and accessibility.[58] Examined through the lens of accountability, the federal enforcement of the CHA is sorely lacking. The CHA reports contain little or no detail regarding provincial noncompliance. The secrecy surrounding federal-provincial discussions reflects the norms of executive federalism, which has long been criticized for shielding public policy decisions from public scrutiny. By comparison, the Auditor General's 1999 report at least gives a vague indication of both the number and nature of instances of provincial noncompliance. The system of federal enforcement is in sore need of reform. Such reform would enhance Medicare's accountability to Canadians. Can we trust the federal government to enforce national standards for health care? To date, public enforcement machinery has centred on the federal government. However, it is fair to say that the federal government has failed to live up to its responsibilities. It may be time to consider other options. One option is the establishment of a Medicare commission that would have a mandate to monitor provincial compliance with national standards. The commission would be independent and nonpartisan, and would be insulated from the political pressures that influence the federal cabinet at present. Information gathering would be active, not passive, and would include a requirement that provinces provide detailed information regarding the actual operation of health care systems. In this connection, the establishment of the Canadian Institute for Health Information (CIHI) is a positive development because it may be able to assist both levels of government in generating the kind of hard data that is required.[59] This supervisory body would report directly to Parliament and be headed by a Medicare commissioner. The commissioner would be assisted by an expert staff of health economists and health service researchers. What is missing from this proposal, of course, is any reference to an individual complaints process, as well as a dispute settlement mechanism. I will now address these issues, in the context of the SUF.

The Social Union

Moving Away From Federal Unilateralism

My proposal for a Medicare commissioner is similar to existing arrangements inasmuch as it is centred on the federal government. However, the constitutional and financial context surrounding the CHA suggests that this sort of regulatory framework for evaluating provincial compliance may be inappropriate. Constitutionally, the understanding of the division of powers

Table 3: Alleged violations of the Canada Health Act subject
to discretionary enforcement mechanism and federal response

Date	Alleged violation	National standard
23/05/84	Bill Blaikie (Winnipeg-Birds Hill, NDP) presents a petition by several hundred northern Ontario residents who must travel to Toronto and Winnipeg to receive medical treatment each year. They call upon the government to uphold the CHA.	Accessibility
21/05/87	Hon. Lloyd Axworthy (Winnipeg-Fort Garry, Lib.) notes the Alberta government's intention to eliminate the coverage of podiatry treatment by medicare and expresses concern that elderly people will suffer.	Comprehensiveness
09/02/88	Women in BC are forced to pay for their own abortions even if a fetus is severely deformed, as BC covers only those abortions where the mother's life is in danger. NDP health critic Marion Dewar asks the federal government to penalize BC.	Comprehensiveness
17/03/88	Marion Dewar (Hamilton Mountain, NDP) claims that the removal of insured coverage for certain health services such as abortion is a threat to the principles underlying the CHA, and calls on the minister of health and welfare to act to ensure accessibility to medicare.	Comprehensiveness
31/03/88	Quebec refuses to join agreement between all provinces that ensures medicare coverage for out-of-province care.	Portability
28/05/90	During consideration of Bill C-69, an act to amend certain statutes to enable restraint of government expenditures, Rod Laporte (Moose Jaw-Lake Centre, NDP) recounts the story of the Attfields, a family from Lanigan, Saskatchewan. Mrs. Attfield's husband Kevin had bone cancer and needed a transplant, but cuts forced Princess Margaret Hospital in Toronto to cancel ten transplants and he died before he could be treated.	Accessibility
02/12/91	Brian L. Gardiner (Prince George-Bulkley Valley, NDP) tells of his father having to go to Seattle to get cancer treatment due to insufficient resources or facilities in Canada.	Accessibility
01/05/92	Quebec cuts out-of-country medicare coverage to $480 per day for hospital costs and $50 for medical expenses.	Portability

Violating province	Public federal response
Ontario, Manitoba	No action.
Alberta	No action.
BC	Federal health minister Jake Epp says he lacks the power to decide that abortions are "medically necessary" under the CHA.
All	Pierre H.Vincent (parliamentary secretary to minister of finance) promises close monitoring of developments in abortion services, and notes that the "determination of reasonable access must take into consideration all aspects related to the provision and delivery of any insured health service by a province. This could include an examination and understanding of provincial health delivery resources, facilities, personnel, as well as a recognition of factors, i.e., geography, that may set practical limits on what health services are provided where."
Quebec	Federal health minister Jake Epp, although aware that Quebec is in violation of the CHA, seeks a "negotiated compromise with Quebec centring on the core of the problem, which is Ottawa-Hull." The government is said to want to avoid "ruffling Quebec's feathers." The province's insurance board is expected to allow Hull doctors to refer patients to Ottawa doctors who will be compensated by OHIP.
All	No action.
All	No action.
Quebec	No action.

Date	Alleged violation	National standard
02/06/92	Dawn Black (New Westminster-Burnaby, NDP) notes that 1,400 abortions are performed on Canadian women in US border states due to lack of access in parts of Canada. She calls on the health minister to make RU–486 available in Canada.	Accessibility
23/01/94	BC refuses to cover those who don't pay medicare premiums.	Universality
15/02/94	Ontario and Quebec negotiate to give Quebecers full medical coverage in Ontario. Critics charge that Quebec has been in contravention of the CHA since 1988, when every province except Quebec agreed to reciprocal coverage.	Portability
11/05/94	Dick Harris (Prince George-Bulkley Valley, Ref) notes that Helga Lopp of Prince George, BC had been waiting for over two years for "vital operation to cure a life-threatening condition" but cutbacks resulted in a backlog of over 300 patients.	Accessibility
18/05/94	Canadian Snowbird Association threatens Ontario government with lawsuit over plan to cut out-of-country hospital stay coverage from $400 to $100 a day.	Portability
01/07/94	OHIP cuts to out-of-country coverage take effect.	
17/08/94	Canadian Snowbird Association launches lawsuit against Ontario.	
23/09/95	Three provinces refuse to pay for out-of-country medical expenses.	Portability
10/06/94	Grant Hill (Macleod, Ref.) raises the issue of a 42-month waiting list for cataract surgery in Ontario (4,662 patients waiting) and asks how this was reasonable access.	Accessibility
04/04/95	Grant Hill (Macleod, Ref.) makes reference to lack of reasonable access to hip replacement in Manitoba (60-week wait), cataract surgery in Saskatchewan (30-week wait), hernia surgery in Quebec (1,460-patient list) and to user fees for stitches, anaesthetic and syringes at Eastern Kings Memorial Hospital in Nova Scotia.	Accessibility
18/10/95	Deborah Grey (Beaver River, Ref.) expresses concern about waiting lists of 61 weeks for hip replacement in Manitoba, 44 days for breast cancer radiation treatment in Ontario, and a 1,200-person heart bypass waiting list in Ontario.	Accessibility
29/10/96	The Canadian Snowbird Association files a lawsuit against the BC government for cutbacks in out-of-country medicare coverage.	Portability

Violating province	Public federal response
All	No action.
BC	No action.
Quebec	No action.
BC	Hon. Diane Marleau says that "the principles and the values of the Canada Health Act will prevail. I do not believe that any Canadian whose life is threatened imminently has had to wait for two years for surgery."
Ontario	On 30 June 1994, Diane Marleau requests delay in plan until after federal-provincial talks in September; Ontario refuses.
	Marleau says there is nothing the federal government can do.
Alberta, BC, Saskatchewan	Marleau begins an investigation.
Ontario	Diane Marleau responds: "We continue to work with the provinces. As a matter of fact, one of the things we did in the last budget was maintain transfer payments in health to give an indication of our commitment toward the funding of proper health care services in the provinces."
Manitoba, Saskatchewan, Quebec, Nova Scotia	Hon. Diane Marleau (Minister of Health, Lib) replies that while "there are pressures from time to time in different areas, ... the Canada Health Act ensures that these pressures are addressed by the individual provinces." Furthermore, she refers to her 6 January 1995 letter to all provinces describing the federal government's position on user fees and the CHA, and says that medical necessity "has been defined by medical associations, provincial governments and in some cases the courts."
Manitoba, Ontario	Diane Marleau says that Ontario announced a transfer of more money into the breast cancer treatment area in order to reduce the waiting time.
BC	No action.

Date	Alleged violation	National standard
14/08/97	Snowbirds call on Health Canada to enforce portability of CHA after losing court battle over BC's $75 out-of-country hospital expense limit.	Portability
09/11/96	Alberta hospitals refuse dialysis to visitors from other provinces, citing cutbacks in medicare for giving priority to Albertans. Private clinics step in to offer these services.	Portability, accessibility
15/01/97	Alberta refuses to pay more than $100 per day plus doctors' fees for premature baby born and hospitalized in Nebraska.	Portability
23/05/97	Halifax couple in court battle to get province to pay for in-vitro fertilization and embryo transplantation claims they were offered $25,000 to keep quiet.	Comprehensiveness
10/09/97	Blue Jays player Ed Sprague, an American covered by private insurance, gets MRI within 24 hours of a shoulder injury, while OHIP patients wait for months. Provincial Liberal health critic Gerard Kennedy claims CHA violation. Provincial Health Minister Jim Wilson disagrees.	Accessibility
16/11/97	Howard Gimbel continues to charge out-of- province patients direct fees for cataract surgery.	Portability
27/03/98	Alberta forces residents who opt out of medicare to do so for a full benefit year rather than restoring medical coverage immediately when an individual resumes paying premiums.	Universality
03/04/99	Class action certification denied to family of a five-year-old autistic boy who launched a lawsuit against the BC government for refusal to cover costs of intensive therapy program, allegedly in violation of the CHA. BC Supreme Court ruled that a single claim would be more efficient.	Comprehensiveness
12/06/99	Ottawa doctor Charles Shaver "crusades" to have the federal government enforce the portability principle of the CHA against Quebec, which refuses, *inter alia*, to pay the difference between its hospital daily rates and those of other provinces.	Portability
07/08/99	Severe staff shortages prompt Montreal hospitals to urge patients to stay away unless they have life-threatening injuries. Universal access to health care is allegedly threatened.	Accessibility
10/05/00	Bill 11 is passed by the Alberta legislature.	Extra-billing, accessibility

This table covers the period from 17 April 1984, when royal assent was given to the Canada Health Act, to the present. Whereas alleged violations are often described by critics or the media as engaging a particular principal of the CHA, the listed national standard has been reformulated wherever necessary to reflect my own understanding of the relevant CHA condition.

Violating province	Public federal response
BC	No action.
Alberta	No action.
Alberta	No action.
Nova Scotia	No action.
Ontario	No action.
Alberta	No action.
Alberta	No action.
BC	No action.
Quebec	No action.
Quebec	No action.
Alberta	The following day, Allan Rock tells the House of Commons: "We are therefore serving notice today that we will monitor closely what may happen on the ground in private for profit facilities permitted under Bill 11 to ensure that queue jumping and other accessibility issues do not arise."

upon which the CHA is premised assumes a degree of *de facto* concurrent jurisdiction (provincial regulatory power, federal financing power) over large areas of social policy. Both the federal and provincial governments have a legitimate role to play in health policy, albeit through radically different policy instruments. An enforcement regime entirely within the hands of the federal government sits uncomfortably with joint federal-provincial responsibility for Medicare. This is all the more true given the policy instrument employed by the federal government—conditional grants. Conditional grants give rise, in political terms, to quasi-contractual relationships because provinces agree to comply with national standards in exchange for federal funding.

In addition, the financial circumstances surrounding the federal role in Medicare suggest that unilateral enforcement is not a realistic option at present. Given that the federal government's standing to serve as standard-setter derives from its fiscal involvement, it is material that that involvement has declined over the last twenty years.[60] The story of declining federal funding began in 1977, with the shift away from 50/50 cost-sharing to a block grant (the Established Programs Financing, or EPF grant) consisting of a mixture of cash and tax points, with the cash component tied to an escalator based on growth in per capita gross national product (GNP). In 1982, the escalator was applied to the entire EPF entitlement, not just the cash component, making the EPF cash transfer strictly residual. The escalator was then eliminated in stages, first in 1986 (when it was reduced to GNP less two percent), then in 1990 (when the EPF per capita transfer was frozen). Finally, the EPF was eliminated in 1995 and replaced by a block grant for health, social assistance and post-secondary education, known as the Canada Health and Social Transfer (CHST).

The CHST has generated an enormous amount of controversy, in part because the provinces claim that it radically reduced the level of federal transfers.[61] And to be sure, the value of the cash component of federal transfers declined dramatically, from $18.5 billion in 1995–96, the last year before the CHST came into force (representing combined cash contributions under the EPF and the Canada Assistance Plan) to a low of $12.5 billion in 1998–99, a decline of $6.0 billion overall. The provinces have emphasized this figure.[62] However, the CHST consists of a mixture of cash transfers and tax points and, over time, the value of those tax points has increased significantly. For example, between 1995–96 and 1998–99, the value of the tax points increased from $11.4 billion to $14.2 billion.[63] The net reduction over this period was therefore $3.2 billion (from $29.9 to $26.7 billion), not the $6.2 billion reduction in cash transfers pointed to by the provinces. Moreover, in the 1999 and 2000 budgets, the federal government did increase cash transfers to the provinces by $11.5 and $2.5 billion over five years, respectively, apparently bringing total cash transfers to $15.5 billion annually by 2000–1. Moreover, the value of the tax points is expected to increase to $17.2 billion in 2003–4 and, as a consequence, the CHST is expected to stand at $29.4 billion in 1999–2000, $30.8 billion in 2000–1, $31.3 billion in 2001–2, $32.0 in 2002–3, and $32.7 billion in 2003–4, compared to $29.9 billion in 1995–96, the last year before the CHST came into force (none of these figures have been adjusted for inflation). However, it is important to note that of the new $14 billion in cash transfers, only $8 billion will be added to the cash base of the CHST, and will be ongoing, which raises serious questions regarding the future stability of federal cash contributions. Nevertheless, let us proceed on the assumption that those one-time supplements constitute part of the CHST.

An additional complication is that it is now difficult to gauge the actual level of federal financial support for health care because the CHST is a block grant for health, postsecondary education and social assistance, which provinces are free to spend as they choose. The federal government has addressed this problem by allocating a portion of the CHST to health expenditures, according to a complex formula described in Table 4 below. Since the provinces have not proposed a formula of their own,[64] I will rely on it here. When these calculations are performed, federal support for health care stood at $15.7 billion in 1995–96, declined to a low of $14.4 billion in 1997–98, and since then has increased, to $15 billion in 1998–99 and $17.5 billion in 1999–2000. It is projected to increase to $18.5 billion in 2000–1, $19 billion in 2001–2, $19.5 billion in 2002–3 and $19.9 billion in 2003–4.

The final piece of the puzzle is the relative contribution of the federal government to provincial health care expenditures. The slight decline in total federal funding has occurred against the background of increasing health care expenditures by the provinces. According to the Canadian Institutes for Health Information, provincial government health expenditures increased from $48.9 billion in 1995–96, to $49.1 billion in 1996–97, $50 billion in 1997–98, and are estimated to have increased to $52.8 billion in 1998–99 and $55.6 billion in 1999–2000. As a percentage of provincial expenditures, then, the federal contribution has declined and then recovered over this period, from 32.1 percent in 1995–96, to a low of 28.4 percent in 1998–99, and then increased to 31.5 percent in 1999–2000. However, federal cash contributions have dropped far more steeply, from 16.3 percent in 1995–96 to a low of 10.1 percent in 1998–99, and climbed back to 13.3 percent in 1999–2000. It is these declining relative levels of federal cash transfers that have led to a loss of moral authority and financial leverage on the part of the federal government with respect to the enforcement of the national standards in the CHA.

The Social Union Framework Agreement

Prior to the current round of discussions on health care, a number of these concerns had already been raised by the provinces, and led to a set of federal-provincial negotiations that culminated in the SUF. Although the negotiations

	CAP/EPF								
	1995 −96	1996 −97	1997 −98	1998 −99	1999 −00	2000 −01	2001 −02	2002 −03	2003 −04
Total CHST	29.9	26.9	25.8	26.7	29.4	30.8	31.3	32.0	32.7
Total CHST cash base	18.5	14.7	12.5	12.5	14.5	15.5	15.5	15.5	15.5
Budget 1998 cash	–	–	–	–	12.5	12.5	12.5	12.5	12.5
"Health" increase to base from 1999 budget	–	–	–	–	–	1.0	2.0	2.5	2.5
1999 supplement	–	–	–	–	2.0	1.0	0.5	–	–
2000 cash supplement	–	–	–	–	0.0	1.0	0.5	0.5	0.5
Total CHST health cash	8.0	6.3	5.4	5.4	7.4	8.1	8.3	8.3	8.3
Total CHST tax points	11.4	12.2	13.3	14.2	14.9	15.3	15.8	16.5	17.2
Total CHST health tax points	7.7	8.3	9.0	9.6	10.1	10.4	10.7	11.2	11.7
National health contribution	15.7	14.6	14.4	15.0	17.5	18.5	19.0	19.5	19.9
Provincial health expenditure	48.9	49.1	50	52.8	55.6				
Total CHST health cash as a per cent of expenditures	16.3%	12.9%	10.8%	10.2%	13.3%				
National health contribution as a per cent of expenditures	32.1%	29.7%	28.8%	28.4%	31.5%				

1 Figures for "Total CHST."

2 The historical (1995–96) share of the CAP/EPF block grant spent by provinces on health was 43% (8.0/18.5). This share is carried over for calculations subsequent to the introduction of the CHST in fiscal 1996–97. However, from fiscal 1999–00 onwards, "Total CHST health cash" is calculated using the following formula: ([Budget 1998 cash] x 0.43) + [Health increase to base from 1999 budget] + [1999 supplement] + ([2000 cash supplement] x 0.75).

The entire "Health increase to base from 1999 budget" and "1999 supplement" is included in "Total CHST health cash," pursuant to an agreement entered into by the federal government with all provinces and territories on 4 February 1999, in which the premiers and territorial leaders agreed to earmark all of the 1999 budget increases in CHST transfers to health funding. See Prime Minister of Canada, news release, "The Federal-Provincial-Territorial Health Care Agreement" (4 February 1999).

The historical share of EPF cash allocated by provinces to health spending was 75%; this is the fraction of the "2000 cash supplement" that is used in the above formula, as per Finance Canada estimates (Interview with Nilar Gyi, Department of Finance, on 26 May 2000).

3 The historical share of CHST tax points apportioned by provinces to health spending is 67.9%, thus "Total CHST health tax points" is this fraction of "Total CHST tax points" (ibid.).

4 The Provincial Government Sector includes health spending from provincial/territorial government funds, federal health transfers to the provinces/territories, and provincial government health transfers to municipal government.

were prompted by the decline in federal financial support, it is important to recognize that other considerations were at play as well. The provinces were still bitter over the manner in which the CHST was introduced, accusing the federal government of having acted unilaterally, without prior notice or consultation. Moreover, the provinces had relied on past promises of federal financial support. They had been induced to create provincial programs and, even though federal funding was declining, they were obliged as a condition of receiving federal funds both to continue those programs and to meet national standards. Additionally, recent initiatives, such as the Millennium Scholarship Fund, suggested that the federal government would expend new monies on direct federal initiatives instead of restoring federal transfer payments. The provinces called for a variety of measures, including provincial consent to the introduction of new shared-cost programs, stable and adequate funding with a long-term commitment from the federal government, the right to opt out with compensation, à la Meech and Charlottetown,[65] and even the devolution of revenue-raising authority to reduce vertical fiscal imbalance. Lurking in the background were national unity concerns, such as the need to demonstrate the viability of nonconstitutional options to renew the federation, and a desire to reassert social policy as an important component of Canadian identity in the face of economic globalization.[66]

The SUF addressed some of these concerns. The specific focus here is Article 6, entitled "Dispute Avoidance and Resolution." Coming into the negotiations, the provinces and social policy commentators had consistently called for the need to institutionalize federal-provincial relations in the social policy arena.[67] Unilateral federal enforcement of the CHA, in particular, was a source of provincial irritation. The provinces accordingly called for the establishment of dispute resolution machinery that was impartial. In the end, SUF did not establish the sort of machinery that the provinces sought. Rather, aside from some scattered specifics, Article 6 establishes a general framework for the creation of dispute settlement machinery in the future. Important details remain underspecified.

What does Article 6 actually say? Signatories committed themselves to "working collaboratively to avoid and resolve intergovernmental disputes." In terms of substantive policy areas, dispute resolution would be applicable, *inter alia*, to the CHA (although Article 6 also states that existing legislative provisions will be respected). Article 6 appears to contemplate three types of processes: dispute avoidance, negotiations and mediation. Dispute avoidance will be encouraged "through information-sharing, joint planning, collaboration, advance notice and early consultation, and flexibility in implementation." Negotiations will be premised on joint fact-finding, which may be conducted by a third party, and which will be made public if one party so requests. In addition, negotiations may be accompanied by mediation; again, mediation reports will be made public if one party so requests. Mechanisms for dispute resolution must respect a list of general principles; they have to be "simple, timely, efficient, effective and transparent," allow for the possibility of nonadversarial solutions, be appropriate for the specific sectors in which the disputes arise and provide for the expert assistance of third parties.

It is difficult to get a handle on what specific procedures would be consistent with Article 6. Indeed, there are many institutional questions surrounding the design of dispute resolution that remain unresolved. With respect to the modes of dispute resolution that are referred to—negotiations and mediation—Article 6 does not address important issues. For example, Article 6 does not stipulate that either negotiations or mediation be obligatory. Without such an obligation, negotiations or mediation may not even be commenced (witness the Bill 11 dispute). As well, the role of the mediator is not addressed. As Guy Tremblay has written in his analysis of Article 6, mediators in the labour relations context can often propose solutions to parties, which may incorporate the interpretation and application of the relevant legal materials to the facts at hand.[68] If a mediator was charged with producing this sort of report, and if such a report were made public, it might carry a normative force that compensated for its lack of legal enforceability.

But the central problem is the failure of Article 6 to refer to dispute settlement mechanisms other than negotiation and mediation. The obvious omission is adjudication. The gap is all the more glaring because compliance with the terms of the CHA is justiciable.[69] An individual could launch a court case in which the issue would be the compliance of a provincial health insurance scheme with the national standards spelled out in the CHA. Similar litigation occurred with respect to the now-defunct Canada Assistance Plan.[70] Indeed, had the federal government sought to challenge Bill 11, it could have proceeded by way of a reference to the Supreme Court of Canada. Alternatively, public interest organizations in Alberta could still launch a court case either in the Alberta superior courts or the federal court, although there are important hurdles to overcome with respect to standing and the review of cabinet discretion.[71] Because negotiations and mediation may fail, it is important that adjudication be available. Indeed, the possibility of adjudication may create the incentives for a negotiated or mediated solution.

What institutions should be vested with adjudicative responsibility? The options are courts, specialist panels or some combination of the two. My preference is for the latter option. Both courts and specialist panels possess institutional advantages over the other that should be harnessed by any dispute settlement system. Specialist panels would possess the requisite expertise to engage in the sort of fact-finding that the criteria of accessibility and comprehensiveness demand. As I mentioned earlier, a variety of data, ranging from information regarding cost-effectiveness to waiting lists and physician-to-patient ratios, will play into the interpretation of these criteria. An additional advantage of specialist panels is the ability to appoint those who are not lawyers but have expertise in health policy and intimate knowledge of the health care system. Finally, specialist panels can be constituted from a list mutually agreeable to the federal and provincial governments, an option constitutionally precluded for courts.

In this scheme, courts would serve a supervisory function, largely confined to ensuring that the panel system conforms to norms of procedural propriety. But courts would also be important in securing access to dispute resolution for citizens. Although I have emphasized the importance of bilateral mechanisms in light of joint federal-provincial responsibility for health care, these should not operate to the exclusion of citizen interests. Medicare is a central part of the Canadian understanding of social citizenship and, ultimately, is concerned less with financial relationships between governments than with providing high-quality medical care to Canadians in the service of fair equality of opportunity. The constitutionally secured independence of courts would ensure that dispute settlement machinery would not fall prey to the political dynamic of executive federalism.

Thus, I contemplate a two-track process whereby either governments, federal or provincial, or citizens could invoke the dispute settlement machinery established under the SUF. A similar arrangement currently exists under the Agreement on Internal Trade,[72] although it would be inappropriate to simply apply that model here.[73] Under the AIT, citizens may launch complaints against provincial or federal laws or practices in one of two ways. A government may act on behalf of a citizen with whom it has a substantial and direct connection or, if a government refuses to act on behalf of a citizen, a citizen may act on her own. Under the latter process, the intergovernmental body created by the AIT, the Internal Trade Secretariat, exercises a gatekeeping function to screen out frivolous complaints. The principal difference between the economic union and social union contexts is that provincial and individual interests are not aligned in the latter, whereas they are in the former. Challenges to provincial measures under the AIT are typically brought by nonresident economic entities (citizens or corporations)—outsiders—that are legally resident in another province, and on whose behalf the home province may have good economic and political reasons for acting. An outsider, for example, may be a large corporate entity that employs individuals and consumes services in the home province. With respect to the CHA, by contrast, aside from barriers to interprovincial mobility, challenges to provincial measures will typically be brought by insiders against their provinces of residence. Other provinces would have no incentive to take up claims on their behalf and, indeed, in order to protect themselves from claims brought by other provinces, might act collusively to impede citizen complaints. Accordingly, citizens should not be required, in the first instance, to convince governments to bring claims on their behalf.

Does Bill 11 Violate the CHA?
The Need for Dispute Settlement Machinery

The SUF was referred to by both the federal and Alberta governments early on in the Bill 11 dispute. Rock invoked the SUF in his initial letter to Jonson of 26 November 1999, as a justification for raising questions regarding Bill 11.[74] Jonson confirmed that Alberta was a signatory to the SUF in his letter to Rock of 10 December 1999, with respect to the SUF's provisions on accountability.[75] However, neither party has referred to the need for dispute settlement machinery or Article 6.

This is extremely disappointing since dispute settlement machinery would have been particularly useful in the Bill 11 challenge. For legal scholars, one of the most interesting features of the Bill 11 dispute is that behind the political rhetoric lies a real legal disagreement. This disagreement was framed around duelling legal opinions commissioned by CUPE and the Alberta government that arrived at opposing answers to this question of the compliance of Bill 11 with the CHA.[76] At its core, this disagreement turns on competing interpretations of both Bill 11 and the program criteria in the CHA. The existence of this sort of legal disagreement suggests both the potential and the need for institutions to resolve it.

So what is the legal dispute? Although far from a model of clear legislative drafting, Bill 11 clearly contemplates that two different categories of surgical services will be available in Alberta. The first consists of surgical services covered by the provincial health insurance scheme. The Act refers to these as "insured surgical services," which it defines as services that are "provided by a physician, or by a dentist in the field of oral surgery, in circumstances under which a benefit is payable under the Alberta Health Care Insurance Act."[77] Where can insured surgical services be received? Section 2(1) of Bill 11 provides that surgical services, not just insured surgical services, can only be received in a public hospital or "an approved surgical facility," the language used by Bill 11 to refer to for-profit clinics. An approved surgical facility is either a facility "designated" to provide insured surgical services, or a surgical facility accredited to provide uninsured surgical services.[78] By implication it appears that insured surgical services can be received at a public hospital or a designated surgical facility. However, there are two restrictions on the kinds of insured surgical services that can be provided at designated surgical facilities. No such facility may provide a "major surgical service," such a service to be defined in bylaws enacted pursuant to the Medical Profession Act.[79] It follows that insured surgical services that are also major surgical services cannot be provided at designated surgical facilities, although what a major surgical service constitutes remains unclear. In addition, only public hospitals may admit patients for medically supervised stays exceeding twelve hours,[80] which suggests that insured surgical services requiring supervised stays of more than twelve hours cannot be provided by designated surgical facilities. With respect to insured surgical services, Bill 11 prohibits queue jumping, i.e. the giving or accepting of money or valuable consideration in order to give any person priority for the receipt of an insured surgical service.[81] Moreover, Bill 11 also prohibits designated surgical facilities from imposing user charges.[82]

Bill 11 also refers to a second category of surgical services which falls within the ambit of a broader category termed "enhanced medical goods or services." These are defined as "medical goods or services that exceed what would normally be used in a particular case in accordance with generally accepted medical practice."[83] The list of enhanced medical goods and services will be defined by the provincial cabinet through regulation.[84] It appears that enhanced medical goods or services can be provided by public hospitals and surgical facilities designated to provide insured surgical services;[85] it is not clear whether surgical facilities that have been accredited to provide uninsured surgical services can provide enhanced medical goods and services as well. Bill 11 accords enhanced medical goods and services and insured surgical services differential treatment in two respects. First, Bill 11 contemplates user charges for enhanced medical goods and services, subject to a disclosure requirement,[86] whereas user charges for insured surgical services are clearly forbidden.[87] Second, it appears that the prohibition on queue jumping in section 3 might be inapplicable to enhanced medical goods or services, because payments for those services would be payments not "for the purpose of giving any person priority for the receipt of an insured surgical service" but for the purpose of bypassing the public system altogether.[88] Taken together, the legality of user charges and the potential legality of queue jumping mean that enhanced medical services and goods will be allocated on the basis of ability to pay.

Given that market forces will determine the distribution of enhanced medical services and goods, what services and goods fall into that category is of critical importance. Indeed, the central disagreement between the Alberta and CUPE opinions is the relationship between enhanced medical goods or services and insured surgical services. Bill 11 is silent on this crucial point but commentators have been willing to offer interpretations. The CUPE opinion suggests enhanced medical goods or services could differ from insured services or goods in one of two ways. First, they may be goods or services that are of higher quality than insured goods or services, but which address the same underlying medical condition. For example, whereas the health insurance plan may provide a basic hearing aid or pacemaker that meets the test of medical necessity, individuals may be able to purchase a hearing aid or pacemaker of higher quality. Second, enhanced medical services may be identical to insured services in every respect except that they are provided more quickly than medical necessity requires. The concern expressed by the CUPE opinion is that the ability of individuals to obtain more quickly the same services available from the public insurance scheme would eviscerate the ban on queue jumping. The Alberta opinion, by contrast, offers a more benign interpretation of enhanced medical goods and services by suggesting those services can only be provided when bundled with insured surgical services. The textual basis for this interpretation of Bill 11 is a provision that stipulates that persons who receive insured surgical services shall not pay for enhanced medical goods or services unless certain disclosure requirements have been met.[89] The implication drawn by the Alberta opinion is that enhanced medical goods and services merely supplement, but do not substitute for, insured surgical services.

Which view is correct? To begin, the Alberta opinion is flawed because there are other provisions in Bill 11 which clearly suggest that the relationship between enhanced and insured services and goods is not one just of supplementation, but also of substitution. In this regard, subsection 5(5)(a) is quite explicit because it refers to a situation where a patient is provided with an enhanced medical good or service *because* the normal medical good or service is not available; presumably, if it were available, it would be unnecessary to receive the enhanced good or service. It would appear, then, that enhanced goods or services may either supplement or substitute for insured goods or services. Does this mean that the CUPE opinion is correct? In the end, a great deal will turn on the implementation of Bill 11 through regulations. But it does seem that Bill 11 is open to implementation in the manner envisaged by CUPE.

If Bill 11 were implemented in this way, would the resulting scheme contravene the CHA? The key national standard is comprehensiveness, which requires that provincial health plans provide all "medically necessary" or "medically required" hospital and physician services. Although it is not entirely clear on this point, the CUPE opinion argues that Bill 11 breaches the comprehensiveness criteria because it provides that provincial health insurance plan will only cover those medical goods that are "minimally" medically necessary, rather than those which are medically necessary. There are a number of difficulties with this argument. First and foremost, Bill 11 does not define what medical goods and services can or will be covered by the provincial health insurance plan. Rather, Bill 11 only defines the content of enhanced medical goods and services that may be offered outside the provincial insurance system.

The CUPE opinion, however, offers a more complex argument that links up Bill 11 with the provincial health insurance plan. Recall that Bill 11 defines enhanced goods and services as those "that exceed what would normally be used in a particular case in accordance with generally accepted medical practice," a phrase that is clearly a benchmark of medical necessity. Indeed, Bill 11 states at one point that enhanced medical goods or services are *not* "medically required."[90] The CUPE opinion (1) reads back this definition of medical necessity into the Alberta Health Care Insurance Act,[91] which defines insured services as those services provided by physicians that are "medically required,"[92] and (2) argues that this definition is merely one of "minimal" medical necessity, which falls short of the comprehensiveness standard in the Canada Health Act. Let us assume that the first point is correct. What about the second point? CUPE's argument is that the standard of medical necessity laid down by Bill 11 falls short of the standard of medical necessity laid down by the CHA. However, the CHA is famously ambiguous on this point. Although medical necessity is the central concept in the CHA, the Act does not define this crucial term. I have argued elsewhere that in the face of this ambiguity, "medical necessity" should be interpreted in a generous manner, to encompass any and all services which restore individuals to a state of normal functioning.[93] However, the definition of "medical necessity" adopted in Bill 11 is another plausible interpretation, particularly because it relies on medical judgement, not cost-effectiveness, as the framework of reference. If that is right, then Bill 11 may not contravene the comprehensiveness requirement. At the very least, the point is unsettled.[94] And, when interpretive disagreements of this sort arise, so does the need for institutions to resolve them.[95]

The better objection to Bill 11 is that the resulting scheme would contravene not the letter but the spirit of the CHA. As the CUPE opinion puts it, "patients with identical medical conditions would receive different standards of care or different waiting times for care, depending entirely on their ability to pay."[96] The genesis of public health insurance schemes in Canada, of course, was a rejection of unregulated markets as the appropriate mechanism for the allocation of medical goods and services. Two-tier medicine sits uncomfortably with the moral premises of Medicare. This is not the first time that events on the ground have pointed to a gap between the ambitions of and the legal framework surrounding Medicare. Indeed, the introduction of explicit bans on user fees and extra-billing in 1984 was a response to the concern that existing program criteria, such as accessibility, were inadequate means for pursuing that end.

As well, although Bill 11 may not violate the CHA, it might set in place a process that creates a state of affairs in Alberta that will contravene the Act. The standard criticism against the creation of a privately funded health care system that exists alongside and in parallel to a publicly funded system is that it will siphon off resources from the public system. A private system, it is argued, will attract the best physicians, which will increase waiting lists for specialist treatments, rather than decreasing them. The availability of a private option will facilitate the exit of the wealthy from the public system, and will eliminate both their incentive to ensure that that system functions effectively, and their desire to contribute financially to that system. In the end, all of these developments would impede accessibility. Defenders of Medicare routinely present these factual propositions as articles of faith, whereas in fact, they are empirical propositions that must be tested against the evidence. Thus, Bill 11 creates the need for effective monitoring machinery that can determine whether threats to accessibility actually materialize.

Is the Social Union Framework Dead?

My suggestion that dispute settlement machinery be established under the SUF suggests that the SUF possesses some normative force and, for that reason, that governments will seek to implement it. But does it? I am afraid here that the limited evidence available suggests that the SUF, with respect to social policy that its framers envisaged, has not had the domesticating or civilizing influence on intergovernmental relations.

Consider two recent examples. The first was the federal government's homelessness initiative, announced in December 1999. This initiative involves rather significant federal government expenditure in an area of provincial jurisdiction: housing. It appears that most of these monies will consist of grants to local governments and nonprofit entities. The relevant point is that under the SUF, the federal government was obliged to give at least three months' notice to provincial governments and to offer to consult with them. It appears that this term of the SUF was not complied with. Indeed, my understanding is that provincial ministers with responsibility for social policy were meeting in Ottawa on the very day of the federal announcement, yet only heard about the federal initiative from the media.

The second example is the controversy surrounding Bill 11 in Alberta itself. The active role of the federal government masks the fact that the SUF has played little or no role in the dispute. Under the SUF, Alberta was obliged to give the federal government advance notice prior to the announcement of Bill 11, and to offer consultations. Neither of these requirements was met. Moreover, as I have discussed, neither party invoked Article 6 and suggested the creation of dispute settlement machinery to determine the compliance of Bill 11 with the CHA.

Conclusion

The reform of Canadian Medicare will be one of the dominant policy issues of the next decade. Canadians are in search of practical solutions that simultaneously satisfy the constraints of costs and justice, and which respond to the changing realities of medical practice. My argument in this paper has been that the role of supervisory institutions is an additional topic that should not be ignored. The crafting of supervisory institutions—whether in the form of a Medicare commission and/or dispute settlement machinery under the SUF—must be responsive both to political realities and the constitutional framework surrounding Medicare. But, above all, since Medicare is constitutive of the Canadian understanding of social citizenship, these institutions must ensure that Medicare is accountable to Canadians.

NOTES

1   R.S.C. 1985, c. C–6 [hereinafter CHA].

2   Canada, *The Budget Plan 2000* (Ottawa: Department of Finance, 2000), online at http://wwwfin.gc.ca/budget00/toce/2000/bud2000e.htm (accessed on 5 July 2000).

3   Bill 11, Health Care Protection Act, 4th Sess., 24th Leg., Alberta, 2000 (assented to 10 May 2000) [hereinafter Bill 11].

4   Financial considerations are certainly central to the federal funding story. But financial considerations are also an important part of the debate over Bill 11. One of the principal concerns with Medicare is that waiting lists pose a risk to the health of individuals in need of rationed medical treatments. The Alberta government has argued that Bill 11 would alleviate this difficulty because the availability of a privately financed option would allow those with the financial means to withdraw from the public queue, thereby freeing up resources for those remaining in the public system. As it turns out, the evidence from other jurisdictions is mixed on whether this would actually occur. See P. McDonald *et al.*, *Waiting Lists and Waiting Times for Health Care in Canada: More Management!! More Money??* (Ottawa: Health Canada, 1998) at 285–6.

5   A Framework to Improve the Social Union for Canadians—An Agreement between the Government of Canada and the Governments of the Provinces and Territories (4 February 1999), online at http://socialuniongc.ca/news/020499_e.html (accessed on 21 June 2000) [hereinafter SUF]. Quebec declined to sign the final document. For the position of the government of Quebec, see *Québec's Political and Constitutional Status: An Overview* (1999) at 33–6. In addition, see Secréteriat aux Affaires intergouvernementales canadiennes, news release, "Joseph Facal rend publiques huit analyses d'experts sur l'Union sociale" (21 June 2000), online at http://www.cex.gouv.qc.ca/saic/c990609.html (accessed on 25 May 2000); the following documents, all analyzing the SUF, were released by the government of Quebec in a single unpublished volume entitled *Entente-cadre sur l'Union Sociale* (1999), online at http://www.cex.gouv.qc.ca/saic/index-etudes.htm (accessed on 21 June 2000): A. Noël, "Étude générale sur l'Entente"; A. Binette, "Étude sur le chapitre 1 de l'Entente-cadre (principes)"; J. Frémont, "Étude sur le chapitre 2 de l'Entente-cadre (mobilité)"; G. Otis, "Étude sur le chapitre 3 de l'Entente-cadre (imputabilité publique et transparence)"; A. Gagnon, "Étude sur le chapitre 4 de l'Entente-cadre (travailler en partenariat pour les Canadiens)"; G. Tremblay, "Étude sur le chapitre 6 de l'Entente-cadre (prévention et règlement des différends)." For commentary on the *SUF*, see M. Young, "The Social Union Framework Agreement: Hollowing Out the State" (1999) 10 *Const. Forum* 120; B. Cameron, "A Framework for Conflict Management" (1999) 10 *Const. Forum* 129; K. Banting *et al.*, "Four Views of the Social Union" (1999) 21:3 *Pol'y Options* 68.

6　In this paragraph, I follow S. Choudhry, "The Enforcement of the CHA" (1996) 41 *McGill L.J.* 461 at 461–76 [hereinafter "Enforcement of the CHA"].

7　Former federal health minister Monique Bégin later recalled that during the drafting of the CHA, "[j]ust before the Committee meetings started, I had a meeting [on 20 January 1984] with the Quebec Minister of Health, Pierre-Marc Johnson … [M]y provincial colleague began by declaring the project unconstitutional": see M Bégin, *Medicare: Canada's Right to Health* (Ottawa: Optimum, 1988) at 163–5.

8　*Canada (AG.) v. Ontario (A.G.)*, [1936] S.C.R. 427 (*Reference re The Employment and Social Insurance Act*) [hereinafter *UI Reference (SCC)*]; *Canada (A.G.) v. Ontario (A.G.)*, [1937] A.C. 355 (P.C.) (*Reference re The Employment and Social Insurance Act, 1935*) at 686 [hereinafter *UI Reference (PC)*].

9　Thus, in the *UI Reference (SCC)*, *supra* note at 451, Rinfret J, for the majority, stated that "[i]nsurance of all sorts, including insurance against unemployment and health insurances, have always been recognized as being exclusively provincial matters under the head 'Property and Civil Rights,' or under the head 'Matters of a merely local or private nature in the Province.'" Later, in the same judgement, he stated that the federal act at issue was *ultra vires* because it was in relation to, *inter alia*, "insurance against unemployment, for aid to unemployed persons, *or other forms of social insurance and security*" [emphasis added], which were "subject-matters falling with the legislative authority of the provinces": *ibid.* at 454. At the Privy Council, Lord Atkin in *UI Reference (PC)*, *supra* note at 365 came to the same conclusion: "There can be no doubt that, prima facie, provisions as to insurance of this kind, especially where they affect the contract of employment, fall within the class of property and civil rights in the Province, and would be within the exclusive competence of the Provincial Legislature."

10　See A. Petter, "Federalism and the Myth of the Federal Spending Power" (1989) 68 *Can. Bar Rev.* 448 at 452 (education, health "and other social services" all fall within provincial jurisdiction).

11　P.W. Hogg, *Constitutional Law of Canada* (Toronto: Carswell, 1996) at 6.8(a).

12　This possibility was spelled out in some detail in *UI Reference (SCC)*, *supra* note at 457, and *UI Reference (PC)*, *supra* note at 366. The constitutionality of the federal spending power was recently confirmed by the Supreme Court in the *Reference Re Canada Assistance Plan*, [1991] 2 S.C.R. 525 [hereinafter *CAP Reference*], where it fell to the court to assess the constitutionality of a federal statute that reduced the level of federal contributions under the Canada Assistance Plan, R.S.C. 1985, c. C–1 [hereinafter *CAP*]. The attorney general of Manitoba argued that Parliament lacked jurisdiction to amend the CAP because that statute intruded on provincial jurisdiction over social policy. The Court rejected this argument in *CAP Reference*, *supra* at 567: The written argument of the Attorney General of Manitoba was that the legislation "amounts to" regulation of a matter outside federal authority. I disagree. The agreement under the Plan set up an open-ended cost-sharing scheme which left it to British Columbia to decide which programs it would establish and fund. The simple withholding of federal money which had previously been granted to fund a matter within provincial jurisdiction does not amount to the regulation of that matter. Still less is this so where, as in this case, the new legislation simply limits the growth of federal contributions. In oral argument, counsel said that the Government Expenditures Restraint Act "impacts upon [a] constitutional interest" outside the jurisdiction of Parliament. That is no doubt true, but it does not make the Act *ultra vires.* "Impact" with nothing more is clearly not enough to find that a statute encroaches upon the jurisdiction of the other level of government. The Court recently confirmed the constitutionality of the federal spending power in *Eldridge* v. *British Columbia (A.G.)*, [1997] 3 S.C.R. 624 at 647.

13 Constitution Act, 1867 (UK.), 30 and 31 Vict., c. 3, reprinted in R.S.C. 1985, App. II, No. 5.

14 Petter, *supra* note at 456–7. The leading cases here are *Canada (A.G.)* v. *Ontario (A.G.)*, [1937] A.C. 326 (P.C.) (international treaties); *Amax Potash Ltd.* v. *The Government of Saskatchewan*, [1977] 2 S.C.R. 576 (Crown immunity).

15 Petter, *supra* note at 463–8.

16 *Porter* v. *Canada*, [1965] 1 Ex. C.R. 200; *Central Mortgage and Housing Corp* v. *Co-op College Residences*, (1975) 13 O.R. (2d) 384 (C.A.); *Winterhaven Stables Ltd.* v. *Canada (A.G.)* (1988), 62 Alta. L.R. (2d) 266 (C.A.), leave to appeal to S.C.C. denied (1989) 55 D.L.R. (4th) viii; *YMHA Jewish Community Centre* v. *Brown*, [1989] 1 S.C.R. 1532.

17 My sense is that the constitutional compromise crafted by the Privy Council has generated a peculiar political dynamic that we see at play in the debate over Bill 11. On the one hand, Alberta argues, with some justification, that the federal role in health care is an incursion on provincial jurisdiction. On the other hand, the federal government argues, also with some justification, that that role has been explicitly sanctioned by the courts.

Constitutional scholars have generated an extensive critical literature on the federal spending power. See Petter, *supra* note; E.A. Driedger, "The Spending Power" (1981) 7 *Queen's L.J.* 124; K. Hanssen, "The Constitutionality of Conditional Grant Legislation" (1966–67) 2 *Man. L.J.* 191; J.E. Magnet, "The Constitutional Distribution of Taxation Powers in Canada" (1978) 10 *Ottawa L. Rev.* 473; G.V. La Forest, *The Allocation of Taxing Power under the Canadian Constitution* (Toronto: Canadian Tax Foundation, 1981); A. Lajoie, "The Federal Spending Power and Meech Lake" in K.E. Swinton and C.J. Rogerson, eds., *Competing Constitutional Visions: The Meech Lake Accord* (Toronto: Carswell, 1988) 175; B. Laskin, "Provincial Marketing Levies: Indirect Taxation and Federal Power" (1959–60) 13 *U.T.L.J.* 1; W.R. Lederman, "Some Forms and Limitations of Co-operative Federalism" (1967) 45 *Can. Bar Rev.* 409; J.E. Magnet, "The Constitutional Distribution of Taxation Powers in Canada" (1978) 10 *Ottawa L. Rev.* 473; F.R. Scott, "The Constitutional Background of Taxation Agreements" (1955) 2 *McGill L.J.* 1; D.V. Smiley, *Conditional Grants and Canadian Federalism* (Toronto, Canadian Tax Foundation, 1963); P.E. Trudeau, *Federalism and the French Canadians* (Toronto: Macmillan, 1968). That body of work has revolved around the question of whether the spending power allows the federal government to circumvent the division of powers. I am sympathetic to these arguments, but in my view, constitutional scholars have ignored a logically prior question—why social policy falls under exclusive provincial jurisdiction. Of course, this proposition is the assumption that underlies the critique of the generous approach to the federal spending power taken by the Privy Council and the modern Supreme Court. This question is one which I examine in a work in progress (tentatively entitled "Recasting Social Canada: A Reconsideration of Federal Jurisdiction over Social Policy.") If the provinces cannot agree with the federal government on the shape of Medicare in the future, the courts may have to confront this question as well.

18   Premier Klein's televised announcement of the release of a health care policy
     statement was made on 16 November 1999: see R. Klein, TV address, "Improving
     Alberta's publicly funded health care system" (16 November 1999), online at http:/
     /www.gov.ab.ca/premier/speech/healthaddress/index.cfm (accessed on 21 June
     2000). The following day, Alberta Health and Wellness released the policy
     statement as well as a document covering questions and answers regarding the
     statement: see Alberta Health and Wellness, news release, "Policy Statement on
     Health Principles Released" (17 November 1999), online at http://
     www.health.gov.ab.ca/whatsnew/1999%20releases/nov17-99.htm (accessed on 24
     June 2000); Alberta Health and Wellness, news release, "Policy Statement on the
     Delivery of Surgical Services" (17 November 1999), online at http://
     www.health.gov.ab.ca/health_protection/questions.htm (accessed on 10 July
     2000); Alberta Health and Wellness, news release, "Policy Statement on the
     Delivery of Surgical Services: Common Questions and Answers" (26 January
     2000), online at http://www.health.gov.ab.ca/Policy/q&a.htm (accessed on 10
     July 2000). In response to the concerns of Albertans, in February 2000 the
     government released another publication that answered questions concerning the
     policy statement: see Alberta Health and Wellness, "We are Listening: Here's
     What We've Heard; A Summary of Albertans' Views on the Policy Statement on
     Surgical Services" (February 2000), online at http://www.health.gov.ab.ca/
     health_protection/index.html (accessed on 24 June 2000)). After tabling Bill 11 on
     2 March 2000, the Alberta government outlined its provisions in a news release
     posted to its website: see Government of Alberta, news release, "Legislation
     Introduced Prohibiting Private Hospitals and Two-Tier Health Care" (2 March
     2000), online at http://www.gov.ab.ca/acn/200003/8843.html (accessed on 21
     June 2000). Alberta capped charges for enhanced medical goods and services
     purchased in hospitals and other health authority facilities on 8 March 2000: see
     Government of Alberta, news release, "Charges for Enhanced Medical Goods and
     Services Capped" (8 March 2000), online at http://www.gov.ab.ca/acn/200003/
     8863.html (accessed on 21 June 2000).

19   Health Canada, news release, "Minister Rock Responds to Premier Klein's Policy
     Statement on the Delivery of Surgical Services" (26 November 1999), online at
     http://wwwhc-sc.gc.ca/english/archives/releases/26nov99e.htm (accessed on 21
     June 2000) [hereinafter "Minister Rock Responds"]. Jonson replied by assuring
     him that Alberta would comply with the CHA (see Alberta Health and Wellness,
     news release, "Health Minister Responds to Federal Government" (10 December
     1999), online at http://www.health.gov.ab.ca/whatsnew/1999%20releases/dec10-
     99.htm (accessed on 24 June 2000)) [hereinafter "Health Minister Responds"].

20   A. Rock, "Canada's Health Care System" (University of Calgary, Faculty of
     Medicine, 10 March 2000), online at http://www.hc-sc.gc.ca/english/archives/
     speeches /10mar2000mine.htm (accessed on 24 June 2000). In response to Rock's
     speech, Jonson initially charged the federal health minister with misleading the
     public: see Alberta Health and Wellness, news release, "Federal Health Minister
     Misleading Canadians" (10 March 2000), online at http://www.health.gov.ab.ca/
     whatsnew/Releases%202000 /mar10b-2000.htm (accessed on 18 May 2000).
     Jonson subsequently sent a letter to Rock on 14 March 2000, in which he accused
     him of speaking on matters within provincial jurisdiction, and demanded that the
     minister state whether Bill 11 complies with the CHA: Government of Alberta,
     Notice to the Editors, "Letter to Allan Rock from Halvar Jonson" (14 March

2000), online at http://www2.gov.ab.ca/healthfacts /PrinterFriendly.cfm?ID=143 (accessed on 24 June 2000). In a reply dated 16 March 2000, Rock denied intruding on provincial jurisdiction, pledged to continue speaking out on "health issues which are of such great importance to all Canadians," and repeated his intention to complete a review of Bill 11 before determining whether it violated the CHA: see Health Canada, news release, "Letter to the Honourable Halvar Jonson, M.L.A." (16 March 2000), online at http://www.hc-sc.gc.ca/english/ archives/letter_16mar2000.htm (accessed on 24 June 2000).

21   Health Canada, "Letter to the Honourable Halvar Jonson" (7 April 2000), online at http://wwwhc-sc.gc.ca/english/archives/letter_07apr2000.htm (accessed on 24 June 2000). Amendments to Bill 11 introduced by the Alberta legislature on 12 April 2000 included, *inter alia*, a strengthening of the queue jumping prohibition, a requirement that "enhanced" medical goods and services be reasonably priced, and an obligation on health authorities to use existing hospital facilities efficiently: see Alberta Health and Wellness, news release, "Government Introduces Amendments to Bill 11" (12 April 2000), online at http://www.gov.ab.ca/acn/ 200004/9004.html (accessed on 24 June 2000). The same day, Allan Rock reiterated, in a letter to Halvar Jonson, that the federal government's standpoint regarding private clinics being considered hospitals under the CHA had not changed since Diane Marleau's letter dated 6 January 1995: see Health Canada, news release, "Letter to the Honourable Halvar Jonson" (12 April 2000), online at http://www.hc-sc.gc.ca/english/archives /letter_12apr2000.htm (accessed on 24 June 2000).

22   In lieu of further action against Alberta, Rock simply promised to "monitor closely what may happen on the ground in private for-profit facilities permitted under Bill 11 to ensure that queue jumping and other accessibility issues do not arise": *House of Commons Debates* (11 May 2000) at 6670 (A. Rock) [hereinafter *Federal Concession*]. See also Health Canada, news release, "Health Minister responds to Bill 11" (11 May 2000), online at http://www.hc-sc.gc.ca/english/ archives/releases/2000/2000_46e.htm (accessed on 24 June 2000).

23   CHA, *supra* note, s. 7.

24   *Ibid.*, ss. 15, 14.

25   *Ibid.*, s. 20. In addition, s. 22(1)(c) of the CHA authorizes the federal cabinet to promulgate regulations that would require, as an additional condition for federal funding, that provinces provide "such information … as the Minister may reasonably require for the purposes of the Act": s. 13(a). Only one regulation has been acted pursuant to this provision. That regulation authorizes the Minister to require that provinces provide information with respect to the type and amount of extra-billing: see Extra-billing and User Charges Information Regulations, S.O.R./86–259.

26   The conclusion that the CHA contemplates enforcement follows not only from its express terms, but also from the very logic of national standards themselves. As Sopinka J. observed in *Canada (Minister of Finance) v. Finlay (no. 3)*, [1993] 1 S.C.R. 1080 at 1125–6 [hereinafter *Finlay (no. 3)*], the national standards laid down by the now-inoperative CAP must have had some minimum content in order for the federal government to be able "to limit its contributions to schemes that were of the general nature it wished to support." If national standards are to be meaningful, and if the federal government is to be able to limit its contributions to provinces that operate health insurance plans that further its policy objectives, an institution

(presumably the federal government) should ensure compliance with those standards.

27   CHA, *supra* note, s. 12(1)(a).

28   Comprehensiveness, which requires that provincial health plans insure all "medically necessary" services (CHA, *supra* note 1, s. 9, read in combination with s. 2), poses different problems, and may accordingly require a different process for interpretation and specification. To be sure, there are important issues of fact to be resolved. Thus, the assessment of medical necessity would require, at the very least, an analysis of the effectiveness of certain medical interventions, an empirical question. However, the definition of "medical necessity" has also bedevilled health services researchers, health lawyers and bioethicists, because it has an inescapable normative component: see E.J. Emanuel, *The Ends of Human Life: Medical Ethics in a Liberal Polity* (Cambridge, Mass.: Harvard University Press, 1991) at 139–44; T.A. Caulfield, "Wishful Thinking: Defining 'Medically Necessary' in Canada" (1996) 4 *Health L.J.* 63. It may be that the specification of the list of insured services should be defined through a process that proceeds from shared premises as to the goals of health care delivery. On the other hand, some have argued that a list-based approach would be insufficiently flexible to take into account new treatments: National Forum on Health, *Canada Health Action: Building On the Legacy—Final Report*, vol. 2. (1997) online at wwwnfh.hc-sc.gc.ca/publicat/finvol2/balance/pubpri4.htm (accessed on 24 June 2000). For the purposes of this paper, I would like to bracket this difficult issue, although in my analysis of Bill 11, I assume that the definition of medical necessity could be the subject of adjudication.

29   Health Canada, *Canada Health Act Annual Report 1998–99* (Ottawa: Supply & Services Canada, 2000) at 9.

30   The 1997–98 report states, in this vein: "[D]uring the year under review, a number of issues related to possible noncompliance were identified and resolved, while others are currently under review": Health Canada, *Canada Health Act Annual Report 1997–98* (Ottawa: Supply & Services Canada, 1998) at 8.

31   Office of the Auditor General, *Report of the Auditor General of Canada to the House of Commons* (Ottawa: Auditor General's Office, 1999) at para. 29.49 [hereinafter *Report, 1999*].

32   *Ibid.* at para. 29.51.

33   *Ibid.* at para. 29.52.

34   *Ibid.* at para. 29.53.

35   Office of the Auditor General, *Report of the Auditor General of Canada to the House of Commons* (Ottawa: Auditor General's Office, 1987) at para. 12.109.

36   Office of the Auditor General, *Report of the Auditor General of Canada to the House of Commons* (Ottawa: Auditor General's Office, 1990) at para. 4.176.

37   *Report, 1999, supra* note at para. 29.58.

38   *House of Commons Debates* (11 May 2000) at 6670 (A. Rock).

39   Letter from D. Marleau to provincial and territorial ministers of health (6 January 1995) [on file with author].

40   *House of Commons Debates* (20 March 1991) at 18728 (P. Beatty).

41   (1995), 124 DL.R. (4th) 426 (Ont. Gen. Div.) [hereinafter *Collett*].

42   [1998] 5 WW.R. 312 (B.C.S.C.).

43 L. Surtees, "Patients to recover out-of-province costs under new agreement," *The Globe and Mail* (31 March 1988) A13; "Quebec won't join interprovincial Medicare deal: Deputy minister," *The Gazette* (Montreal) (8 December 1988) A5; A. Riga, "Deal covering medical costs in the works with Ontario," *The Gazette* (15 February 1994) A6.

44 *House of Commons Debates* (11 May 1994) at 4208 (D. Harris); *House of Commons Debates* (10 June 1994) at 5160 (G. Hill); *House of Commons Debates* (4 April 1995) at 11484–5 (G. Hill); *House of Commons Debates* (18 October 1995) at 15525 (D. Grey). For further references, see Table 3 of this article.

45 Sheila Copps (Hamilton East, Lib.) asked Hon. Jake Epp (minister of national health and welfare) about the Auditor General's conclusion, at s. 12.146 of his report, that the minister was negligent in not responding to specific requests from Members of Parliament to report on instances in which provinces violated the CHA by charging user fees. Epp responded that there are no provinces currently reporting extra-billing, and that the ministry had made annual reports in compliance with the CHA: see *House of Commons Debates* (28 October 1987) at 10484–5.

46 On 30 November 1999, Judy Wasylycia-Leis (Winnipeg North Centre, NDP) confronted the Hon. Allan Rock regarding the Auditor General's conclusion that "the government has no idea whether or not the provinces are complying with the Canada Health Act." Rock responded that "the Auditor General has made some very helpful suggestions, all of which we accept and many of which we are already implementing to ensure that the best information possible is given to parliament annually from the Minister of Health with respect to the status of the Canada Health Act throughout the country": see *House of Commons Debates* (30 November 1999) at 1950. On 1 December 1999, Deborah Grey (Edmonton North, Ref.) repeated the criticism levelled by the Auditor General that "the federal government has no idea whether its health care spending ever makes it to the waiting lines or the emergency rooms." Rock responded once again that the recommendations were "useful" and were already being implemented: see *House of Commons Debates* (1 December 1999) at 1991. On 27 March 2000, Alexa McDonough (Halifax, NDP) reported that "[a]ccording to the Auditor General, even before the federal government cash transfers for health, the government has never taken action to protect the five principles of Medicare. Let me quote: 'Health Canada does not have the information it needs to monitor compliance with the act. The only departmental evaluation undertaken was limited, and it was five years before its results were reported to parliament.'" The Right Hon. Jean Chretien replied that in a recent meeting with Ralph Klein, he insisted that Alberta "would have to respect the five conditions of Medicare," *House of Commons Debates* (27 March 2000) at 5254–5.

47 Former federal health minister and Liberal MP Diane Marleau, without explicitly referring to the Auditor General's report, contended in a 13 March 2000 interview that the federal government has the power to stop Alberta's Bill 11 and alleged violations of the CHA but never passed regulations to support the Act: see D. Bueckert, "Ottawa can stop Alberta: Ex-minister," *The Toronto Star* (13 March 2000) A6. Diane Marleau again derided government inaction regarding Bill 11 and other alleged CHA violations in a subsequent interview dated 6 April 2000: see M. MacKinnon, "Ex-minister blasts PM on Medicare: Marleau assails her own party's inaction," *The Globe and Mail* (6 April 2000) A1. Subsequently, federal Health Minister Allan Rock wrote in A. Rock, Letter to the Editor, *The Globe and Mail* (17 April 2000) A12:

In his report of Nov. 29, the Auditor-General of Canada recommended that Health Canada strengthen its ability to enforce the provisions of the Canada Health Act and improve on its ability to report on matters relating to the act. On May 11, I announced Health Canada's intention to devote new resources in order to respond directly to the Auditor-General's recommendations.

48   "Enforcement of the CHA," *supra* note; C.M. Flood, "The Structure and Dynamics of Canada's Health Care System" in J. Downie and T. Caulfield, eds., *Canadian Health Law and Policy* (Toronto: Butterworths, 1999) at 26.

49   *Report, 1999, supra* note at para. 29.57.

50   *Ibid.* at para. 29.50.

51   For a history of Quebec's stance on the federal spending power, see Secréteriat aux Affaires intergouvernementales canadiennes, "Québec's Historical Position on the Federal Spending Power 1944–1998" (July 1998), online at http://wwwcex.gouv.qc.ca/saic/english.htm (accessed on on 24 June 2000). See also Quebec, *Report of the Royal Commission of Inquiry on Constitutional Problems*, vol. 2 (Quebec: Royal Commission of Inquiry on Constitutional Problems, 1956) (Chair: T. Tremblay).

52   For references, see *infra* note.

53   *Federal Concession, supra* note.

54   J.J. Arvay and T.M. Rankin, "Canada Health Act and Alberta Bill 11" Legal Opinion, 8 (March 2000) [unpublished, on file with the author] [hereinafter "CUPE Opinion"].

55   A. McIlroy, "Rock plans urgent drive to overhaul health care; patient waiting lists, national home care top his agenda," *The Globe and Mail* (27 January 2000) A1.

56   Federal-Provincial Fiscal Arrangements Act, R.S.C. 1985, c. F–8, ss. 13(3), as am. by Budget Implementation Act, S.C. 1995, c. 17, s. 48 [hereinafter Federal-Provincial Fiscal Arrangements Act]; T.J. Courchene, "ACCESS: A Convention on the Canadian Economic and Social Systems" (Ontario: Ontario Ministry of Intergovernmental Affairs, 1996).

57   C.M. Flood, "Accountability, Flexibility and Integration" (2000) 21:4 *Pol'y Options* 17 at 17–19.

58   "Enforcement of the CHA," *supra* note.

59   The Canadian Institute for Health Information, a national, nonprofit organization, was launched in 1994 following its approval by federal, provincial and territorial ministers of health in September 1992. Its mandate is "to improve the health of Canadians and the health system by providing quality and timely health information." See Canadian Institute for Health Information, "What We Do," online at http://www.cihi.ca/ wedo/do.htm (accessed on 24 June 2000).

60   This summary is taken from Finance Canada, "A Brief History of Federal Transfers" (2000), online at http://wwwfin.gc.ca/FEDPROVE/hise.html (accessed on 22 June 2000).

61   The figures in the following two paragraphs are taken from Canada, *Backgrounder on Federal Support for Health in Canada* (Ottawa: Finance Canada, 2000) at 5, online at wwwfin.gc.ca/activty/pubs/Health_e.pdf (accessed on 6 July 2000) [hereinafter *Federal Support*].

62 The provinces have accordingly called for cash transfers to be restored immediately to the levels where they stood in 1994–95 ($187 billion dollars). According to the provinces, this would require an increase of $4.2 billion, which suggests that they are relying on the 2000–1 cash base of $14.5 billion. See Provincial and Territorial Ministers of Health, "Understanding Canada's Health Care Costs: Interim Report" (June 2000), online at http://www.gov.on.ca/health/english/pub/ministry/ptcd/ptcd_doc_e.pdf (accessed on 10 July 2000) at 19 [hereinafter Provincial and Territorial Ministers of Health]. In addition, the provinces have called for the adoption of "an appropriate escalator to ensure that funding for health through the CHST keeps pace with the economic trends, social factors, and changing health technology": see *ibid.* at 1. At present, CHST levels are set by s. 14 of the Federal-Provincial Fiscal Arrangements Act, *supra* note.

63 The provinces continue to question the legitimacy of counting CHST tax points as a form of federal transfer payment, *inter alia*, because the tax transfer does not appear in the federal government's public accounts, because it does not appear as an expenditure in federal budgets, because increases in federal personal and corporate income taxes have offset the tax room vacated by the federal government in 1977, and because the tax room was originally transferred by the federal government to the provinces in 1942: see *Provincial and Territorial Ministers of Health, supra* note at 10–13. However, the same report acknowledges that the provinces agreed to the adoption of the EPF arrangement in 1977, which included tax points as part of the federal contribution: *ibid.* at 5. Moreover, the provinces "were not unhappy with the block fund concept (*including the tax transfer component*)": *ibid.* at 6 [emphasis added].

64 The closest the provinces come to addressing the issue is in a recent report where they refused to count federal tax transfers: *ibid.*

65 Proposed constitutional amendments contained in the Meech Lake Accord and the Charlottetown Accord would have dramatically altered the legal framework surrounding the exercise of the federal spending power: Canada, *Constitutional Accord 1987* (Ottawa: Queen's Printer, 1987) at cl 7.; Canada, *Charlottetown Accord: Draft Legal Text* (Ottawa: Queen's Printer, 1992) at s. 16. These amendments would have allowed a province to opt out from shared-cost programs established after the coming into force of the amendment in areas of exclusive provincial jurisdiction, and to receive "reasonable compensation" if that province carried on "a program or initiative" that was "compatible with national objectives." These amendments were criticized by some for not going far enough in disciplining the exercise of the federal spending power; because they only applied to new and not existing shared-cost programs, for example, those relating to health, welfare and education; because they applied to transfers to provinces, for example, the CHST, but not transfers to individuals; and because they required that provinces operate programs that were compatible with national objectives. In addition, Quebec sovereignists argued that the adoption of the amendment would have amounted to a victory for the federal government because it formally recognized the existence of the federal spending power. Conversely, some argued that the amendments attached too many restrictions on the exercise of the federal spending power because they would have made it extremely difficult for the federal government to introduce new national programs with minimum national standards, thereby eliminating shared-cost programs as instruments of national unity, and because the threat of provincial nonparticipation would have forced the federal government to propose much looser and more general national standards. For a collection of these views, see K.

Banting, "Political Meaning and Social Reform" in K.E. Swinton and C.J. Rogerson, eds., *Competing Constitutional Visions: The Meech Lake Accord* (Toronto: Carswell, 1988) 163; R.W. Boadway, J.M. Mintz and D.D. Purvis, "Economic Policy Implications of the Meech Lake Accord" in Swinton and Rogerson, *supra*, 225 at 229–32; Canada, *Report of the Special Joint Committee on the 1987 Constitutional Accord* (Ottawa: Supply and Services Canada, 1987) ch. 7; D. Coyne, "The Meech Lake Accord and the Spending Power Proposals: Fundamentally Flawed" in M.D. Behiels, ed., *The Meech Lake Primer: Conflicting Views of the 1987 Constitutional Accord* (Ottawa: University of Ottawa Press, 1989) 245; P. Fortin, "The Meech Lake Accord and The Federal Spending Power: A Good Maximum Solution" in Swinton and Rogerson, *supra*, 213; P.W. Hogg, "Analysis of the New Spending Power (Section 106A)" in Swinton and Rogerson, *supra*, 155.

66　See R. Boadway, "Delivering the Social Union: Some Thoughts on the Federal Role" (1998) 19:9 *Pol'y Options* 37; T.J. Courchene, "In Praise of Provincial Ascendency" (1998) 19:9 *Pol'y Options* 30; D. Cunningham, "Ontario's Approach to Improving Canada's Social Union" (1998) 19:9 *Pol'y Options* 14; J. Facal, "Pourquoi le Québec a adhéré au consensus des provinces sur l'union sociale" (1998) 19:9 *Pol'y Options* 12; D. Hancock, "Designing a New Social Framework for Canadians" (1998) 19:9 *Pol'y Options* 17; M. Jérôme-Forget, "Canada's Social Union: Staking Out the Future of Federalism" (1998) 19:9 *Pol'y Options* 3; H. Lazar, "The Social Union: Taking the Time to Do It Right" (1998) 19:9 *Pol'y Options* 43; A. McLellan, "Modernizing Canada's Social Union: A New Partnership Among Governments and Citizens" (1998) 19:9 *Pol'y Options* 6; K. Ng and D.R. Sloan, "Reforming Canada's Social Union: The Territorial Perspective" (1998) 19:9 *Pol'y Options* 23; A. Noël, "Les trois unions sociales" (1998) 19:9 *Pol'y Options* 26; R. Romanow, "Reinforcing 'The Ties That Bind'" (1998) 19:9 *Pol'y Options* 9; C. Thériault, "New Brunswick's Perspective on the Social Union" (1998) 19:9 *Pol'y Options* 20; F. Vaillancourt, "Alter the Federal-Provincial Powers Mix to Improve Social Policy" (1998) 19:9 *Pol'y Options* 50.

67　Canadian Intergovernmental Conference Secretariat, news release, "Framework Agreement on Canada's Social Union" (6 August 1998), online at http://wwwscics.gc.ca/cinfo98/85007010_e.html (accessed on 25 May 2000); J. Richards, "The 'Unholy Alliance' Versus 'Securing Our Future Together'" (1998) 19:9 *Pol'y Options* 40 at 41; K.G. Banting, "Social Citizenship and the Social Union in Canada" (1998) 19:9 *Pol'y Options* 33 at 36; L. Johnson, *Behind the "Social Union"* (Toronto: Ontario Legislative Library, 1999), online at http://www.ontla.on.ca/library/b29tx.htm (accessed on 24 June 2000); D. Schwanen, *More Than the Sum of Our Parts: Improving Mechanisms of Canada's Social Union* (Toronto: C.D. Howe Institute, 1999) at 27–8.

68　Tremblay, *supra* note. Tremblay refers to a consensus document agreed to by all the provinces in Victoria on 29 January 1999, which would have made mediation obligatory, and in the event of an impasse, would have required the report to be made public.

69　In fact, the funding criteria in the CHA have been interpreted in a handful of cases: *Lexogest Inc v. Manitoba (A.G.)* (1993), 101 D.L.R. (4th) 523 (Man. C.A.); *Collett, supra* note.

70　*Canada (Minister of Finance) v. Finlay*, [1986] 2 S.C.R. 607 and *Finlay (no. 3), supra* note.

71　I discuss these at length in "Enforcement of the CHA," *supra* note.

72　Canada, Agreement on Internal Trade, (Ottawa: Industry Canada, 1994) [hereinafter AIT].

73　For a discussion of the dispute settlement mechanisms under the AIT, see R.J. Howse, "Between Anarchy and the Rule of Law: Dispute Settlement and Related Implementation Issues in the Agreement on Internal Trade" in M.J. Trebilcock and D. Schwanen, eds., *Getting There: An Assessment of the Agreement on Internal Trade* (Toronto: C.D. Howe Institute, 1995) 170.

74　"Minister Rock Responds," *supra* note.

75　"Health Minister Responds," *supra* note.

76　"CUPE Opinion," *supra* note; J.C. Levy, "Canada Health Act and Alberta Bill 11" Legal Opinion, 27 March 2000 [unpublished, on file with the author]. Halvar Jonson relied on this opinion in a news release dated 5 April 2000, in which he reasserted his claim that Bill 11 did not in any way violate the CHA: see Government of Alberta, news release, "Bill 11 Consistent with Canada Health Act" (5 April 2000), online at http://www.gov.ab.ca/ acn/200004/8976.html (accessed on 22 June 2000).

77　Bill 11, *supra* note, s. 29(i).

78　*Ibid.*, s. 29(b), read in combination with s. 16.

79　*Ibid.*, s. 2(2).

80　*Ibid.*, s. 29(m), read with s. 1.

81　*Ibid.*, s. 3.

82　*Ibid.*, s. 4(b).

83　*Ibid.*, s. 29(f).

84　*Ibid.*, s. 25(1)(g). Note that this provision does not require the provincial cabinet to exercise its regulation making power in accordance with the CHA.

85　*Ibid.*, s. 5(1).

86　*Ibid.*, ss. 5(1), 5(2).

87　However, s. 5(1.1), *ibid.*, caps the rate for enhanced medical goods or services as "cost plus a reasonable allowance for administration." This language was introduced into Bill 11 to limit the price for uninsured services. However, given that the cost of enhanced goods and services will in part be a function of factors of production that are supplied by markets that are not covered by public health insurance, this may prove to be an illusory limit on prices.

88　However, s. 3, *ibid.*, does prohibit persons from paying or accepting payment "for enhanced medical goods or services ... for the purpose of giving any person priority for the receipt of an insured service," which arguably does extend the prohibition against queue jumping to enhanced medical goods and services.

89　*Ibid.*, s. 5(1).

90　*Ibid.*, s. 5(2)(b)(iii).

91　R.S.A. 1980, c. A–24.

92　*Ibid.* at s. 1(n).

93　"Enforcement of the CHA," *supra* note at 485–6.

94　In this vein, Charles *et al.* have observed that "the concept of medical necessity has taken on diverse, implicit and subtextual meanings over time to accommodate the different policy interests of specific groups": Charles *et al.*, "Medical Necessity in Canadian Health Policy: Four Meanings and ... a Funeral?" (1997) 75 *Milbank Q.* 365 at 367. Included in this list of meanings is "what physicians and hospitals do," which is roughly equivalent to the standard laid down by Bill 11. For an argument that medical necessity should be re-oriented away from comprehensiveness toward reasonable access, and that attempts to define a concise and operational definition of medical necessity are futile, see J. Hurley *et al.*, *Defying Definition: Medical Necessity and Health Policy Making*, Centre for Health Economics and Policy Analysis, Working Paper 96–16.

95   But even if the definition of "medical necessity" in Bill 11 does contravene the comprehensiveness requirement, it does not follow that Alberta's health care system has violated the CHA. What counts in the end is the list of covered services and goods on the provincial health insurance scheme. Bill 11 does not purport to amend this list. If, for example, the list of insured goods and services exceeds the minimum set by the provincial legislation, and the federal legislation sets a higher standard that Alberta meets, the CHA would have been complied with.

96   "CUPE Opinion," *supra* note at 29.

3

Fiduciary Law and For-Profit and Not-For-Profit Health Care

MOE M. LITMAN

> That any sane nation, having observed that you could provide for
> the supply of bread by giving bakers a pecuniary interest in baking
> for you, should go on to give a surgeon a pecuniary interest in
> cutting off your leg, is enough to make one despair of political
> humanity.
>
> —George Bernard Shaw, *The Doctor's Dilemma* (1913)

Everyone wants to make a buck, even physicians. And that's fine within limits. Some of these limits are prescribed by a strict body of law called fiduciary law. Fiduciary law, though increasingly prominent, remains somewhat obscure. Except at the highest level of generality, it is not well understood. Physicians do understand that as fiduciaries they owe a considerable duty of loyalty to their patients.[1] Overwhelmingly, no doubt, they discharge this duty with conscience and integrity. Some, however, do not. I believe that most physicians, and for that matter many lawyers, do not fully comprehend just how far a doctor's legal duty of loyalty goes and the degree of legal jeopardy faced by physicians who breach this duty. Exacting compliance with the duty of loyalty is critical to our medical system. To the degree that the legal system tolerates disloyalty, it erodes patient/physician trust which is central to an effective and efficient health care system. And, if the law tolerates disloyalty, there is good reason for this erosion. If infidelity is permitted, patients need to be on guard with their doctors. Patients must assess whether the information and advice they receive is intended to promote their best interests or the best interests of their physicians or third parties. Neither efficiency nor the therapeutic goals of the health care system are advanced when patients distrust their physicians.

Fiduciary law is the basis for sanctioning a failure of loyalty by persons whose loyalty is essential to the efficacy and integrity of important but diverse relational institutions such as the physician/patient relationship.[2] In general terms, fiduciaries are actors who are required to look after the interest(s) of another or others with vigilance, dedication and selflessness. The idea of "fiduciary duty" has contributed to and become an integral part of the culture of fidelity to which the medical community professes abiding commitment.[3] Current pressures for change in the health care system, in particular privatization and cost-containment initiatives, may well test this commitment.[4] Some proposals for change, if they come to pass, could, and based on the experience in the United States, will likely influence health care providers to conduct themselves on the basis of considerations other than the best interests of their patients.[5] When a patient's best interest is not the exclusive touchstone of health care decisions, not only is there a real and substantial danger of erosion of the quality of health care, but a potential for legal liability for breach of fiduciary duty.[6]

Health care services are profoundly important but exceedingly expensive. Fee-for-service remuneration of physicians contributes significantly to the costs of health care, in part because this form of remuneration harbours within it an incentive to provide more care and more expensive care, rather than less care and less expensive care. In Canada and the United States concern over affordability of an acceptable level of health care has spawned cost-containment and privatization strategies intended to reduce costs to manageable levels. The rationing of health care is central to these strategies and, in the United States, where for-profit health care is pervasive, financial rewards are employed extensively to limit costs and thereby increase the bottom line. From the perspective of fiduciary law, incentives which inhere in both fee-for-service systems and cost-containment and privatization mechanisms are, at the very least, provocative. Fiduciary law requires single-minded attention and exclusive and selfless fidelity to the best interests of patients. It is intolerant of anything which might cause a health care provider to provide more care than is needed (the fee-for-service system) or less care than is needed (the cost-containment and privatization systems). At first glance, therefore, it appears that health care providers discharge their roles in chronic violation of fiduciary obligation.

The purpose of this chapter is to explore the implications of fiduciary law to both for-profit and nonprofit health care providers. In the course of this task, the fiduciary obligations of physicians and other individual health care providers will be examined, as will the fiduciary obligations of health care institutions including hospitals, health care facilities, health care authorities or boards and the health management organizations (HMOs) of the United States. After briefly surveying the source of fiduciary obligation of these actors, the nature of fiduciary duty will be explored, including the murky but important relationship between fiduciary law and tort law. Tort law includes the law of negligence or, as it is often described, malpractice law. In the course of analyzing fiduciary law, the multi-faceted concept of conflict of interest will be broken down into its component parts and then utilized as a benchmark to evaluate the conduct of the various fiduciary actors who are engaged in the delivery of health services.

Given the trend towards cost-containment and the continuing and persistent pressure to permit for-profit institutions into the health care field in Canada, it is instructive to examine the American experience with fiduciary law's regulation of private for-profit health service providers. In the recent, important and controversial decision of *Pegram* v. *Herdrich*, the US Supreme Court concluded that even if inadequate treatment provided by an HMO fiduciary is improperly and exclusively motivated by a self-interested desire to cut costs with a view to enhancing profit, an injured patient's only recourse is malpractice law.[7] Given the extreme disloyalty involved in such a treatment decision, the *Herdrich* decision has in the United States effectively eliminated fiduciary law as a check and balance against the perfidiousness of for-profit HMOs. In rationalizing this result, the Court in the *Herdrich* case suggested that fiduciary law offers little of practical value to complainants in malpractice suits which is not already provided by tort law. This important assertion, with transboundary implications, will be assessed in the light of Canadian case law.

Basic Fiduciary Law and Its Relationship to the Law of Malpractice: The Legal Background

A. The Fiduciary Status of Health Service Providers

First principles of Canadian law suggest that health care providers are either fiduciaries or agents of fiduciaries. Physicians are presumed to be fiduciaries and, though their fiduciary status is not inevitable, both theory and long-standing judicial pronouncements suggest that where physicians discharge their traditional role of steward of their patients' health, their fiduciary status is all but inevitable.[8] On the other hand, where physicians are charged with or undertake promoting the interests of third parties such as employers, insurers or even the state (in criminal or administrative proceedings), the fiducial character of the relationship is much more debatable. But even where physicians appear to owe their loyalties to third parties, there is authority for the proposition that they are the fiduciaries of the "patients" whom they examine.[9]

Nonphysicians who deliver health care services, both individual and institutional, are charged with the same fundamental mandate as physicians, namely the protection and promotion of the health interests of their patients. Hence, it should come as no great surprise that many of these health service providers—hospitals, health care authorities, HMOs, dentists, physiotherapists and others—are fiduciaries. In the case of HMOs, US legislation deems them to be fiduciaries. From a Canadian perspective, the fiduciary status of HMOs is not a stretch. As will be suggested below, Canadian fiduciary law principles, if applied to "comparable" Canadian institutions (nonprofit hospitals and health authorities), appear to support the conclusion that they are fiduciaries.

The principles of fiduciary law explain why physicians are fiduciaries and why many other health service providers are also likely fiduciaries. The Courts have identified *indicia* or identifying characteristics of fiduciary relationships on which they routinely rely in assessing whether relationships are of a fiducial character. Fiduciaries have scope for the exercise of some discretion or power; they can unilaterally exercise their power or discretion so as to affect the beneficiaries' legal or practical interests; and beneficiaries are peculiarly vulnerable to or at the mercy of the fiduciary holding the discretion or power.[10] While the precise nature and limits of the elastic and interrelated concepts which form the various *indicia* have yet to be judicially fixed,[11] they clearly support the assertion that both institutional and individual health care providers are fiduciaries. There is a considerable power imbalance between health care providers and typical patients. The power differential is a product of a complex interaction of factors, including the profound psychological anxiety patients have over matters pertaining to health, the disparity of knowledge and skill between the health care providers and their patients, consciousness of this disparity, the role of health care providers as gatekeepers of critically important therapies and procedures and the deeply felt and pervasive conviction of patients that health service providers are dedicated to protecting and promoting their health interests.[12] Physicians, in particular, are possessed of the kind of power and influence which lies at the core of the *indicia*. This is illustrated by the common practice of patients seeking out and then embracing or deferring to the opinions of their health care providers regarding treatment options.[13]

More significant than the *indicia*, which do no more than suggest or evidence the existence of fiduciary relationships, are the various tests deployed by the Supreme Court of Canada for determining whether a relationship is fiduciary. These tests are vitally important because the prevailing judicial view appears to be that even if all the *indicia* are present, a relationship may not be fiduciary, and conversely, if none are present, a relationship may nevertheless be fiduciary.[14] The various tests are highly interrelated, though they are often articulated and applied as discrete tests. Pursuant to these tests, a relationship is fiduciary if there is either (i) an undertaking by a party (whether unilateral or as part of an agreement, or even legislatively imposed) to selflessly and exclusively dedicate oneself to the interests of another;[15] (ii) a reasonable expectation of such dedication;[16] or (iii) a reasonable basis for reliance on such a dedication.[17] Naturally, undertakings of fidelity beget reasonable expectations of fidelity and such expectations, in turn, beget reasonable reliance by the intended beneficiaries of undertakings on the parties making the undertaking. Moreover, entry into a profession that has engendered public expectations of dedicated and selfless service to others can in itself be regarded as a pledge or undertaking to provide such service. In other words, there is an intimate, overlapping and interactive connection between the dynamics of the various touchstones (tests) of the existence of fiduciary relationships.

Fiduciary undertakings are rarely explicit. They are almost always tacit and capable of discernment only from contextual sources. When the circumstances surrounding a relationship suggest that service providers are committing themselves to "look after" the interests of others,[18] not only with skill and attention, but with selfless and exclusive dedication, it is appropriate to attribute to the undertaking a fiducial character. Contextual analysis suggests, unequivocally, that physicians pledge to devote themselves exclusively and selflessly to the interests of their patients. The Hippocratic Oath,[19] applicable codes of ethics and the standard practices of physicians are replete with both explicit and implicit promises of this form of fidelity.[20] These sources establish that the paramount obligation of physicians is to promote the best interests of patients.[21] The Hippocratic Oath includes an explicit pledge to abstain from exploitive behaviour. Though the pledge emphasizes the duty to refrain from sexually exploiting patients, it is clear that what is proscribed is exploitive behaviour generally.[22] These various sources also mandate both avoidance of conflicts of interest and the strict maintenance of the privacy interests of patients.[23] Most health care professionals, including nurses, physiotherapists and dentists, through applicable codes of ethics and the standard norms of their practices, make similar pledges and commitments to their patients.[24] Hence they are fiduciaries or, at least, agents of fiduciaries who must live up to fiduciary standards. It has previously been suggested, in support of the judicial finding that a hypnotherapist is a fiduciary, that "any individual who places himself in a position as a medical advisor will be subject to the same duty of utmost good faith and fiduciary status that is owed by a physician or surgeon."[25] In addition, based on the reasonable expectation test, there is a strong case to be made that hospitals and health authorities are also fiduciaries. The pervasive use by these institutions of fiduciary actors to provide health services to patients, checks and balances within institutional environments designed to promote the best interests of patients, policies which implicate fidelity to patients and protection of their privacy interests, as well as legislative mission statements which focus on the responsibility of hospitals and health care authorities to promote and protect the health of patients, all support the conclusion that these health care institutions are fiduciaries.[26]

The origins and nature of HMOs and the manner in which they finance their operations are succinctly described in the *Herdrich* case as follows:[27]

> Beginning in the late 1960s, insurers and others developed new models for health-care delivery, including HMOs. ...The defining feature of an HMO is receipt of a fixed fee for each patient enrolled under the terms of a contract [or plan] to provide specified health care if needed. The HMO thus assumes the financial risk of providing the benefits promised: if a participant never gets sick, the HMO keeps the money regardless, and if a participant becomes expensively ill, the HMO is responsible for the treatment agreed upon even if its cost exceeds the participant's premiums.

HMOs are regulated by a unique, complex and far-reaching US federal statute called the Employee Retirement Income Security Act (ERISA).[28] Given the critical nature of the role played by HMOs, it is not surprising that ERISA deems them to be fiduciaries. Through their employee-physicians, HMOs make insurer-like eligibility (coverage) decisions and, as well, make treatment or medical decisions in respect of plan beneficiaries. Looked at from a Canadian perspective, the frontline use of fiduciary actors by HMOs implicates fiduciary law, in part, because of pronounced public expectations about the fiducial role played by physicians in the delivery of health care. Even though HMOs function as insurers and not merely as health service providers in making eligibility decisions, and, like insurers, stand to gain or lose in making such decisions, there is widespread judicial agreement that in making coverage decisions insurers are under a fiduciary-like, though not a fiduciary obligation of good faith.[29] While it is true that Canadian courts have, in the context of insurance cases, indicated that it is "conceptually difficult to apply fiduciary law to parties who are inherently in a conflict of interest,"[30] it would be a mistake to regard inherent conflict between parties as an insuperable hurdle to a fiduciary relationship. In the case of a permitted or inescapable conflict of interest, the common law rule is that a fiduciary must resolve the conflict in favour of the beneficiary.[31] Implicit in this rule is the notion that a relationship may be fiduciary notwithstanding the existence of inherent conflict of interest. Interestingly, and perhaps not so coincidentally, ERISA in effect embraces the rule that fiduciaries must resolve conflict of interest in favour of duty.[32] Given the nature of the hybrid role of HMOs—they are both insurers and health providers—and the profound importance of the services which they provide, it is conceivable that even absent legislation deeming them to be fiduciaries, they would nevertheless, under the principles of common law, have this status.

B. The Nature of Fiduciary Duty and Breach of Fiduciary Duty

Loyalty is the core value of fiduciary relationships and hence the focus of fiduciary law.[33] Whether loyalty is the only concern of fiduciary law is an important question. If it is, then wrongs committed by fiduciaries which do not entail disloyalty are not fiduciary wrongs. They are simply wrongs committed by fiduciaries. The distinction is significant, given that the most common form of failure by fiduciaries is a failure of skill and judgement, a defalcation which often does not involve disloyalty. If the exclusive focus of fiduciary obligation is fidelity, then the failure to provide reasonable care and skill would fall, at least ordinarily, outside of the scope of fiduciary law and into the purview of contract and tort law. Surprisingly, notwithstanding the antiquity of this body of law, there is current ambiguity in the case law on this very point. Certain passages in recent Supreme Court of Canada judgements can be read, and have been read, as supporting the notion that a failure of skill or competence by a fiduciary is a breach of fiduciary obligation.[34] The most explicit of these passages is found in Justice La Forest's majority judgement in *Hodgkinson* v. *Simms* where he reasoned:[35]

> [F]iduciary duty is different in important respects from the ordinary duty of care. ... [W]hile both negligent representation and breach of fiduciary duty arise in reliance-based relationships, the presence of loyalty, trust, and confidence distinguishes the fiduciary relationship from a relationship that simply gives rise to tortious liability. *Thus, while a fiduciary obligation carries with it a duty of skill and competence*, the special elements of trust, loyalty, and confidentiality that obtain in a fiduciary relationship give rise to a corresponding duty of loyalty [emphasis added].

Much turns on whether this and the other passages alluded to are intended to suggest that simple negligence is a breach of fiduciary duty. If so, then very favourable fiduciary doctrine may be available to beneficiaries of fiduciary relationships in ordinary negligence cases. This doctrine includes extended limitation periods applicable to fiduciary wrongs,[36] relaxed rules of causation,[37] and compensation principles unfettered by the limits of forseeability.[38] Fiduciary law's causation rules can be of particular advantage to patients who sue their physicians for failure to disclose material risks. Tort law's approach to causation, especially its insistence that patients—the plaintiffs—bear the burden of proving causation, is widely regarded to be a very significant impediment to a successful lawsuit.[39] Fiduciary law takes the opposite approach. It reverses the burden of proof by requiring that physicians—the defendants—establish that had their patients been fully and properly informed, they would nevertheless have chosen to undergo the same treatment which they actually received and which ultimately led to the harm suffered by them.[40] Discharging this burden of proof is extremely difficult to do.[41]

My view is that the Supreme Court of Canada did not intend to suggest that negligence, without disloyalty, is a breach of fiduciary obligation. It makes little sense to confer special juristic advantage on beneficiaries of fiduciary relationships in the absence of fiduciary disloyalty. Extended limitation periods and the other special rules which favour beneficiaries of fiduciary relationships have been developed, and can only be justified, as a response to the egregious wrongs of abuse or violation of trust. Part of this response is the strict and unremitting policy of equity of deterring fiduciary infidelity.[42] From the perspective of policy, there is no warrant in extending the very significant advantages provided by fiduciary law to plaintiffs who complain of ordinary wrongs just because they happen to be perpetrated by fiduciaries. If the substance of a complaint is a failure of skill, then why should it make a difference whether the perpetrator is a fiduciary or a nonfiduciary? What is important in such a case is that a duty of care is owed, not the source of the duty, and that the defendant has failed to live up to an appropriate standard of care. It would be surprising and unfortunate, therefore, if Justice La Forest's statement was intended to mean anything other than that fiduciaries have tort-based duties of care. As to the other Supreme Court of Canada cases which are capable of being interpreted as supporting the notion that negligence perpetrated by a fiduciary is *per se* a breach of fiduciary duty, when read contextually it is clear that each of the wrongs described in these cases as "fiduciary wrongs" involved a failure of loyalty.[43] The true position is set out in the Australian High Court case of *Breen* v. *Williams* where Dawson and Toohey JJ. stated that "what the law exacts in a fiduciary relationship is loyalty, often of an uncompromising kind, but no more than that."[44]

The notion that mere negligence is not a breach of fiduciary duty was underscored by Justice Southin of the British Columbia Supreme Court in the well-known case of *Giradet* v. *Crease*.[45] In that case a lawyer was sued by his client for both negligence and breach of fiduciary duty. In the course of emphatically rejecting the plaintiff's fiduciary theory, Southin J. stated that "to say that simple carelessness in giving advice is … a breach [of fiduciary duty] is a perversion of words. … [A]n allegation of breach of fiduciary duty carries with it the stench of dishonesty—if not of deceit, then of constructive fraud."[46]

Though breach of fiduciary duty often involves dishonesty by a fiduciary, it seems clear that fiduciary liability is not dependant on proof of such dishonesty.[47] In *Guerin* v. *The Queen,* the Supreme Court imposed liability on the federal Crown for breaching its fiduciary duty owed to the First Nation plaintiff.[48] The Crown had leased the plaintiff's lands on terms which were less favourable than those specified by the plaintiff when it surrendered its land to the Crown for the purpose of facilitating the intended lease. The Crown received no benefit from the actual lease it entered into and was not guilty of attempting to confer improperly a benefit on the third-party lessee. Accordingly, the Crown's behaviour could not even remotely be described as dishonest.

In *Guerin*, the precise nature of the Crown's breach of fiduciary duty was described, in the majority judgement in the case, in the following terms:[49]

> After the Crown's agents had induced the band to surrender its land on the understanding that the land would be leased on certain terms, it would be unconscionable to permit the Crown simply to ignore these terms. When the promised lease proved impossible to obtain, the Crown, instead of proceeding to lease the land on different, unfavourable terms, should have returned to the band to explain what had occurred and seek the band's counsel on how to proceed. The existence of such unconscionability is the key to a conclusion that the Crown breached its fiduciary duty. Equity will not countenance unconscionable behaviour in a fiduciary, whose duty is that of utmost loyalty to his principal.

This passage reaffirms that the gravamen of breach of fiduciary obligation is disloyalty. In *Guerin*, disloyalty was evidenced by unconscionability, but in other cases it could be evidenced by dishonesty or even, it is suggested, moral turpitude. The existence and nature of a fiduciary's wrong would have to be assessed in light of the fiduciary's undertaking(s) or the reasonable expectations of the beneficiary of the fiduciary relationship.[50] As will be seen below, the fiduciary concept of disloyalty provides broad scope for liability for breach of fiduciary duty, but it does have its limits.

Negligence is not *per se* a breach of fiduciary duty because it does not necessarily entail disloyalty. Where it does, it may be such a breach.[51] A simple failure by a physician, for example, to communicate a material risk is mere negligence and typically has been so regarded. However, a physician's failure to disclose a material personal interest, such as a research interest or an economic interest related to the patient's course of treatment, is a failure of loyalty.[52] Such a failure is a breach of fiduciary duty, though it also violates the principle of informed consent and thereby implicates negligence.[53] If an act or omission is a breach of fiduciary duty, irrespective of whether it is also a tort, fiduciary doctrine, including the reverse onus provisions of fiduciary law, are available to a plaintiff in a lawsuit.[54]

C. Classic Fiduciary Disloyalty: Conflict of Interest

Central to the concept of fiduciary loyalty is the requirement that fiduciaries act with an "eye single to the interests of ... beneficiaries."[55] It follows that conflict of interest is strictly prohibited. This prohibition is anchored in practical and not merely moral considerations, a point developed in the following colourful passage extracted from *Breen* v. *Williams*, a decision of the High Court of Australia:[56]

> The law of fiduciary duty rests not so much on morality or conscience as on the acceptance of the biblical injunction that "[n]o man can serve two masters"... Duty and self-interest, like God and Mammon, make inconsistent calls on the faithful. Equity solves the problem in a practical way by insisting that fiduciaries give undivided loyalty to the persons whom they serve.

Equity's uncompromising intolerance of divided loyalties is based on a recognition that human beings are driven by self-interest. This point lies at the heart of Lord Herschell classic statement in *Bray* v. *Ford* that "human nature being what it is, there is danger ... of the person holding a fiduciary position being swayed by interest rather than duty, and thus prejudicing those whom he was bound to protect..."[57] And it is not at all implausible that fiduciaries who are earnest about duty may subconsciously be influenced by self-interest. This point may explain or even justify those conflict of interest cases where the propriety, honesty and dedication of fiduciaries are not only unquestioned but affirmed, yet liability is nevertheless imposed.[58] In its unremitting protection of beneficiaries, equity must not only be alive to deception but also self-deception.[59]

The fiduciary concept of undivided loyalty is multi-faceted and hence has spawned a number of proscriptions and prescriptions. Collectively they provide considerable, but of course far from perfect protection for beneficiaries of fiduciary relationships. First, and perhaps foremost, amongst the proscriptive duties of fiduciaries is the obligation to avoid conflict of interest.[60] Classically, this means that fiduciaries must avoid situations in which their personal interests, most often, but not always economic interests, might interfere with their duty of loyalty. Conflict of interest also arises if an interest of a third party to whom a fiduciary has allegiance is advanced through the discharge of fiduciary duty or exercise of fiduciary power.[61] For this reason, referral of a patient to a diagnostic facility in which a physician's spouse has a financial interest is clearly an impermissible conflict of interest. Fiduciaries must provide single-minded attention to the best interests of those they serve and therefore fiduciary law is properly intolerant of circumstances in which the conduct of a fiduciary might be fashioned by personal agenda rather than fiduciary duty.

One author has described the obligation to avoid conflict of interest as a duty to "scrupulously avoid placing ... [oneself] in a possible or potential conflict of interest."[62] The significance of putting the matter this way is that it suggests that it is wrong *per se* for fiduciaries to enter into potential conflicts of interest whether or not these conflicts become operative and ultimately damage the interests of beneficiaries of fiduciary relationships.[63] The duty to avoid possible or potential conflict of interest has a prophylactic justification. Beneficiaries are better protected if fiduciaries are required to avoid temptation and not merely resist it. The significance of the duty to avoid potential conflict should not be underestimated. It means, for example, that even absent statutory regulation, physicians and other health care fiduciaries must refrain from acquiring financial interests in diagnostic or "surgical facilities" which may service their patients. Of course, this prohibition binds health care professionals whether or not they personally ply their services in such facilities. Though strict enforcement of the rule against conflict of interest provides patients with a significant measure of protection, both experience with and the inherent limitations of the conflict of interest rule suggest that one should not be sanguine about the degree of protection provided by the rule. Conflict of interest behaviour is extremely difficult to detect.[64] There are an infinite variety of ways, some of which are very subtle, for both corporations and physicians to circumvent bans against this type of behaviour.[65]

Classic conflict of interest focusses on selfish or disloyal behaviour by fiduciaries. However, the seeds of a broader notion of conflict of interest can be found in Canadian jurisprudence, albeit in only a single case. The Ontario High Court case of *Cox* v. *College of Optometrists of Ontario* stands for the proposition that health service providers, who are constrained by conflict of interest regulations under the then-operative Health Disciplines Act, must avoid an appearance of conflict of interest, even when there is neither actual nor potential conflict in the classic sense.[66] In *Cox*, an optometrist, Dr. Cox, located his clinic in part of an optical company's retail space in a shopping mall. The relationship between Dr. Cox and the optical company was purely that of landlord and tenant. Rent was not tied into fees earned from Dr. Cox's patients and Dr. Cox was not under any obligation to refer patients to the optical company, nor subject to any financial or other incentive for doing so. The holding that Dr. Cox was in conflict of interest was based squarely on the notion that there was a reasonable apprehension of or appearance of conflict.[67] Extending the concept of conflict of interest beyond cases where there is an actual or possible conflict of interest and duty may seem an unwarranted incursion into the personal freedom of fiduciaries. But it can be justified. The enlarged notion of conflict of interest adopted in the *Cox* case has the effect of maintaining and perhaps even enhancing public confidence in the integrity of an important health-service institution where both loyalty and a perception of loyalty are essential to the efficacy of the institution.[68] To burden fiduciaries with the obligation of supporting the fabric of the fiduciary institutions which provide them with their livelihoods is not draconian.

The obligation of a fiduciary to disclose a conflict of interest is a classic and familiar fiduciary duty.[69] This duty is triggered by the fact of conflict, irrespective of whether the conflict arises from breach of the threshold duty to avoid conflict of interest or from circumstances beyond the control of a fiduciary.[70] In either event, a fiduciary's ongoing duty of loyalty impels appropriate disclosure of the conflict. Appropriate disclosure means that fiduciaries report fully, frankly and on a timely basis the nature and extent of any conflict.[71] Disclosure must be detailed and sufficiently ample so as to allow beneficiaries to realistically assess the risk posed to them by the divided loyalties of their fiduciaries.[72] This may mean, for example, that physicians who are rewarded on a per-patient basis for recruiting participants into drug trials must disclose the amount of compensation they receive, not just on a per-patient basis, but on a global basis.[73] In some very limited circumstances, where a conflict of interest is both tolerated in law and is a matter of widespread public knowledge, as is the case with the conflict associated with the fee-for-service model of physician remuneration, active disclosure, it is suggested, is probably not required. In respect of many such conflicts, appropriate disclosure will be "deemed" to have been made.[74] But it is important not to assume that merely because a conflict of interest is legally tolerated there is no duty to disclose the fact of the conflict. In the United States, notwithstanding that ERISA explicitly permits divided loyalties by those who deliver managed health care,[75] it has been held that a failure to disclose financial incentives under which a physician operates is a breach of fiduciary duty.[76]

It would also be a mistake to assume, and I believe this assumption is often made, that disclosure by a fiduciary of a conflict of interest *ipso facto* cures or reverses the conflict and thereby frees the fiduciary to pursue self-interest with impunity.[77] Such an assumption confuses, or at least wrongly equates, the duty of disclosure with the defence of patient consent. No doubt disclosure can give rise to *bona fide* consent by a patient to conduct which, absent such consent, would be a breach, even a flagrant breach, of fiduciary duty. But this form of consent should not be assumed as proved by the mere fact of appropriate disclosure. Judicial and legislative reticence about equating disclosure with waiver of rights is warranted given that patients to whom disclosure is made often have "few real options."[78] Disclosure should be presumptively regarded as no more than the conscientious discharge by physicians of their obligation to warn patients that circumstances exist in which they may be influenced by self-interest rather than patient welfare. And even where a physician's disclosure of a conflict of interest is regarded as giving rise to a waiver of rights by a patient, the waiver ought ordinarily to be interpreted restrictively as authorizing the physician to operate within a conflict-of-interest environment and not as an authorization to actually pursue self-interest at the expense of the patient. In the context of a pharmaceutical trial this latter point would mean that a physician's research agenda would be permitted to co-exist with his or her duty of patient loyalty but that the physician would continue to be under a strict duty to promote the best interests of the patient, even if the effect of doing so would be to completely undermine the physician's scholarly endeavour.

A third duty spawned by the overarching obligation of fiduciary loyalty is a corollary of the threshold duty to avoid conflict of interest. Given the existence of the threshold duty, logic suggests that fiduciaries who find themselves in impermissible conflict are duty bound to speedily eliminate both personal and, where possible, third-party interests which conflict with their duty. The only alternative to jettisoning an interest which conflicts with duty is obtaining the informed consent of the beneficiary of the relationship to what otherwise would be a breach of fiduciary duty.

Fourthly, as previously observed, fiduciaries who find themselves in conflict of interest, whether legally tolerated or not, must conduct themselves exclusively in the best interests of those to whom they owe fiduciary obligations. This rule is set out explicitly in ERISA,[79] but it is also the common law rule.[80] In the Australian High Court case of *Breen* v. *Williams*, the common law was described by Brennan C.J. in the following terms: "Equity requires that a person under a fiduciary obligation should not put himself or herself in a position where interest and duty conflict or, if conflict is unavoidable, should resolve it in favour of duty and except by special arrangement, should not make a profit out of the position."[81] Though Justice Brennan's statement does not specifically address the duty of a fiduciary whose conflict of interest is legally tolerated, either by statute or common law, there is little doubt that such a fiduciary is also bound to resolve conflict in favour of duty.[82]

The stringency of fiduciary law's conflict of interest rules suggests that most physicians are chronically in conflict of interest. Under a fee-for-service model of remuneration, physicians are enriched each time they provide a fiduciary service. This means that physicians have a personal interest in providing fiduciary services, particularly services for which there is generous compensation.[83] Importantly, it has been pointed out that "[i]n a fee-for-service system, a physician's financial incentive is to provide more care, not less, so long as payment is forthcoming."[84] Though the incentive to provide more care will generally enure to the advantage of patients, this is not inevitably the result. Excessive and inappropriate treatment, especially invasive treatment such as surgery, is not in the patient's best interest.[85] From a broader perspective, the provision of unnecessary services which flow from the incentive to provide more rather than less care, contributes to the burdensome costs of contemporary health care systems. In Canada these costs have lead to the paring down of health care,[86] presumably to the disadvantage of the patient population.

The early common law prohibited trustees, the original and prototypical fiduciaries,[87] from being paid on a fee-for-service basis.[88] Today trustees may charge out their services on this basis because legislation has been enacted which overrides the relatively strict common law prohibition to the contrary.[89] More generally, today both statute and the common law tolerate or authorize conflicts of interest which implicate fiduciaries, including fiduciaries who are important actors in the delivery of health care.[90] In the United States, for example, the Employee Retirement Income Security Act explicitly permits divided loyalties in the delivery of managed health care plans which are central to the operation of HMOs.[91] Similarly, provincial health insurance statutes in Canada, by tying physician fees into negotiated fee-for-service schedules, appear to legitimize, at least implicitly, the conflict of interest that is inherent in such fee-for-service schemes.[92] Recently, the controversial Alberta Health Care Protection Act, better known as Bill 11, extended legislative tolerance of fee-for-service systems to fees charged by physicians for "enhanced medical goods or services."[93]

Legislative or common law tolerance of fee-for-service-based physician remuneration does not mean that physicians who are paid in this way are free of conflict of interest. Legislation which permits conflict of interest does not alter the reality of the conflict; it alters only the legal consequences which flow from it. Legislation which contemplates the payment of physicians on a fee-for-service basis implicitly authorizes physicians to benefit, at least incidentally, from the provision of fiduciary services. But this form of legislation does not provide physicians with carte blanche immunity to all of fiduciary law's conflict-of-interest rules. Physician conduct which is fee-driven, rather than patient-driven, continues to be an impermissible conflict of interest and a serious, though not easily detected or proved, breach of fiduciary duty.[94]

Fiduciary Law And For-Profit Medicine: The US Supreme Court Decision in the *Herdrich* Case

Fiduciary theory requires courts to meticulously scrutinize the conduct of fiduciaries who are permitted to operate in conflict of interest in order to assess whether they have improperly succumbed to temptation. Until the much heralded and provocative decision in *Pegram* v. *Herdrich*[95] in late 2000, it appeared beyond question that fiduciary law would play an important role in the United States in protecting patients from the risks associated with privatization and cost-containment in health care. Left undisturbed, the decision of the US District Court of Appeals in *Herdrich* would have served to warn fiduciaries who are permitted to operate in conflict of interest that the slope between permissible conflict of interest and impermissible fiduciary misconduct is both short and slippery.[96] Unfortunately, the decision was overturned by no less than a unanimous panel of the Supreme Court of the United States. In Canada, where the pressures for cost-containment and, to some extent, privatization, are substantial, the *Herdrich* case and its implications warrant close study.[97]

In *Herdrich*, Cynthia Herdrich initiated proceedings against her physician Lori Pegram, the Carle Clinic Association and various "Carle-" related institutional and corporate operators of a health insurance plan of which Herdrich was a beneficiary. Collectively, the defendants functioned as an HMO, owned by its physician/operators. Herdrich had been diagnosed by Dr. Pegram as having an inflamed and enlarged appendix and was advised that she needed further diagnostic work in the form of an ultrasound. Dr. Pegram determined that there was no emergency and therefore no need for, and no coverage for, immediate diagnosis. Accordingly, rather than the ultrasound taking place immediately at a local hospital, it was delayed for eight days in order that it could occur at a Carle-staffed facility situated some fifty miles away. During the waiting period the plaintiff's appendix ruptured and she contracted peritonitis.

Herdrich's lawsuit alleged negligence and state fraud, but the point at issue before the District Court of Appeals was her allegation that various of the defendants had breached their ERISA-based fiduciary duties. The specific question before the Appeal Court was whether Herdrich's complaint supported a cause of action for breach of fiduciary duty. Dissenting Justice Flaum concluded that it did not. He regarded Herdrich's complaint as amounting to nothing more than an allegation that within the Carle HMO scheme there existed structural incentives to deny and reduce care to patients covered by the plan. The purpose of providing less care to patients would be to collect "large year-end bonuses" that were available if costs could be kept down and profits enhanced.[98] In Justice Flaum's view, Herdrich's allegations were "insufficient to make out a cause of action for breach of fiduciary duty under ERISA" because the "mere existence of the asserted conflict" is specifically contemplated and explicitly permitted under ERISA.[99] Accordingly, in dissent, Justice Flaum concluded that the conflict of interest alleged by Ms. Herdrich was not a legal wrong and, therefore, her complaint did not disclose a cause of action for breach of fiduciary duty.

In finding for the plaintiff, the majority of the Court of Appeal rejected Justice Flaum's dissenting analysis in the following terms:[100]

> Our point is not that a fiduciary may not have dual loyalties; it is that the tolerance of dual loyalties does not extend to the situation like the case before us where a fiduciary jettisons his responsibility to the

physical well-being of beneficiaries in favour of "loyalty" to his own financial interests. Tolerance, in other words, has its limits.

What is particularly interesting about the majority judgement is that it appears to infer that Herdrich's complaint contains an allegation to the effect that the undue delay in providing diagnostic services to the complainant stemmed from or was caused by the incentive structure operative at the Carle HMO. This point is made in the following somewhat ambiguous and, perhaps, even confusing extract:[101]

> Our decision does not stand for the proposition that the existence of incentives *automatically* gives rise to a breach of fiduciary duty. Rather, we hold that incentives *can* rise to the level of a breach where, as pleaded here, the fiduciary trust between plan participants and plan fiduciaries no longer exists (i.e., where physicians delay providing necessary treatment to, or withhold administering proper care to, plan beneficiaries for the sole purpose of increasing their bonuses).

Justice Flaum's dissenting criticism, that it is improper for courts to make their own "determination about appropriate incentive levels in managed care" and that "no standards" exist for making such determinations, did not sway the majority.[102] The stain of self-interest was too strong to ignore, especially in light of what may have been a clinical judgement made by Dr. Pegram that was devoid of medical justification.[103] Accordingly, in the view of the majority, "the direct and inferential allegations contained in Herdrich's complaint ..." raise a triable issue about whether the clinical judgement of Dr. Pegram was overwhelmed by self-interest in the form of substantial reward.[104] Of course, whether Dr. Pegram succumbed, wittingly or unwittingly, to the promise of reward, would have to be determined in a hearing on the merits.[105] Such a hearing would consider, amongst other things, just how divorced from appropriate clinical judgement was Dr. Pegram's conclusion that Herdrich was not in need of immediate attention.

The judges comprising the majority of the Court of Appeal did not comment on the important question of whether it would be appropriate to extend the inferential mode of reasoning utilized in *Herdrich* beyond the pre-trial technical issue of whether the allegations contained in Herdrich's complaint could, as a matter of law, support an action for breach of fiduciary duty.[106] In cases like *Herdrich*, utilizing inferential reasoning as an aid to resolving the actual merits of fiduciary claims in the course of a trial may well be warranted. After all, "hard evidence" of self-interested behaviour by physicians will rarely exist and if it does, the evidence is unlikely to see the light of day.[107] It should not be forgotten that what makes fiduciary conduct impermissible is the intangible of improper (usually self-interested) motivation, hardly the subject matter of public pronouncement or disclosure. Judicial insistence on hard evidence of improper motivation would make it well-nigh impossible to succeed in fiduciary-based lawsuits against physicians who are permitted to operate in conflict of interest. And while courts should be extremely cautious about drawing pivotally important inferences from circumstantial evidence, doing so would hardly be breaking new ground. For centuries courts have drawn pivotal inferences from suspicious circumstances, albeit in entirely different contexts.[108] Where circumstances are consistent with a breach of fiduciary duty and no other rational explanation, inferring a breach of fiduciary duty is entirely legitimate. Making such an inference, on a selective basis, does not undermine the scheme of divided loyalties permitted by ERISA.

In reversing the decision of the District Court of Appeals, the Supreme Court did not reject the appellate Court's finding that structural incentives in the Carle HMO system caused delays in the provision of proper care. Indeed, Souter J., writing the opinion of the Supreme Court, affirmed the existence of these incentives when he stated, "[I]n an HMO system, a physician's financial interest lies in providing less care, not more."[109] The basis for reversing the Court of Appeals' holding in *Herdrich* was the adoption of the Magistrate judge's opinion at first instance that Carle was not involved [in the impugned events] as "an ERISA fiduciary."[110] Specifically, Souter J. stated that HMOs, despite being ERISA fiduciaries, are not engaged in a fiduciary function when they act through their physicians to make either eligibility or treatment decisions (including diagnostic decisions) or "mixed eligibility decisions" which entail both eligibility and treatment considerations.[111] In other words, when making these important decisions, HMOs, through fiduciaries, do not wear their fiduciary hats. Of course, decisions which are not fiduciary decisions cannot implicate fiduciary liability, even if they are dripping with self-interest. It follows from the conclusion of the Supreme Court that decisions which impact profoundly on the health care of ERISA plan participants are as much constrained by fiduciary law as are decisions made by HMOs about the landscaping of their properties and the furnishing of their offices.

Just how did Souter J. justify the seemingly extraordinary conclusion that coverage, treatment or hybrid decisions made by HMOs are not fiduciary in character? In broad outline the argument takes the following form. First, he expresses doubt about whether Congress would ever have conceived of these decisions as being fiduciary decisions. Second, he seeks to resolve the doubt by examining the consequences, both for HMOs and for plan beneficiaries, of treating these decisions as being fiduciary. Startlingly, he asserts that for-profit HMOs could not survive if these decisions are seen to be fiduciary decisions.[112]

Surprisingly, and less than persuasively, Justice Souter also suggests that the survival of nonprofit HMOs might be in jeopardy if Herdrich's theory were adopted.[113] He then goes on to conclude that even if coverage, treatment and mixed eligibility decisions are seen as fiduciary decisions, subjecting these decisions to the scrutiny of fiduciary law would be of little practical advantage to plan beneficiaries.[114] This is because, despite the application of fiduciary law, liability issues would ultimately be resolved on the basis of the malpractice principles of tort law.[115] Malpractice law, according to Souter J., with a couple of narrow and inconsequential exceptions, affords complainants the same protections and benefits as fiduciary law.[116] Not surprisingly, given the Supreme Court's perception that the consequences of Herdrich's theory would be devastating for for-profit HMO's and that denying fiduciary liability has innocuous implications for plan beneficiaries, and further, given Congress's long-standing and ongoing commitment to HMOs, Souter J. concludes that "Congress did not intend Carle or any other HMO to be treated as a fiduciary to the extent that it makes mixed eligibility decisions acting through its physicians."[117] For emphasis, he adds that "the judiciary has no warrant to precipitate the upheaval that would follow a refusal to dismiss Herdrich's ERISA claim."[118]

In my respectful opinion, Justice Souter's analysis is fundamentally flawed in a number of important respects. Some of these are of broad import to the entire body of fiduciary law. Others are significant to the operation of fiduciary law within the ERISA context. Particularly suspect is the "doubt" expressed by Justice Souter on behalf of the Supreme Court "that Congress would ever have thought of a mixed eligibility decision as fiduciary in nature."[119] Interestingly and tellingly, Justice Souter does not advert to anything in the text of ERISA to substantiate this doubt. Instead, he relies on the analogical point that "mixed eligibility" decisions bear "only a limited" resemblance to "the usual business of traditional trustees."[120] There is actually little to dispute in this point. No doubt, that which trustees do in their employ and seek to do differs very considerably from the conduct and goals of HMO fiduciaries or, for that matter, other fiduciaries such as business partners, lawyers and physicians.

The critical question which flows from Justice Souter's observation is why are these differences of any moment? Certainly, the differences in fiduciary function do not put into question the fiduciary status of these various actors, all of whom, despite their differential mandates, are dedicated to protecting and promoting the interests of another or others. If this is correct, then it follows that the difference which is so material to Justice Souter's analysis serves only to highlight that fiduciaries have differential missions and, accordingly, diverse job descriptions. In other words, the divergence between the usual business of trustees and that of HMO fiduciaries flows inexorably from their very different callings. The real question is not and cannot sensibly be whether

ERISA fiduciaries engage in activities which are similar to the usual activities of trustees. The real question is whether the conduct of ERISA fiduciaries can be said to come within the scope of the fiduciary responsibility assumed by them or imposed on them by ERISA. While the mandate of ERISA fiduciaries who administer and manage medical benefit plans is complex, it seems indisputable that, at least in part, this mandate includes tending to, through HMO physicians, the medical requirements of plan beneficiaries and covering the costs of these requirements. Hence, through these physicians, a considerable portion of HMO activities tend to be medical in nature, though they necessarily implicate financial decisions.[121]

Justice Souter's judgement proceeds under the assumption that conduct by an HMO fiduciary which does not bear much resemblance to the proprietary conduct of trustees is appropriately characterized as nonfiduciary conduct by a fiduciary, rather than fiduciary conduct.[122] There is nothing compelling or even persuasive about this assumption. That trust law is "merely the baseline for determining the scope of fiduciary duty" is a well-established proposition in the law of the United States and, in all probability, Canada.[123] This proposition implies that trust law may be a source for understanding and delineating the scope of fiduciary responsibility of a nontrustee fiduciary, but it also implies that the content and limits of fiduciary obligation and function may be informed by sources other than trust law.[124] It seems peculiar that Souter J., given the existence of ERISA, would utilize the common law of trusts as a barometer of what is and what is not fiduciary conduct of a nontrustee fiduciary. It is ERISA which confers on HMOs their fiduciary status and which defines their fiduciary mandate. Had Justice Souter focussed on ERISA rather than the common law of trusts, as he should have, he would have concluded, without a shred of doubt, that mixed eligibility decisions are fiduciary decisions.

Looked at through the lens of ERISA, the proposition that coverage, treatment and mixed eligibility decisions are not fiduciary decisions is bewildering. How can it be that a person (or organization) who undertakes to administer and manage a health care benefits plan, whose fiduciary status is derived from this undertaking and who, in the discharge of the undertaking, exercises discretionary authority,[125] is not engaged in fiduciary administration? Justice Souter himself, quoting, in part, from ERISA, points out that an ERISA fiduciary is someone who plays the role of "manager, administrator or financial advisor" to "any plan, fund, or program ... established ... for the purpose of providing ... medical, surgical or hospital care or benefits" and who, in this role, "exercises discretionary authority or discretionary responsibility ...."[126] It follows from this description of an ERISA fiduciary that unless eligibility and treatment decisions have nothing to do with the management or administration of medical, surgical or hospital care or benefits under plans established for this purpose, Justice Souter's analysis is misconceived. Without doubt, mixed eligibility decisions, of the type made by Dr. Pergam in relation to Herdrich, lie at the very heart of the provision of medical, surgical and hospital services under ERISA-recognized medical benefit plans. Indeed, if coverage, treatment or hybrid determinations are not fiduciary decisions, it is difficult, if not impossible, to conceive of decisions made by HMOs that are. That actors declared to be ERISA fiduciaries would have no fiduciary responsibilities relating to the interests of plan beneficiaries or, at least, no important fiduciary responsibilities, could hardly have been what Congress had in mind when it imposed fiduciary responsibility on managers and administrators of medical benefit plans.

From the perspective of Canadian law, it is unimaginable that under a legislative scheme like that of ERISA, treatment and eligibility decisions made by an HMO functionary would be regarded as anything but a fiduciary decision. In Canadian law, what qualifies as fiduciary conduct is ascertained by the content of both the undertaking made by a fiduciary actor, in this case the statutorily defined undertaking of the HMO to provide, administer and manage a plan for the payment for and delivery of health services to plan beneficiaries, and the reasonable expectations of those to whom fiduciary duty is owed, again, the plan beneficiaries.[127] Given that HMO fiduciaries must, under the explicit terms of ERISA, discharge their duties with respect to a plan "solely in the interest of the participants and beneficiaries,"[128] it seems clear that the reasonable expectations of plan beneficiaries are that eligibility and treatment decisions are made with their best interests in mind.

It follows from the foregoing that there should not have been any doubt about whether mixed eligibility decisions by ERISA fiduciaries are fiduciary decisions. The issue before the US Supreme Court should have been whether Flaum J. was correct in his dissent in suggesting that the majority of the District Court of Appeals improperly inferred, from the mere existence of the incentive structure operative at the Carle HMO, that there had been a breach of fiduciary duty. The doubt invented by the Supreme Court, about the legal nature of mixed eligibility decisions, was extremely important because it legitimized the next step in its reasoning process—an inquiry into the consequences which likely flow from regarding these decisions as fiduciary in nature.

Was Souter J. correct in suggesting that for-profit HMOs would not be viable if mixed eligibility were treated in law as fiduciary decisions? He reasoned that the *raison d'etre* of for-profit HMOs is, of course, profit.[129] A critical element of realizing profit is controlling the costs of providing care to plan beneficiaries.[130] One method for controlling costs is the utilization of financial incentives which reward physicians if health delivery costs are kept low and penalize them if these costs are high.[131] Souter J. points out that the "relationship between sparing medical treatment and physician reward is not a subtle one" and asserts that "no HMO organization could survive" without rewarding physicians for rationing treatment.[132] Rationed treatment "necessarily raises some risk" beyond the ordinary risk patients endure in a nonrationed system.[133] Accordingly, when plan beneficiaries are harmed or become ill in the course of treatment provided by an HMO provider, there is a high probability that the self-interest of the provider will be implicated as an improper influence in the coverage, diagnostic and treatment decisions that were made.[134] Given fiduciary law's strict prohibition of conflict of interest, the application of fiduciary law to mixed eligibility decisions would put HMOs in legal peril.[135] Their liability would be chronic and, hence, unaffordable.[136]

In exploring the question of whether the exclusive loyalty standard of fiduciary law threatens the very existence of for-profit HMOs, Souter J. made the following explanatory remarks:[137]

> [W]e need to ask how this fiduciary standard would affect HMOs if it applied as Herdrich claims it should be applied, not directed against any particular mixed decision that injured a patient, but against HMOs that make mixed decisions in the course of providing medical care for profit. Recovery would be warranted simply upon showing that the profit incentive to ration care would generally affect mixed decisions, in derogation of the fiduciary standard to act solely in the interests of the patient without possibility of conflict.

Two points made in this passage invite response. First, it is unfair to characterize Herdrich's complaint as alleging some sort of at-large breach of fiduciary duty. A balanced reading of the allegations, and most certainly a generous one,[138] leaves no doubt that Herdrich's focus was the decision by Carle to not cover the costs of an immediate diagnostic procedure. Implicit in this very specific complaint is the extremely serious allegation that the pivotal determination made by Dr. Pegram, that Herdrich was not in immediate peril, was driven or unduly influenced by the pecuniary interests of both the Carle HMO and Dr. Pegram. Of course, whether these various allegations could be proved in a trial on the merits was not an issue before the Court.

Second, and more importantly, it is clear from the above-quoted passage that Justice Souter's thesis (that HMOs could not survive the application of fiduciary law) assumes that when HMOs make fiduciary decisions, they must satisfy the common law standard of "act[ing] solely in the interests of the patient without possibility of conflict."[139] No doubt, in practice this common law standard would be fatal to for-profit HMOs. Souter J. appears to go even further by suggesting, in effect, that HMOs and fiduciary law are inherently incompatible. In his view the system of rewarding physicians for rationed care is essential to the survival of HMOs, yet repugnant to fiduciary law.[140] Even accepting, *arguendo*, that HMOs can only survive if they are permitted to utilize structural incentives to ration care, Souter's J. analysis is flawed. The error lies in the assumption that the common law fiduciary standard of exclusive dedication to the interests of patients is the applicable standard of review of the fiduciary decisions made by HMOs. This assumption ignores the impact of ERISA. By explicitly permitting ERISA fiduciaries to operate in conflict of interest, ERISA leaves no room for the application of the common law standard of fiduciary behaviour. Because ERISA permits conflict of interest, a complaint that HMOs have dual loyalties is essentially a political complaint which is appropriately addressed to the legislature. So, in effect, by permitting dual loyalties, ERISA has embraced for its own purposes a modified version of fiduciary law. It follows that in evaluating the consequences of the Herdrich theory to HMOs, Souter J. should not have referred to the common law principles of fiduciary law. Erroneous resort to these principles was pivotal to the critical and exaggerated conclusion that the survival of HMOs is dependant upon coverage, treatment and mixed eligibility decisions being free of the scrutiny of fiduciary law. Had the consequences to HMOs of the Herdrich theory been evaluated on the basis of ERISA's modified principles of fiduciary law, as they should have been, the conclusion would have been that these modified principles do not inherently imperil HMOs.

Though ERISA permits fiduciaries to have dual loyalties, it does not authorize them to abandon their responsibilities for the physical well-being of plan beneficiaries. On the contrary, ERISA explicitly recognizes the primacy of beneficiary interests. It provides that fiduciaries must discharge their duties in relation to medical benefit plans "solely in the interest of the participants and beneficiaries, ... for the exclusive purpose of providing benefits to participants and their beneficiaries."[141] On the surface, reconciliation of the right of an HMO to pursue self-interest and its duty to act solely in the interests of plan beneficiaries seems intractable. This is because, in apparent contradiction to the right to pursue self-interest, the duty of exclusive dedication to the interests of plan beneficiaries implies selflessness. However, if the duty is viewed as a limitation of the right, a sensible accommodation is possible. HMOs may make a profit by advancing the legitimate interests of plan beneficiaries, but may not profit at the expense of these beneficiaries. This form of accommodation of right and duty is not unprecedented. It will be recalled that at common law, if a conflict of interest is either unavoidable or permitted, "it ... [must] be resolved in favour of duty."[142] In effect, this means that fiduciaries who have legal authority to operate in conflict of interest are permitted to garner personal benefit from the provision of services so long as these services appropriately advance or protect the interests of their beneficiaries. This, I would suggest, is the law of Canada.

Determining what is an proper balance between the right of HMOs to make a profit and the dedication which they owe to plan beneficiaries is facilitated by an appreciation of the historic purpose of HMOs. In large part, these organizations evolved as cost-containment mechanisms intended to curb the very considerable, if not intolerable, costs associated with excessive services provided by traditional medical practitioners operating in fee-for-service systems.[143] By permitting HMOs to operate in conflict of interest, ERISA legislatively supports both the HMO strategy of cost-containment through the elimination of unwarranted tests and treatments, and the use of reward systems designed to make this strategy a success. But in mandating that HMOs act exclusively in the interest of plan beneficiaries, ERISA clearly limits the lengths to which HMOs may go in pursuing reward. HMOs may not jettison treatments which are medically indicated in order to save money and improve their bottom line. Similarly, HMOs may not deny coverage in order to promote pecuniary self-interest.

Justice Souter argues that the duty "to act exclusively in the interest of a beneficiary ... translates into no rule readily applicable to HMO decisions or those of any other variety of medical practice."[144] As is apparent in my preceding comments, I disagree. Looking at the text of ERISA in the context of the historic evolution of HMOs, rules can readily be discerned which sensibly accommodate both the rights and obligations of HMOs. A fair balance between HMO rights and duties is struck if HMOs are permitted to pursue profit while observing the following rules: (1) coverage decisions must be made in good faith, (2) treatment decisions must be made in accordance appropriate professional standards of medical practice, and (3) mixed decisions must be made both in good faith and in accordance with reasonable and customary medical practice. Not only does this approach reconcile in a balanced way the interests of both HMOs and plan beneficiaries, but importantly, it also provides the necessary room for HMOs to pursue the profits essential to their existence. It follows, then, that the question that Souter J. should have asked in *Herdrich* is what are the consequences for HMOs if their coverage, treatment and mixed eligibility decisions must meet the standards of good faith and professional competence. Whatever may be the fulsome answer to this question, it cannot be said that the burden of meeting these standards threatens the survival of HMOs. After all, both insurers and practitioners of medicine presently live with these standards and not only survive, but live rather well.

The preceding analysis provokes an obvious question. Given that malpractice law, quite independently of fiduciary law, imports a duty of professional skill and competence and, also, that contract/insurance law imports an obligation to make coverage determinations in good faith,[145] is it not wise to avoid the complexity, severity and uncertainty of fiduciary law? In other words, if justice can be done utilizing conventional and familiar legal rules, is there a legitimate role for fiduciary law to play? Justice Souter explores these themes and concludes that fiduciary law, in the context of a *Herdrich* type of claim, is surplusage and, hence, that if fiduciary relief is unavailable to complainants, it will not be missed. On the first of these points, Souter J. observes that the allegation of breach of fiduciary issue will ultimately be resolved by malpractice principles. He notes:[146]

> [T]he defense of any HMO would be that its physician did not act out of financial interest but for good medical reasons, the plausibility of which would require reference to standards of reasonable and customary medical practice in like circumstances. ... Thus, for all practical purposes, every claim of fiduciary breach by an HMO physician making a mixed decision would boil down to a malpractice claim, and the fiduciary standard would be nothing but the malpractice standard traditionally applied in actions against physicians.

On the second point, that fiduciary law will not be missed, Souter J. acknowledges that in some states, complainants would be better off if they were able to enlist fiduciary law to assist them in their legal proceedings.[147] But he ultimately concludes that the advantages flowing from fiduciary law do not operate "across the board," are not of great moment and, in any event, have nothing to do with Congress's motivation for imposing fiduciary obligation on HMOs.[148]

Though Souter J. is quite correct in suggesting that fiduciary claims founded on allegations of inadequate care traditionally have been resolved on the basis of the standards of malpractice law (at least in the Canadian context), it is not accurate to suggest that fiduciary law has no meaningful and independent value to complainants. As noted earlier in this chapter, Canadian fiduciary law affords complainants important advantages which are not available elsewhere in private law.[149] These advantages can make the difference between success and failure in a lawsuit and, in the event of success, may have a significant impact on the level of recovery. Extended limitation periods, reverse onus provisions, more generous remedial rules and, perhaps, more forgiving causation rules, are examples of highly beneficial doctrinal benefits which are available to complainants in fiduciary cases. In addition, though at first blush this may not appear to be a practical benefit, fiduciary law is capable of capturing much more accurately than tort or contract law the gravity of certain types of wrongs perpetrated by physicians on their patients.[150] There is a gulf of difference between poor medical practice *simpliciter* and either physician misconduct or poor medical practice which emanates from a profound breach of trust. The latter implicates morally improper and dishonourable behaviour and for this reason can be regarded as far more serious than mere negligence. Characterizing misconduct as a breach of fiduciary duty, rather than a tort or breach of contract, is not just a taxonomical matter which has an impact on the theoretical coherence of law. Inherent in liability for breach of fiduciary duty is the strong moral reprobation of the law. In other words, the idea of a fiduciary wrong is a way for society to censure or condemn a certain type of egregious conduct. Moreover, it may well be that conceptualizing the role of health care providers in fiduciary terms has a desirable symbolic and psychological impact on health care providers themselves. Though it is a subtle point which is not easily susceptible of proof, intuition suggests that patients may well be better off if their health care providers conceptualize themselves as being both ethically and legally bound to protect others, rather than as free actors who may be liable to others if they misstep. Accordingly, at least from a Canadian perspective, there is a very considerable advantage to complainants in being able to resort to fiduciary law, as arcane as it may be—even when tort and contract law hold out the promise of recovery.

Implications of the *Herdrich* Analysis for Canada

It is instructive to consider whether Justice Souter's opinion that nonprofit HMOs may not be able to survive the application of fiduciary law has implications for the delivery of health services in Canada. Canadian hospitals and health authorities operate almost exclusively on a nonprofit basis. If fiduciary law threats the viability of nonprofit HMOs, it is worth considering whether it jeopardizes nonprofit Canadian health-service institutions. It should be noted that there is no basis in law for even suspecting that the public or private character of a fiduciary actor in and of itself has differential impact on the nature of fiduciary duty owed by each type of actor.[151] What determines the content of fiduciary duty is the content of the fiduciary undertaking and not, *per se*, the attributes of the fiduciary. Both private and public fiduciaries who provide and/or manage health care services are duty bound to exclusively serve the best interests of their patients and cannot, in discharging their fiduciary role, be influenced by personal or third-party interests.

Case law has identified two potential problems for nonprofit fiduciaries who are engaged in the provision of health services. In the *Herdrich* case Souter J. focusses on one of these. He states:[152]

> Herdrich's theory might well portend the end of nonprofit HMOs as well, since those HMOs can set doctor's salaries. A claim against a nonprofit HMO could easily allege that salaries were excessively high because they were funded by limiting care, and some nonprofits actually use incentive schemes similar to that challenged here....

Most physicians who work for hospitals or health authorities in Canada are not salaried. Hence, the scale of the potential problem identified by Souter J. is not as great in Canada as it may be in the United States. In any event, the notion that payment of "excessive" salaries to physicians is a breach of fiduciary duty because it diminishes the resources available to provide health services, is not persuasive, at least not as a general proposition. Though interesting from a theoretical perspective, it would be extremely difficult to establish that enhanced remuneration of physicians caused significant diminution of care below that which could be expected from physicians whose compensation was "standard." Moreover, from a theoretical perspective it can be argued that enhanced physician salaries actually benefit patients by attracting highly qualified practitioners to the job. Perhaps in the extremely rare, if not hypothetical, case, where physician salaries are demonstrably out of all proportion to the value received, and impact both palpably and detrimentally on patient care, it can be said that, at the point of hiring of the "over-paid" physician, fiduciary law has been transgressed. As to Justice Souter's other suggestion, that some nonprofit HMOs utilize physician incentive schemes similar to those utilized by for-profit HMOs, no doubt such schemes, in cases where they impact detrimentally on patient care, should be scrutinized by fiduciary law, notwithstanding the nonprofit context. Where a profit motive has been constructed by a nonprofit HMO to operate within its system of health delivery, the not-for-profit character of the HMO is immaterial. What is material and of interest to fiduciary law is the profit motive of the individual physician. That profit motive puts the physician in conflict of interest. Moreover, it should not be forgotten that the mere existence of a scheme which rewards physicians for cost-containment is not *per se* a breach of the ERISA-modified standard of fiduciary obligation. It follows that neither of the phenomenon identified by Souter J. as being problematic for nonprofit HMOs—excessive remuneration and reward for cost-containment—are inevitably part of nonprofit operations. Legally requiring nonprofit HMOs and similar nonprofit institutions to meet fiduciary standards does not *per se* threaten the existence of these institutions.

A potentially more serious problem posed by fiduciary law to nonprofit HMOs, hospitals or health authorities, stems from the universal practice of cost-containment. From the perspective of an individual patient, treatment decisions driven or influenced by cost-containment considerations are highly improper because they violate the basic fiduciary tenet that fiduciaries may consider only the interests of their beneficiaries in the discharge of their fiduciary responsibilities. That cost-containment, in the form of a physician's decision to ration services, may not be a defence to a legal claim brought against a physician and has been recognized both in the United States and in Canadian jurisprudence, though only in the context of negligence actions.[153]

In the US case of *Wickline* v. *State of California*, the California Appeals Court concluded that it was simply improper for physicians to permit cost-containment programs to "corrupt medical judgement."[154] A similar patient-oriented approach was adopted in British Columbia in *Law Estate* v. *Simice*,[155] a case in which a physician was sued for failing to make a timely diagnosis of a patient's aneurism. The physician defended himself, in part, on the basis that he was reluctant to utilize a CT scan because of budgetary constraints. Justice Spencer rejected this defence in the following terms:[156]

> If it comes to a choice between a physician's responsibility to his or her individual patient and his or her responsibility to the Medicare system overall, the former must take precedence in a case such as this. The severity of the harm that may occur to the patient who is permitted to go undiagnosed is far greater than the financial harm that will occur to the Medicare system if one more CT procedure only shows the patient is not suffering from a serious medical condition.

A contrary view, to the effect that financial considerations may, in some circumstances, be taken into account in determining a physician's standard of care, was hinted at in the Newfoundland Supreme Court case of *McLean* v. *Carr*.[157]

It can be argued that whatever may be the destiny of the cost-containment defence in malpractice suits, it is less likely to get a sympathetic hearing in fiduciary law. After all, fiduciary law regards divided loyalties as anathema. It follows that an assertion by a physician that a medical decision was influenced by interests, pecuniary or otherwise, of anyone other than his or her patients is not a defence. Indeed, it appears to be an admission. But is it? My view is that fiduciary law does not preclude nonprofit fiduciaries from engaging in cost-containment considerations. The problem with the foregoing analysis, which suggests otherwise, is that it fails to take into account that fiduciary duty is owed not just to particular individual patients, but to all persons, present and future, who form the class of patients. In a nonprofit system of health care, cost-containment can legitimately be seen as part of the process of allocating limited resources to the at-large patient population for the purpose of maximizing benefits to the individuals who form this population.[158]

Cost-containment and even specific allocation decisions are compatible with the fiduciary obligations of health care institutions because they incorporate the pre-relational understanding of both treatment providers and patients that considerations such as efficacy, patient prognosis and just plain "affordability" will affect decisions about the nature, incidence and timing of medical services provided.[159] To suggest that health care providers have an duty to expend, without limitation, the finite resources of a health care system on particular patients, implies that health expenditures may be made without regard to the consequences to other patients, even those who may be better candidates for successful treatment. It must not be forgotten that these latter patients are also owed and will be owed fiduciary duties.[160] Hence, in my view, it is inappropriate to view allocation decisions made by nonprofit health care providers in terms of the conflict of interest. Allocation decisions driven by cost-containment considerations are more properly viewed as justifiable, if not essential, distributions of limited resources amongst the class of fiduciary beneficiaries. In technical legal terms the appropriate paradigm through which to assess the fiduciary law implications of cost-containment strategies is the concept of "keeping an even hand amongst beneficiaries." Though this maxim often imports an obligation to treat all beneficiaries equally, it cannot and should not be understood literally.[161] If allocation decisions are made on a nonpersonalized, relatively objective basis, in accordance with appropriate principles intended to maximize the health care of patients, the evenhanded principle is satisfied.

It is tempting to relegate the *Herdrich* decision to the pile of mostly American cases which, though of interest, have no particular significance to the jurisprudence of Canada. After all, *Herdrich* focusses on a uniquely American institution, the HMO, and its regulation by a uniquely American statute, ERISA. However, dismissing *Herdrich* as containing no lessons for Canada would be a mistake. It contains both doctrinal and policy lessons which are important to and have currency in the Canadian context.

From a doctrinal point of view, *Herdrich* illustrates the importance of and confusion surrounding the often overlooked issue of scope of fiduciary responsibility. There is no doubt that fiduciary duty is circumscribed and that it is legitimate for courts, in appropriate cases, to reject fiduciary claims on the basis that the fiduciary's misconduct which is impugned lies outside the scope of fiduciary responsibility. The problem with the *Herdrich* analysis is not its recognition that fiduciary responsibility has its limits, but the manner in which it delineates those limits. Rather than circumscribing fiduciary duty by reference to the fiduciary undertaking, *Herdrich* engages in inappropriate analogical reasoning which can only yield the result that "mixed eligibility decisions" are not fiduciary decisions. In Canada, and more broadly the Commonwealth, the scope issue has also been problematic. In *McInerney* v. *MacDonald,* the Supreme Court of Canada concluded that the fiduciary duty of "utmost good faith and loyalty" is the basis of the fiduciary duty of physicians to provide patients with access to their own health records.[162] The contrary view was adopted by the High Court of Australia in the case of *Breen* v. *Williams.*[163] In ruling that physicians have no fiduciary responsibility to provide their patients with access to their own medical records, the High Court criticized, scathingly, Justice La Forest's reasoning in *McInerney* v. *MacDonald* as being "assertion" and not "analysis."[164] Though, on the merits of the issue, I regard the Canadian view as being correct, there is no doubt that the concept of loyalty and good faith is simply too open-ended to provide meaningful compass to the issue of scope. What is clear is that there is confusion in the case law about what is an appropriate and principled basis for determining the scope of fiduciary responsibility. Given the state of confusion in the case law, this thorny and pivotal issue can easily give rise to the wrong conclusion, as it did in *Herdrich*. Though it is beyond the purview of this chapter to elaborate on this point, it is suggested that scope of fiduciary responsibility can only be properly ascertained from the content of fiducial undertaking. Unfortunately, as I have already pointed out, such undertakings are not usually explicit and can only be discerned through contextual analysis. There is inherent vagueness in contextual analysis and, therefore, ascertaining the scope of fiduciary responsibility will continue to be plagued by some degree of uncertainty.

The US Supreme Court's implausible ruling on the scope issue in *Herdrich* appears to have been driven by the desire to avoid the application of fiduciary law. Convinced that it was impossible for HMOs to comply with the exacting behavioural standards of fiduciary law and further convinced that patients could be adequately protected by malpractice law, the Court in effect eliminated the spectre of fiduciary liability of HMOs. I have suggested that neither of these convictions are themselves convincing. But they do reflect a concern about the severity of fiduciary law, a concern which six years earlier found expression in Canadian case law. In *Canson Enterprises Ltd.* v. *Broughton & Co.*, a case which focussed on a breach of fiduciary duty by a solicitor, a sharply divided Supreme Court of Canada debated the extent to which the plaintiff-friendly remedial rules of fiduciary law should be substantively fused with certain rules of tort law.[165] A slim majority of judges in the case, though not a majority of the Court, expressed views similar to those expressed by Souter J. in the *Herdrich* case. In concluding that the remedial principles of the tort of deceit were appropriate for determining the extent of fiduciary liability of the defendant solicitor, La Forest J's majority judgement rejected the application of the traditional remedial principles of fiduciary law in the following terms:[166]

> It was said ... that the [traditional fiduciary] approach is necessary to sustain fiduciary relationships. I do not accept that there is a need to strengthen the fiduciary position *to the point of unnecessary harshness*. Both the common law [that is, tort law] and equity sufficiently support the fiduciary position by compensating the victim of the breach of confidence. Damages equivalent to those for deceit would seem sufficient to meet both these ends [emphasis added].

A minority of judges, whose opinions were expressed by McLachlin J. (as she then was), the present Chief Justice of the Court, argued strongly for the application of the more stringent remedial principles of traditional fiduciary law. In the view of McLachlin J., given the difficulty of detecting and proving a breach of fiduciary duty and the critical importance of "keep[ing] persons in a fiduciary capacity up to their duty," these onerous principles should ordinarily be applied.[167] Though six years have passed since the *Canson* decision was rendered, it is difficult to predict the extent to which fiduciary principles will be maintained in cases where tort law principles may be resorted to.[168]

We have reached a critical juncture in the development of fiduciary law. There is much to be said in favour of the notion expressed in *Canson* that "the same basic claim, whether framed in terms of a common law [tort] action or an equitable remedy [for breach of fiduciary duty], should give rise to ... [the same] levels of redress."[169] But Canadian courts are well advised to resist any temptation to completely eliminate fiduciary law based redress, as did the US Supreme Court in the *Herdrich* case. Over the centuries, fiduciary law has been constructed by equity judges through their sharp observation of human nature. The human urge to pursue self-interest is powerful, even in cases where solemn pledges have been made to protect and promote exclusively and selflessly the interests of another or others. Fiduciary law has been fashioned for the specific task of enforcing fiducial undertakings and, in the noble course of its work, protects vulnerable persons and maintains the integrity of critically important societal institutions—including those whose profound mission is the provision of health care to members of society. In principle, there is nothing wrong with leaving the task of maintaining the integrity of these institutions to bodies of law which are less arcane than fiduciary law, but only if these bodies of law are up to the challenge. In some instances at least, fiduciary law allows plaintiffs whose legitimate complaints do not resonate in tort law, both to succeed and to succeed more amply.[170] In my respectful opinion, it would be a mistake of considerable significance for Canadian courts, either under present circumstances or more especially in any new era of for-profit medicine,[171] to adopt the *Herdrich* solution. The notion that an HMO is every bit a fiduciary but can never be liable as one is both ironic and risky.

Conclusion

Most health service providers, both individual and institutional, are fiduciaries or agents of fiduciaries. As such, they are duty bound to look after the interests of their patients (and clients) with exclusive dedication. This duty of loyalty means that health care providers may not, in the provision of services, be swayed by their own personal interests or the interests of third parties. A long-standing exception to this rule of selflessness is that service providers may be compensated on a fee-for-service basis. More recently, in both Canada and the United States, health service institutions have been permitted to profit from the delivery of health services. The right to profit and to charge on a fee-for-service basis must be understood as being no more than a right to incidentally benefit from the proper discharge of fiduciary obligation. Health service providers are not permitted to sacrifice or materially jeopardize the interests of their patients in order to garner personal benefit or to confer benefits on third parties. Hence, first principles suggest that any cost-containment strategy designed to enhance institutional profit, but which materially increases patient risk, is a breach of fiduciary duty. On this point Canadian law would be wise to embrace fiduciary law's traditional intolerance of conduct which does not meet the standard "single minded attention to the beneficiaries interest." A profit-driven cost-containment strategy which endangers patients is an odious breach of trust. It should not be sanitized and the wrong involved should not be diminished by treating it merely as a species of substandard care. On the other hand, cost-containment practices in a nonprofit context, intended to achieve the best therapeutic outcome for patient populations as a whole, are an entirely different matter. They must be regarded for what they are: part of an unfortunate but necessary process of juggling resources so as to maximize patient benefit. Context is everything and, in a nonprofit context, cost-containment, given the reality of limited health care budgets, is an act of loyalty and not disloyalty. The profoundly important problem of limited budgets should not be visited upon the frontline workers in Canada's not-for-profit health system. Fiduciary law should not be used inappropriately and opportunistically to challenge considered public policy decisions about the level to which health care is funded. That is a political and electoral question.

NOTES

1   Council on Ethical and Judicial Affairs Report on "Sale of Non-Health-Related Goods From Physician's Offices" (1998) 280:6 *JAMA* 563. See also "Symposium: Solicitor/Client Privilege and the Mentally Incapable Older Client" (2000) 19 Estates, *Trusts & Pension J.* 171, in particular the comment by Dr. Michael Gordon at 177 where he states that "[f]rom a geriatrician's perspective, I have no difficulty with the concept of acting on the patient's behalf to protect him/her from harm. I consider that part of my fiduciary responsibility."

2   Business partners are fiduciaries. So too, at least ordinarily, are the parties to the following relationships: lawyer-client, guardian-ward, trustee-principal, director-corporation, and principal-agent. See *Lac Minerals Ltd.* v. *International Corona Resources Ltd.*, [1989] 2 S.C.R. 574 at 597, 35 E.T.R. 1, 61 D.L.R. (4th) 14 [hereinafter *Lac Minerals* cited to S.C.R.]; M. Gillien and F. Woodman, *The Law of Trusts: A Contextual Approach* (Toronto: Emond Montgomery, 2000) at 742.

3   Gordon, *supra* note 2 at 177. In addition, the codes of ethics of various health service providers make it clear that the first and foremost obligation of the health care providers is promoting the best interests or well-being of patients. See, for example, s. 1 of the Canadian Medical Association, "Code of Ethics" (15 October 1996), online at http://www.cma.ca/inside/policybase/1996/10-15.htm; Canadian Nurses Association, *Code of Ethics for Registered Nurses* (Ottawa: Canadian Nurses Association, 1999) at 20, s. 8; Canadian Physiotherapy Association, *Code of Ethics*, June 1989, preamble; Canadian Association of Occupational Therapists, *CAOT Code of Ethics*, January 1996, online at http://www.caot.ca/ default.cfm?ChangeID=50&pageID=35, article 1, 2 (accessed on 28 November 2000).

4   See Health Care Protection Act, S.A. 2000, c. H–3.3 (assented to 30 May 2000), popularly known as Bill 11, which permits essential services and enhanced services to be offered in a single facility. For an analysis of Bill 11, see T.A. Caulfield, C.M. Flood and B. von Tigerstrom, "Comment: Bill 11: Health Care Protection Act" (2000) 9:1 *Health L. Rev.* 22. As to cost-containment, see T. A. Caulfield and G. Robertson, "Cost Containment Mechanisms in Health Care: A Review of Private Law Issues" (1999) 27 *Man. L.J.* 1 (1999) and T.A. Caulfield and D.E. Ginn, "The High Price of Full Disclosure: Informed Consent and Cost Containment in Health Care" (1994) 22 *Man L. J.* 328.

5   See A. Farber Walsh, "The Legal Attack on Cost Containment Mechanisms: The Expansion of Liability For Physicians and Managed Care Organizations" (1997) 31 *John Marshall L. Rev.* 207 and cases cited therein, as well as W.A. Chittenden III, "Malpractice Liability and Managed Health Care: History and Prognosis" (1991) 26 *Tort & Insurance L. J.* 451 and cases cited therein.

6   J. Carlisle "Conflict of Interest, The Fiduciary Metaphor," dialogue (1996) May–June, online at College of Physicians and Surgeons of Ontario Dialogue at http:/ /www.cpso.on.ca/articles.asp?ArticleId=60056929 (accessed on 27 November 2000), where he states: "The physician-patient relationship is based on trust. This is not simply a quaint tradition of the medical profession but recognition that such a relationship of trust between the doctor and patient is necessary for the proper function of the doctor-patient relationship."

7   *Pegram* v. *Herdrich*, 120 S.Ct. 2143 (2000), rev'g 154 F. 3d 362 (7th Cir. 1998) [hereinafter *Herdrich*, all citations refer to the decision of the Supreme Court unless otherwise indicated].

8   The earliest Canadian case to recognize the *fiduciary* nature of the physician-patient relationship is *Rowe* v. *Grand Trunk Railway Co.* (1866), 16 U.C.C.P. 500 at 506. Modern authorities subscribe to the theory that physicians, at least ordinarily, are fiduciaries. See also *Norberg* v. *Wynrib*, [1992] 2 S.C.R. 226 at 271 where McLachlin J. states: "But perhaps the most fundamental characteristic of the doctor-patient relationship is its fiduciary nature. *All the authorities agree that the relationship of physician to patient also falls into that special category of relationships which the law calls fiduciary*" [emphasis added]. As to the possibility of a physician not being a fiduciary, see *infra*, note 10 and accompanying text.

9   In *Parslow* v. *Masters*, [1993] 6 W.W.R. 273, Hunter J. of the Saskatchewan Court of Queen's Bench concluded that a physician-patient relationship was a fiduciary relationship even though, on the facts of that case, the physician, Dr. Masters, was hired by a third-party insurer to provide an assessment about the medical condition of the insured, Ms. Parslow.

10 *Frame v. Smith*, [1987] 2 S.C.R. 99 at 136 *per* Wilson J. These *indicia* are very heavily relied on in the case law.

11 The focal point of disagreement is the meaning of the term "vulnerability." In *Hodgkinson v. Simms*, [1994] 3 S.C.R. 377, 117 D.L.R. (4th) 161, 5 E.T.R. (2d) 1 [hereinafter *Hodgkinson* cited to S.C.R.] Sopinka and La Forest JJ. vigorously debate the degree of vulnerability which must exist before it can be said that one is "vulnerable" at law.

12 See e.g., S. Shortell *et al.*, "Physicians as Double Agents" (1998) 280 *JAMA* 1102 and Carlisle, *supra* note 7 at 1.

13 While I do not have empirical data to support this assertion, my personal practice, as well as an informal survey of friends and physicians, suggests that this form of reliance is commonplace, if not routine. Physicians included in my survey were Joanne Caulfield (Edmonton), Leonard Sternberg (Toronto), Eric Burke (Knoxville, Tennessee) and David Schiff (Edmonton). See also G. Robertson, *infra* note 42.

14 Another view is that vulnerability is essential to the existence of a fiduciary relationship. See Justice Sopinka's views in *Lac Minerals*, *supra* note 3 at 599 and *Hodgkinson*, *supra* note 12 at 409.

15 *Guerin et al. v. The Queen*, [1984] 2 S.C.R. 335 at 384, 13 D.L.R. (4th) 321, [1984] 6 W.W.R. 481 [hereinafter *Guerin* cited to S.C.R.] quoted in both *McInerney v. McDonald*, [1992] 2 S.C.R. 138 at 154, 93 D.L.R. (4th) 415 [hereinafter *McInerney* cited to D.L.R.] and *Hodgkinson*, *supra* note 12 at 408. See also *Norberg v. Wynrib*, *supra* note 9 at 273.

16 *Lac Minerals*, *supra* note 3 at 658, 662, La Forest J. and *Hodgkinson*, *supra* note 12 at 412.

17 *Hodgkinson*, *ibid.* at 413.

18 *Norberg v. Wynrib*, *supra* note 9 at 292, McLachlin J.

19 The Oath of Hippocrates, online at http://www.humanities.ccny.cuny.edu/ history/reader/hippoath.htm (accessed on 29 November 2000):

> The regimen I adopt shall be for the benefit of my patients ... and not for their hurt or for any wrong. ...Whatsoever house I enter, there will I go for the benefit of the sick, refraining from all wrongdoing or corruption, and especially from any act of seduction, of male or female, of bond or free.

20 That these sources may evidence of a fiduciary undertaking and the reasonable expectations which such an undertaking engenders is apparent from the following observations made by La Forest J. in his judgement in *Hodgkinson*, *supra* note 12 at 412. He states:

> The existence of a fiduciary duty in a given case will depend upon the reasonable expectations of the parties, and these in turn depend on factors such as trust, confidence, complexity of subject matter, and community or industry standards. For instance in Norberg, *supra*, the Hippocratic Oath was evidence that the sexual relationship diverged significantly from the standards reasonably expected from physicians by the community. This inference was confirmed by expert evidence to the effect that any reasonable practitioner in the defendant's position would have taken steps to help the addicted patient, in stark contrast to the deplorable exploitation which in fact took place....

21 *Supra* note 4.

22 *Supra* note 20.

23 With respect to conflict of interest, see J. Carlisle, "Doctors' Notes" (July–August 1994) College of Physicians and Surgeons of Ontario Dialogue, online at http://www.cpso.on.ca/articles.asp?ArticleId=611583129 (accessed on 27 November 2000); The College of Physicians and Surgeons of Alberta, *Conflict of Interest*, December 1994, online at http://www.cpsa.ab.ca/policyguidelines/conflict.html (accessed on 28 November 2000). With respect to both conflict of interest and privacy, see Canadian Medical Association, *supra* note 4; J. Carlisle, *supra* note 7; Canadian Nurses Association, *supra* note 4, Confidentiality, ss. 1–3 at 15; Canadian Physiotherapy Association, *supra* note 4; Canadian Association of Occupational Therapists, *supra* note 4, articles 2, 6; Canadian Association of Speech-Language Pathologists and Audiologists, CASLPA Canon of Ethics, online at http://www.caslpa.ca/english/membership/ethics.html (accessed on 1 October 1999), articles 6, 7, 13.

24 Canadian Nurses Association, *supra* note 4, Health and Well Being, s. 1, at 8; Canadian Physiotherapy Association, *supra* note 4, Preamble, Premise Statement and ss. 1.10, 3.7 and 3.8.

25 M.V. Ellis, *Fiduciary Duties In Canada*, looseleaf (Scarborough, Ont.: 2000) at 10–20 citing the case of *Tannock* v. *Bromley* (1979), 10 B.C.L.R. 62 (S.C.).

26 The Regional Health Authorities Act, S.A. 1994, c. R–9.07, s. 5, sets out the responsibilities of regional health authorities in Alberta. They include "promot[ing] and protect[ing] the health of the population in the health region" and providing "health services in a manner that is responsive to the needs of individuals and communities. ..." Policy directives of the various health authorities evidence a fiduciary undertaking. See, for example, the following "Directives" of the Capital Health Authority: "Conflict of Interest," Number 1.3.1, 5 May 1997; "Confidentiality," Number 1.3.2, 3 July 1997; "Patient/Client/Resident Abuse," Number 1.3.5, 15 December 1997. Hospitals which operate in a nonregionalized setting also operate on the basis of similar guidelines. See the St. Joseph's Hospital (Brantford, Ontario) policy statements on "Conflict of Interest." Number IV–44–00, October 1999, and "Confidentiality," IV–08–00, November 1985, revised, November 1992.

27 *Herdrich*, *supra* note 8 at 2149, Souter J.

28 U.S.C. ss. 1104(a)(1).

29 A. Legrand, "Insurers Beware? A Survey of Bad Faith claims Against Insurers in Canadian Law" (1999) 17 Can. J. Ins. L. at 85.

30 *Ibid.* at 87, citing *Fredrickson* v. *Insurance Corp. of B.C.* [1990] 4 W.W.R. 637 at 667.

31 *Infra* note 82 and accompanying text.

32 *Breen* v. *Williams*, *infra* note 45, quoted in text at 25.

33 P.D. Finn, "The Fiduciary Principle" in T.G. Youdan, ed., *Equity, Fiduciaries and Trusts* (Toronto: Carswell, 1989) 1 at 28. See also *Breen* v. *Williams* (C.A.), *infra* note 45 at 549, Kirby J.

34 As to "can be read," see *Hodgkinson*, *supra* note 12 at 405, *Norberg* v. *Wynrib*, *supra*, note 9 at 285, *Blueberry River Band* v. *Canada* [1995] 4 S.C.R. 344 at 401 and 405–6 [hereinafter *Blueberry*]. As to "has been read," see M. Morellato, "The Crown's Fiduciary Obligation Toward Aboriginal Peoples" (September 1999) Pacific

Business & Law Inst. 4.1 at 4.8 where the author, referring to the fiduciary status of the Crown *vis à vis* aboriginal persons, states: "Accordingly, it is clear that the crown's fiduciary obligations not only comprise duties of good faith and loyalty, but also include duties of skill and competence in managing the affairs of aboriginal peoples."

35 *Hodgkinson, supra* note 12 at 405.

36 For a useful introduction to the limitation of action rules pertaining to breach of fiduciary duty, see *M.K.* v. *M.H.*, [1992] 3 S.C.R. 6 at 59–61, (1992) 96 D.L.R. (4th) 289.

37 W.M.C. Gummow, "Compensation for Breach of Fiduciary Duty" in T.G.Youdan, ed., *Equity, Fiduciaries And Trusts* (Toronto: Carswell 1989) 57 at 88–91. In *Canson Enterprises Ltd.* v. *Boughton Co.*, [1991] 3 S.C.R. 534, 85 D.L.R. (4th) 129, 1 W.W.R. 245 [hereinafter *Canson* cited to S.C.R.] the Supreme Court of Canada brought the causation requirement of fiduciary law somewhat into line with tort law notions. However, it is not clear the extent to which there has been fusion of common law notions of causation (tort and contract law's approach) with equity (fiduciary law). The Court was very divided on the question of whether common law and even statutory notions such as "mitigation" and "contributory negligence" ought to impact on fiduciary analysis.

38 See *Guerin, supra* note 16 at 360; *Canson, ibid.* at 545, McLachlin J., where she attributes the same view to the majority ("La Forest has avoided one such pitfall in indicating that compensation for breach of fiduciary duty will not be limited by foreseeability.") and *Blueberry, supra* note 35 at 401, where McLachlin J. comments on an aspect of the trial judges decision in the following terms: "This concern is misplaced. It amounts to bringing forseeability into the fiduciary analysis through the back door. This constitutes an error of law."

39 Tort law requires that patients establish that they would have engaged in a different course of conduct than the one which lead to their loss had they been properly informed about the material risks. See, L. Klar, *Tort Law*, 2d ed. (Toronto: Carswell, 1996) at 308–9 and see generally E. Picard and G. Robertson, *Legal Liability of Doctors and Hospitals in Canada*, 3d ed. (Toronto: Carswell, 1996) ch. 3.

40 The reverse onus rule is explained in the case of *Brickenden* v. *London Loan & Savings Co.*, [1934] 3 D.L.R. 465, a decision of the Judicial Committee of the Privy Council on appeal from the Supreme Court of Canada. In that case a solicitor breached his fiduciary duty by acting for both parties to a lending transaction without revealing that he had a personal interest in two mortgages that were part of the transaction. In rejecting the solicitor's appeal, Lord Thankerton stated at 469:

> When a party, holding a fiduciary relationship, commits a breach of his duty by nondisclosure of material facts, which his constituent is entitled to know in connection with the transaction, he cannot be heard to maintain that disclosure would not have altered the decision to proceed with the transaction, because the constituent's action would be solely determined by some other factor, such as the valuation by another party of the property proposed to be mortgaged. Once the Court has determined that the nondisclosed facts were material, speculation as to what course the constituent, on disclosure, would have taken, is not relevant.

See *Commerce Capital Trust Co.* v. *Berk* (1989), 57 D.L.R. (4th) 759 for a more recent application of the reverse onus principle. This case involved a lawyer, acting on both sides of a mortgage transaction, who failed to fully disclose to the mortgagee information that went to the value of the asset underlying the mortgage transaction. The trial judge concluded that Commerce Capital had not proved that had it been fully informed, it would not have advanced the mortgage monies. This finding was reversed on the basis that, given the fiduciary relationship between the parties, the onus of proof was on the defendant, not the plaintiff.

41   In tort law, it is the patient/complainant who bears the burden of proof. It is apparent from the last sentence in Privy Council's reasoning in the *Brickenden* case just why it is so difficult to discharge the burden of proof, *ibid*. The *Commerce Capital Trust Co.* case, *ibid.*, illustrates the importance of this burden. See 763–6 where the Ontario Court of Appeal sets out its reasons for overturning the trial judge's finding based on the reasoning in the *Brickenden* case, *ibid*. See also G. Robertson, "Informed Consent Ten Years Later: The Impact of *Reibl* v. *Hughes*," (1991) 70 *Can. Bar Rev.* 423 at 428 and 435 where he states that "plaintiffs in informed-consent cases are almost always unsuccessful, and often this is because of the requirement of causation."

42   *Hodgkinson, supra* note 12 at 453, LaForest J.: "The law of fiduciary duties has always contained within it an element of deterrence." In *Soulos* v. *Korkontzilas*, [1997] S.C.R. 217 at 235, 146 D.L.R. (4th) 214 [hereinafter cited to S.C.R.], McLachlin J., after quoting this passage, goes on to state:

The constructive trust imposed for breach of fiduciary relationship thus serves not only to do the justice between the parties that good conscience requires, but to hold fiduciaries and people in positions of trust to the high standards of trust and probity that commercial and other social institutions require if they are to function effectively.

See also *Canson, supra* note 38 at 543, where McLachlin J. states: "[E]quity is concerned, not only to compensate the plaintiff, but to enforce the trust which is at its heart."

43   In all three cases referred to in note 35—*Hodgkinson, supra* note 12, *Norberg* v. *Wynrib, supra* note 9 and *Blueberry, supra* note 35—the description of the defalcations of the fiduciaries should be understood in light of the conflicts of interest they were in. In *Norberg*, what lay at the root of Dr. Wynrib's failure to meet an appropriate standard of care was his pursuit of personal gratification. In *Blueberry*, the Crown's "fiduciary liability" for failing to act with "reasonable diligence" (at 405), must be understood in light of the Crown's ulterior motives. These are described by McLachlin J. at 379 as follows:

The Crown, facing conflicting political pressures in favour of preserving the land for the band on the one hand, and making it available for distribution to veterans on the other, may be argued to have been in a position of conflict of interest.

In other words, in none of these cases is breach of fiduciary duty based upon negligence, *simpliciter*.

44   *Breen* v. *Williams* (1996), 138 A.L.R. 259 (H.C. Aus.) at 274, aff'g (1994), 35 N.S.W.L.R. 522 (N.S.W.C.A.) [hereinafter *Breen*, all citations refer to the decision of the High Court unless otherwise indicated]. See also Finn, *supra*, note 34 at 28.

45   (1987), 11 B.C.L.R. (2d) 362.

46   *Ibid.* at 362.

47 *Canson, supra* note 38 at 549 where McLachlin J. points out that:

> Guerin [*supra* note 16] was not concerned with abuse of trust prop-
> erty in the classic sense. There were no assets on the property which
> had been misappropriated. The wrong was the failure to adhere to the
> conditions of surrender ...

See also, Canson note 38 at 573 where La Forest J. rejects the theory recently
advanced by McEachern C.J. in *C.A.* v. *Critchely* [1998] 155 D.L.R. (4th) 475 at 500,
to the effect that breach of fiduciary duty necessarily entails a defendant who takes
advantage of a relationship of trust or confidence for his or her direct or indirect
personal advantage.

48 *Guerin, supra* note 16.

49 *Ibid.* at 388.

50 In *Horsman Bros. Holdings Ltd.* v. *Panton & Panton,* [1976] 3 W.W.R. 745 (B.C.S.C.),
Craig J. noted that even innocent conduct can be a breach of trust if it violates the
terms of a trust. Specifically, at 750 he states, "If a person deals with the funds [of
a trust] ... in a manner inconsistent with the trust, he breaches the trust, even
though he may do so 'innocently'." The terms of a trust are an expression of the
specific undertaking made by a trustee. Hence, the focus of the concept of breach
of trust is the content of the trustees undertaking.

51 This point is well illustrated in the United States District Court case of *Donovan*
v. *Bierwirth*, 538 F. Supp. 463 (1981), aff'g 680 F. 2d 263 (2nd Cir. 1982) at 471. In that
case the fiduciary failure of trustees of a pension fund is described in negligence
terms; that is, "acting imprudently in purchasing" securities "without [making]
sufficient inquiry into the facts upon which they based their decisions." However,
the failure of loyalty that rendered the trustees' defalcation a breach of fiduciary
duty was the conflict of interest that the trustees were in when they purchased the
stock. The trustees were corporate officers of the company whose stock was
purchased and the purchase of the stock appeared to be driven by the
corporation's efforts to ward off a hostile takeover attempt. As Mishler J. stated at
471, in referring to the trustees "[w]e find that their conduct was solely motivated
by their all-consuming desire to defeat the tender offer."

52 *Moore* v. *Regents of the University of California*, 793 P.2d 479, 271 Cal. Rptr. 146 (S.
Ct. 1990) [cited to Cal. Rptr.]. See particularly at 150, where Pannelli J. states: "[A]
physician must disclose personal interests unrelated to the patient's health, whether
research or economic, that may affect the physician's professional judgment ...."

53 L. Klar, *Tort Law*, (Toronto: Carswell, 1991) at 248ff.

54 *Canson, supra* note 38 at 565, La Forest J. He states: "Where concurrent liability lies
in tort and contract and in equity (fiduciary law), the appellants may sue in
whatever manner they find most advantageous." See *ibid.* at 570 to the same effect.

55 *Pegram* v. *Herdrich*, 7th Circ., 1998, *supra* note 8 per Wood and Coffey J.J. citing
Donovan v. *Bierwirth, supra* note 52.

56 *Supra* note 45 at 285, Gaudron and McHugh JJ.

57 [1896] A.C. 44 at 51–2, emphasis added, quoted with approval in *Public Trustee* v.
Toronto Humane Society (1987), 60 O.R. (2d) 236 at 247–8 (H.C.).

58 In the classic case of *Keech* v. *Sanford* (1726), 25 E.R. 223, a trustee renewed a lease,
which was the subject matter of a trust, for his own personal benefit. The landlord
refused to renew the lease in favour of the trust beneficiary who was an infant. In
ordering the trustee to assign the lease to the infant, the Court stated at 223: "I

must consider this as a trust for the infant; for I very well see, if a trustee, on the refusal to renew, might have a lease to himself, few trust estates would be renewed to the ... [beneficiary]; though not say there is a fraud in this case, yet he should rather have let it run out, than to have had the lease to himself. ..." To the same effect see *Re Lithwick* (1976), 61 D.L.R. (3d) 411 at 416 where Grange J. responds as follows to the request that costs be awarded against an executer whom the Justice has removed from office by reason of conflict of interest:

> I do not think that is an appropriate order. While he has placed himself in a position ... which necessitates his removal as executor, there is no suggestion of dishonesty or impropriety in the conduct of his trust, and his conflict of interest arose in part through services to his late brother which may have been voluntary and for which I doubt that he will ever be properly compensated.

See *Zwicker et al.* v. *Standury et al.*, [1953] 2 S.C.R. 438 at 440, Kellock J. and *Canadian Aero Service Ltd.* v. *O'Malley* (1973), 40 D.L.R. (3d) 371, both of which stand for the proposition that breach of fiduciary duty does not depend upon proof of *mala fides*. On the other hand, some Courts have been willing to assess the good faith and reasonableness of fiduciaries who appear to have profited from their fiduciary role. See also D. W. M. Waters, *Law of Trust In Canada*, 2nd (Toronto: Carswell, 1984) at 711 and cases referred to therein.

59 Deception and self-deception play an important role in the theory of evolutionary biology. See O.D. Jones, "Evolutionary Analysis In Law: An Introduction and Application To Child Abuse" (1997) 75 *North Carolina L. Rev.*, 1117 at 1151 and references cited therein in footnotes 90–2. See also M. Surbey and J. McNally, "Self-Deception as a Mediator of Cooperation and Defection in Varying Social Contexts Described in the Iterated Prisoner's Dilemma" (1997) 18 *J. Evolution and Human Behavior* 417.

60 Ellis, *supra* note 26 at 1–4 and *Breen*, *supra* note 45 at 274, Brennan J.

61 The purpose of the rule against conflict of interest is to promote strict allegiance to the beneficiary of the fiduciary relationship. Hence, first principles suggest that if third parties, to whom fiduciaries are duty bound or whose interests fiduciaries would reasonably be presumed to wish to promote (e.g., a spouse), have their interests advanced through the discharge of fiduciary duty or the exercise of fiduciary power or simply through the transmission of valuable fiduciary information, the rule against conflict of interest is implicated. See *Soulos* v. *Korkontzilas*, *supra* note 43 where a real estate broker arranged for his wife to purchase property which his client was attempting to purchase. The broker withheld important information from his client and provided it to his wife, who purchased the property in the joint names of herself and her husband. The fiduciary wrong in that case was corrected by the legal remedy of constructive trust. The Supreme Court of Canada focussed on the wrong of failing to transmit the "counteroffer" to the client, but clearly there were further breaches of fiduciary duty, including the transmission of the details of the counteroffer to the broker's wife.

62 Ellis, *supra* note 26 at 1–4.

63 *Ibid.* and see also B.M. Dickens, "Conflict of Interest in Canadian Health Care Law" (1995) 21 *Am. J. L. & Med.* 259 especially at 262–4.

64 Rodwin, *supra* note 1 at 55–96.

65 *Ibid.* at 94–6.

66 (1988), 65 O.R. (2d) 461 (Ont. Div. Ct.).

67 *Ibid.* at 469–70.

68 See Dickens, *supra* note 64 at 268–71 for a more in depth discussion of the *Cox* case.

69 See Ellis, *supra* note 26 at 1–5 – 1–6 where the duty of disclosure is introduced as a general fiduciary duty. See also 10–3 – 10–12 where the duty of disclosure of physicians is discussed. See also the recent comments of the Supreme Court of Canada on the duty of disclosure of lawyers, *Canson, supra* note 38 at 571.

70 Conflict of interest can arise unavoidably through the conduct of third parties. For example, if a physician has a large shareholding in a company that happens to take over or merge with another company that owns and operates diagnostic facilities to which the physician refers patients, the physician is in a conflict of interest. It is instructive to think of the duty to disclose as being a secondary and contingent duty which arises when a fiduciary has failed in his or her threshold obligation to avoid conflict of interest or finds him or herself unavoidably in conflict. As will be elaborated below, the duty of disclosure exists whether or not the conflict is legally tolerated. See *infra* note 77 and accompanying text.

71 As to the duty to disclose, the rule is that all material matters which may affect the loyal discharge of fiduciary obligation must be disclosed. The scope, scale and nature of disclosure required of a fiduciary is set out in *R. v. Kelly*, [1992] 2 S.C.R. 170. Though *Kelly* is a case which focusses on the criminal liability of a financial advisor for receiving secret commissions, the reasoning in the case is applicable to a civil claim based on fiduciary theory. The duty of disclosure is described in a number of ways in *Kelly* including, at 190, a duty to make "adequate and full" disclosure, "full, frank and fair disclosure" and "adequate and timely disclosure." See also the contents of note 74 for an elaboration of these concepts. See also *Halushka v. University of Saskatchewan* (1965), 53 D.L.R. (2d) 436 (Sask. C.A.) which sets out the standards of disclosure in a medical research and experimentation context.

72 *R. v. Kelly, ibid.* at 190, where Cory J., on behalf of the majority of the Court states:

> The policy motivating the prohibition of secret commissions is the protection of vulnerable principals and the preservation of the integrity of the agency relationship. A requirement that disclosure of a commission be made by the agent promotes the objective of this section. *Indeed, disclosure is essential to alert the principal to the existence of conflict of interest situations. In the absence of disclosure, the principal has no way of knowing if the agent is truly acting in the principal's best interests and cannot determine whether the advice of the agent should be accepted* [emphasis added].

> See also the contents of footnote 74, following, for an elaboration of the rationale for a fulsome duty of disclosure.

73 In *R. v. Kelly, ibid.* at 190–1, Cory J. states:

> A general and vague disclosure that the agent is receiving commissions will not meet the objective of this section. The agent must disclose the nature of the benefit which is being received, the amount of that benefit calculated to the best of the agent's ability and the source of the benefit. It may not be possible for the agent to be exact as to the amount of commission which will be received. It will suffice if a reasonable effort is made to alert the principal as to the approximate amount and the source of commission to be received. Obviously, the

principal will be influenced by the amount of benefit the agent is receiving. The greater the benefit to the agent, the greater the agent's conflict of interest, and commensurately the greater the risk for the principal. The disclosure must be timely in the sense that the principal must be made aware of the benefit as soon as possible. Certainly the disclosure must be made at the point when the regard may influence the agent in relation to the principal's affairs. It is essential then that the agent clearly disclose to the principal as promptly as possible the source and amount or approximate amount of the benefit.

It is only if the disclosure is both adequate and timely that the agency relationship would be protected. With this knowledge, the principal would then be able to determine whether, and to what extent, to rely upon the advice by the agent. It would be preferable if the disclosure was made in writing.

74 Sheer necessity requires this; otherwise the delivery of medical services would virtually grind to a halt.

75 See *Herdrich* (7th Cir.), *supra* note 8 at 373–4, where the majority acknowledges that dual loyalties of physicians are tolerated under ERISA.

76 See *Shea* v. *Esensten*, 107 F 3d at 628 (8th Cir. 1997), cert. denied, – U.S. –, 118 S.Ct. 297, 139 L.Ed. 2d 229 (1997) and *Ries* v. *Humana Health Plan Inc.*, No. 94 C 6180, 1995 WL 669583 (N.D, Ill. Nov, 8, 1995), referred to by the dissenting judgement in *Herdrich*, *ibid.* at 383. Presumably, the rule in *Reis* would also apply to a situation where physicians have disincentives to provide services.

77 See the following comment made by Dickens, *supra* note 64 at 266–7 and authorities cited by him. He states: "The implication that prior disclosure resolves a conflict of interest is consistent with a number of respected approaches to the issue, but may fail to appreciate how few real options a patient has when disclosure is made."

78 *Ibid.*

79 *Supra* note 29, s. 1104(a)(1).

80 See also *Herdrich* (7th Cir.), *supra* note 8 at 371 where it is stated that an ERISA fiduciary in a permitted conflict of interest "breaches its duty of care ... whenever it acts to benefit its own interests."

81 *Supra* note 45 at 274.

82 Any other rule would render the fiduciary a fiduciary by name only. The duty of loyalty which lies at the heart of fiduciary obligation could hardly be attributed to an individual who is free to pursue self-interest at the expense of a beneficiary. And, though legislation or informed and free consent by a beneficiary can free a fiduciary of the fetter of fiduciary responsibility, elimination of the duty of loyalty leaves the relationship devoid of anything that can even remotely be described as fiduciary. In all likelihood the elimination of fiduciary responsibility requires that the legislature or the beneficiary "plainly and clearly" manifest an intent to this effect.

83 See M. Rachlis and C. Kushner, *Strong Medicine: How to Save Canada's Health Care System* (Toronto: HarperCollins, 1994) at 55, 165–7; *Second Opinion: What's Wrong With Canada's Health Care System and How To Fix It* (Toronto: HarperCollins, 1989) at 131–5. By analogy, see also A. Wazana, "Physicians and the Pharmaceutical Industry" (2000) 283 *JAMA* 373.

84 *Herdrich*, *supra* note 8 at 2149.

85 *Ibid.* at 2157.

86 See J.K. Iglehart, "Revisiting the Canadian Health Care System," (2000) 342 *New Eng. J. Med.* 2007, online at http://www.nejm.org/content/2000/0342/0026/2007.asp. (accessed on 27 November 2000). Iglehart observes that in Canada there has been "a dramatic loss of public confidence in the 1990s as a result of sharp cutbacks in the federal budget." He goes on to state:

> These cutbacks have led to restricted access to specialists, longer waiting times for nonemergency surgery, and the closing or merger of many hospitals, resulting in a loss of beds. The reductions, a central feature of the federal government's successful effort in recent years to eliminate the large annual budget deficit, are now being partially reversed, but the system remains shaken by the decline in public support, reduced morale among physicians and nurses, and increased tension between the federal government in Ottawa and Canada's disparate provinces and territories. ... The federal government began to reduce its contribution to the provincial health insurance plans more than 20 years ago, but the reductions became larger in the 1990s.

See also R. Deber, "Getting What We Pay For: Myths and Realities about Financing Canada's Health Care System," paper prepared for the Dialogue on Health Reform: Sustaining Confidence in Canada's Health Care System, online at http://www.utoronto.ca/hlthadmn/dhr/pdf/atrevised3.pdf. (accessed on 11 April 2000). In particular, see Figure 5 at 17 entitled "Canadian Health Spending in 1992 $ per capita, 1975 to 1999."

87 Trustees are archetypal fiduciaries. They have title to and, ordinarily, manage property belonging to others. In this role they are fiduciaries who must serve the interest of others faithfully and selflessly. See Ellis, *supra* note 26, ch. 2, which focusses on trusteeship. This chapter, interestingly, is entitled "True Fiduciaries."

88 Waters, *supra* note 59 at 716.

89 *Ibid.* at 716–18, 952–4.

90 See the text following for an elaboration of the legislative tolerance of conflict of interest in the health services context. As to the degree to which the common law tolerated conflict of interest arising from remuneration of fiduciaries, see Waters, *ibid.* at 717. Importantly, Waters discusses authority, authority which he describes as somewhat "illogical," for the proposition that trustees are not prohibited from accepting remuneration from third parties. See *Meighen* v. *Buell* (1878), 25 Gr. 604 (C.A.). This is significant in Canada where physicians are primarily paid by the state under provincial health care plans.

91 See *Herdrich* (7th Cir.), *supra* note 8 at 373–4 which acknowledges that dual loyalties of physicians are tolerated under ERISA.

92 See, for example, Alberta's Health Care Insurance Act, R.S.A. 1980, c. A–24, ss. 4 and 7, and Ontario's Health Insurance Act R.S.O., 1990, c. H.6, ss. 17.1(1), 17.1(3) and 17.1(5).

93 See s. 1.1 of the Amendments to Bill 11, s. 5(2) of the Health Care Protection Act, *supra* note 5 which provides that "[n]o person shall charge or collect a rate for enhanced medical goods or services that is greater than cost plus a reasonable allowance for administration."

94 This form of conflict of interest is difficult to detect and enforce because there are an infinite variety of ways, some of which are very subtle, for both corporations and physicians to circumvent bans against conflict of interest (Rodwin, *supra* note 1, particularly at 94–6). As well, avoidance tactics are constantly metamorphasizing

(Rodwin, *supra* note 1, particularly at 96). Moreover, avoidance behaviour is aided and abetted by the specificity of conflict of interest guidelines promulgated by the very persons whom it is sought to regulate. I am not alone in suggesting that it is a mistake for these guidelines to focus on "the specific organizational form" of conflict-of-interest behaviour and not the "general problem" (Rodwin, *supra* note 1, particularly at 96). The College of Physicians and Surgeons of Alberta Conflict of Interest Guidelines, *supra* note 24, do not contain a general prohibition on the practice of conflict of interest. Rather, specific practices, some set out in rather broad language, are prohibited. These include self-referral, seeking or receiving benefits from a third-party referral to a facility in which a registered practitioner holds an interest, investment by a practitioner in a treatment and/or diagnostic facility and sale by a registered practitioner of medical or health care products. It does not appear that any of these guidelines would prohibit the investment in securities in medical equipment or pharmaceutical companies. Though it is true that in respect of large publicly held companies the actions of a single practitioner cannot realistically affect share price, the situation is otherwise with respect to "small cap" companies which are attempting to break into a market. The announcement that a single piece of equipment has been sold to a reputable hospital or facility can cause shares in a company to go up considerably. Moreover, the language in the Alberta guidelines does not clearly prohibit physician conduct which can benefit spouses, close relatives or friends, though it is possible that in some circumstances the prohibition on seeking or receiving benefits from a third party could catch this form of conduct. Moreover, under rule 5 of the guidelines, physicians may earn money by selling medical or health care products to their patients in the form of "a reasonable handling cost."

95 *Supra* note 8.

96 *Ibid.*

97 Much has been written on the *Herdrich* case. See, for example, R.J. Herrington, "*Herdrich* v. *Pegram*: ERISA Fiduciary Liability and Physician Incentives to Deny Care" (2000) 71 *U. Colo. L. Rev.* 715; C.M. Hedgeman, "The Rationing of Medicine: *Herdrich* v. *Pegram*" (2000) 10 *Albany L.J. Sci & Tech.* 305; D.H. Johnson, "ERISA Fiduciary Duty Claim and Managed Care Liability: Implications of *Herdrich* v. *Pegram*" (1999) 11 *Health Lawyer* 1; S.L. Burke, "Suing HMOs: State Your Case (*Pegram* v. *Herdrich*: state suits)" (2000) 16 *New Jersey L.J* 17 pS–9; E.H. Morreim, "Confusion In The Courts: Managed Care Financial Structures and Their Impact On Medical Care" (2000) 35 *Tort & Ins. L.J.* 699; D.T. Bogan, "Protecting Patient Rights Despite ERISA: Will The Supreme Court Allow States To Regulate Managed Care?" (2000) 74 *Tul. L. Rev.* 951.

98 *Herdrich* (7th Cir.), *supra* note 8 at 381, Flaum J. (in dissent). The majority, at 379, describes year-end bonuses as being "relatively substantial."

99 *Ibid.* at 381 per Flaum J.

100 *Ibid.* at 373.

101 *Ibid.* What is ambiguous in this statement is the precise level to which incentives must rise before they are regarded as evidencing a breach. Moreover, it is not at all clear how this statement counters Justice Flaum's assertion that the mere existence of an asserted conflict is not a legal wrong, presumably irrespective of the level of the conflict which is asserted.

102 *Ibid.* at 383.

103 Clearly, the opinion of the majority, Wood, Jr. and Coffey JJ. proceed under the assumption that, given Herdrich's symptoms, ultrasound should have been

"administered with all speed...." *Ibid.* at 374. The lower court's findings of negligence also support this conclusion.

104 *Ibid.* at 371, Coffey J. for the majority. Pulling no punches, at 372 Coffey J. firmly states: "With a jaundiced eye focussed firmly on year-end bonuses, it is not unrealistic to assume that the doctors rendering care under the Plan were swayed to be most frugal when exercising their discretionary authority...."

105 *Ibid.* at 380 where Coffey J. states: "The ultimate determination of whether the defendants violated their fiduciary obligations ... must be left to the trial court."

106 In *Herdrich, ibid.*, the issue was whether the complainant's pleadings, assuming the allegations in them are proven, reveal a cause of action. This kind of procedure is called a demurrer and is designed to terminate unworthy lawsuits in their early stages.

107 On the difficulty of detecting and proving a breach of fiduciary duty, see Cooter and Freedman, "The Fiduciary Relationship: Its Economic Character and Legal Consequences" (1991) 66 *N.Y.U.L. Rev.* 1045, quoted, seemingly, with approval by McLachlin J. in her minority judgement in *Canson, supra* note 38 at 544.

108 In succession law, suspicious circumstances that a will does not express the intent of the will-maker gives rise to presumption that the will-maker did not know and understand of the contents of the will. See the classic case of *Barry* v. *Butlin* (1838), 2 Moo. P.C. 480, 12 E.R. 1089 (J.C.P.C.). See also *Eady* v. *Waring* (1974), 2 O.R. (2d) 627, 43 D.L.R. (3d) 667 (C.A.).

109 *Supra* note 8 at 2149. He also states at 2149:

> In this case, one could argue that Pegram's decision to wait before getting an ultrasound for Herdrich, and her insistence that the ultrasound be done at a distant facility owned by Carle, reflected an interest in limiting the HMO's expenses, which blinded her to the need for immediate diagnosis and treatment.

110 *Ibid.* at 2148.

111 For an elaboration of the concept of "mixed eligibility decisions" see *Herdrich, ibid.* at 2154–5. As to the conclusion that mixed eligibility decisions are not fiduciary decisions, see *Herdrich, ibid.* at 2155–6.

112 Referring to the complainant in *Herdrich, ibid.* Souter J. states at 2156, "Since the provision for profit is what makes the HMO a proprietary organization, her remedy in effect would be nothing less than elimination of the for-profit HMO."

113 *Ibid.* at 2156. For a critical analysis of this suggestion, see text below in Part III, "Implications of the Herdrich Analysis for Canada."

114 *Ibid.* at 2158.

115 *Ibid.*

116 *Ibid.*

117 *Ibid.* at 2155. Souter J. regards Herdrich's theory as incompatible with the survival of HMO's, *ibid.* at 2156. At 2156 he underscores Congress's commitment to HMOs by observing that Congress has promoted the formation and operation of HMOs, including for-profit HMOs, for twenty-seven years.

118 *Ibid.* at 2156.

119 *Ibid.* at 2155.

120 *Ibid.* at 2155. Trustees are, of course, archetypal fiduciaries, see *supra* note 88.

121 For a thoughtful and comprehensive discussion of the nature and implications of mixed medical and economic decisions, including those made by HMOs, see E.H. Morreim, *Balancing Act: The New Medical Ethics of Medicine's New Economics* (Washington, D.C.: Georgetown University Press, 1995).

122 *Supra* note 8 at paras. 34–6.

123 For the US position, see *Varity Corp. v. Howe*, 516 U.S. 489, 496–97, 116 S.Ct. 1065 134, L.Ed. 2d 130 (1966), cited by Faulk J. in his dissent in *Herdrich, supra* note 8 at 381, in support of the proposition that "the common law of trusts ... is merely the baseline for determining the scope of fiduciary duty under ERISA." In Canada, the extent to which nontrust fiduciaries ought to be regulated by trust law principles is controversial. See the majority and minority judgements in *Canson, supra* note 38 for divergent views on this issue. At this point it seems fair to suggest that courts are both willing to embrace trust law analogies (see *Guerin, supra* note 16 at 360 and to depart therefrom in favour of tort law analogies (see La Forest J.'s majority judgement in *Canson, supra* note 38 at 585–7).

124 This certainly is the Canadian position: *Canson, ibid.*

125 *Supra* note 8 at 2151 where Souter J. states that the "fiduciary function addressed by Herdrich's ERISA count ... [is] the exercise of 'discretionary authority or discretionary responsibility in the administration of [an ERISA] plan'." In Canada it has been recognized that the "hallmark of a fiduciary relationship is that ... one party is at the mercy of the other's discretion." See E. Weinrib, "The Fiduciary Obligation" (1975) 25 *U.T.L.J.* 1 at 7, quoted in *Guerin, supra* note 16 at 384.

126 *Herdrich, supra* note 8 at 2151.

127 See text below and also, for a contemporary approach to this issue, see *Terra Energy Ltd. v. Kilborn Engineering Alberta Ltd.*, (1997) 198 A.R. 245 at 278, where Cairns J. states that "[t]he scope of the fiduciary obligation is determined by examining the nature of the fiduciary undertaking."

128 29 U.S.C. s. 1104(a)(1).

129 *Supra* note 8. This point is not made explicitly, but underlies much of Souter J's commentary. See especially 2156 where Souter J. states that "the provision for profit is what makes the HMO a proprietary organization. ...."

130 *Ibid.* at 2149.

131 *Ibid.*

132 *Ibid.* at 2150.

133 *Ibid.*

134 *Ibid.* Again, this point is largely implicit, but see particularly 2156–7.

135 *Ibid.* at 2157.

136 *Herdrich, supra* note 118.

137 *Herdrich, supra* note 8 at 2156.

138 It is trite law that in a proceeding to strike out a statement of claim on the grounds that it does not reveal a cause of action "the complaint should ... be construed generously. ..." See *Herdrich, ibid.* at 2155 footnote 10. See also the decision of the Federal Court of Appeal (7th Cir.), *supra* note 8 at 372 where Coffey J. states: "[W]e are obligated to view complaints in the light most favorable to the nonmoving party...."

139 *Herdrich, supra* note 8 at 2156.

140 *Ibid.* at 2156–7.

141 *Supra* note 129, s. 1104(a)(1), quoted by Souter J., *supra* note 8 at 2151, and above in text at part I.A. "The Fiduciary Status of Health Service Providers."

142 *Supra* note 82 and accompanying text.

143 *Supra* note 8 at 2157, where Souter J. states:

> After all, HMOs came into being because some groups of physicians consistently provided more aggressive treatment than others in similar circumstances, with results not perceived as justified by the marginal expense and risk associated with intervention....

144 *Ibid.* at 2157.

145 Insurers who make eligibility or coverage decisions must do so in good faith and, hence, have fiduciary-like obligations: *supra* note 30.

146 *Supra* note 8 at 2158.

147 *Ibid.* at 2158 and in text above at part I.B. "The Nature of Fiduciary Duty and Breach of Fiduciary Duty." Souter J. concedes that some states do not permit malpractice claims against HMOs and also that in some cases HMOs have deeper pockets than physicians. He also acknowledges that fiduciary claims if successful, presumably unlike malpractice claims, permit complainants to seek reimbursement for attorney fees.

148 *Ibid.* at 2158.

149 See text above at part I.B. "The Nature of Fiduciary Duty and Breach of Fiduciary Duty," and related footnotes.

150 McLachlin J. makes this point both in *Canson, supra* note 38 at 543 and in *Norberg* v. *Wynrib, supra* note 9 at 268–9. In the latter case at 274 she states:

> The fiduciary relationship has trust, not self-interest, at its core, and when breach occurs, the balance favours the person wronged. The freedom of the fiduciary is limited by the obligation he or she has undertaken—an obligation which "betokens loyalty, good faith and avoidance of a conflict of duty and self-interest": Canadian Aero Service Ltd. v. O'Malley, [1974] S.C.R. 592, at 606. To cast a fiduciary relationship in terms of contract or tort (whether negligence or battery) is to diminish this obligation. If a fiduciary relationship is shown to exist, then the proper legal analysis is one based squarely on the full and fair consequences of a breach of that relationship.

151 While it is true that the Crown's fiduciary duty to First Nations under s. 35 of the Constitution Act, 1982 is tempered by its obligations to the larger Canadian polity (See *R.* v. *Sparrow* [1990] 1 S.C.R. 1075), the Crown's private law fiduciary obligations are not diluted by its political, social and economic duties to Canadians at large. See *Guerin, supra* note 16 where the Supreme Court of Canada holds the Crown liable for breach of its private law fiduciary obligations to the Musqueam First Nation. See also *Authorson* v. *Canada* [2000] O.J. No. 4779 (S.C.T.D.), where the Crown is held to be a fiduciary in respect of its obligation to administer certain pensions and allowances for war veterans.

152 See *Herdrich*, supra note 8 at footnote 11 in the judgement.

153 For academic commentary, see Caulfield and Ginn, *supra* note 5.

154 8 Cal. Rptr. 661 at 672 (Cal. App. 1986), aff'd 741 P. 2d 613 (Cal. S.C. 1987).

155 (1994), 21 C.C.L.T. (2d) 228 (B.C.S.C.), aff'd [1996] 4 W.W.R. 672 (B.C.C.A.).

156 *Ibid.* at 240.

157 (1994), 363 A.P.R. 271 (T.D.). The Court expressed the following opinion at 289:

> The question is one of the cost effectiveness of precautions which

could have been taken. It was allegedly too costly in 1987 to do a CT scan on all head-injured patients. I was not, however, provided any evidence to establish that the cost would be prohibitive to scan not all, but just patients whose skulls had considerable force applied and who had a resulting skull fracture.

158 L. Gostin, "Managed Care, Conflicts of Interest, and Quality" (2000) 30 *Hastings Center Rep.* 27 at 28 where he states:

> There is nothing inherently wrong (and much that is right) in taking cost as well as quality into account when allocating medical resources and care. Reduced cost will enable more people to have access to health care and will free more resources to benefit larger populations.

159 Even when a financially driven decision to withhold medical services is justified, that which is being withheld and the reasons for the withholding, as well as the alternatives open to the patient, must be communicated.

160 It can be argued that the State has a constitutional obligation to put its resources at the disposal of health care providers for the provision of medical services. Though there is some division of opinion about this matter, the preponderance of scholarly opinion is that there is no right to health care. See, for example, Canadian Bar Association Task Force, *What's Law Got To Do With It? Health Reform in Canada* (Ottawa: Canadian Bar Association, 1994) at 26. See also M. Jackman, "The Regulation of Private Health Care Under the Canada Health Act and the Canadian Charter" (1995) 6 *Constitutional Forum* 54 at 56–8.

161 The Courts have recognized that departure from the literal strictures of the evenhand principle is justifiable in some circumstances. See *In Re Baden's Deed Trusts*, [1970] 2 W.L.R. 1110 at 1127 (H.L).

162 *Supra* note 16 at 425.

163 *Supra* note 45.

164 *Ibid.* at 275.

165 *Supra* note 38.

166 *Ibid.* at 589.

167 *Ibid.* at 544 adopted by McLachlin J. from the judgement of Lord Dunedin in *Nocton v. Lord Ashburton* [1914] A.C. 932 at 936.

168 The pulse of the Court on this issue is difficult to gauge. The *Canson* Court was deeply divided; its majority ruling was rendered by less than an absolute majority of the nine judges which compose the Supreme Court of Canada and the composition of the Court has been altered significantly with the addition of six new judges since the *Canson* case was decided. Iacobucci, Major, Bastarache, Binnie, Arbour and LeBel JJ. are "new." Moreover, even the majority agreed that some traditional principles of fiduciary law which expand recovery beyond that which is possible in tort law should be maintained, namely the rule that recovery is not limited by the principle of reasonable forseeability: *Canson, supra* note 38 at 545, per McLachlin J. commenting on the views of La Forest J.

169 *Ibid.* at 581.

170 See the reverse onus rule, *supra* note 41 and the text above at part I.B. "The Nature of Fiduciary Duty and Breach of Fiduciary Duty." Absent the constraints of the principle of reasonable forseeability, awards can be larger.

171 If, of course, that era materializes.

4

MOVING MEDICARE HOME
THE FORCES SHIFTING CARE
OUT OF HOSPITALS AND INTO HOMES

COLLEEN M. FLOOD

ome care has recently become a significant policy issue in Canada and many other developed countries.[1] In Canada's medical care system (Medicare) rich and poor alike are equally entitled to hospital and physician services on the basis of need, as opposed to ability to pay.[2] By contrast, in the social services system, services are generally targeted at people whose earnings put them below a certain income level. The shift from caring in hospitals and institutions to home care poses a significant policy challenge in Canada since home care straddles the divide between the medical care system and the social services system. The current structure of the system means that the shift to home care has resulted in a significant passive privatization of Canada's health care system. In other words, care that was once fully publicly funded in a hospital is, when delivered in the home, much more likely to be paid for privately or delivered by unpaid family members.

This paper focusses on the factors that have fuelled and are fuelling the recent and rapid shift from the provision of care in hospitals and institutions to home care. The goal is to analyze which members of society will bear the costs of this shift and to explain why the distribution of these costs has not been given sufficient weight in policymaking. Unpacking the larger forces causing the shift to home care will help Canadian citizens better understand why this shift is occurring and its likely impact on their lives. Having this information should also assist in the critical analysis of different home care policies.

There are six sections to this chapter. The first section describes the hospital closures that have occurred in Canada. The second section outlines the forces contributing to the process of hospital closures and the shift to home care. In particular, this section focusses on how an economic analysis of health care markets and a "determinants of health" approach has fuelled the shift from caring in institutions to caring in the home. The third section describes the public/private mix of funding for home care services. The fourth section tackles the issue of what is encompassed by the phrase "home care." The fifth section of this paper discusses the distributional implications of the shift to home care, which members of society will bear increased costs as a result, and why the distribution of these costs has not been given sufficient weight. Finally, this chapter concludes with some thoughts on advocacy for an equitable and efficient home care program.

Description of Hospital Closures

The shift from caring in institutions to caring in the home is occurring throughout Canada and, indeed, in most other developed countries. The proportion of total health care spending on hospitals has declined in the last twenty years from 42.5 percent in 1979 to (an estimated) 31.6 percent in 1999.[3] In terms of bricks and mortar, between 1986–87 and 1994–95 the number of public hospitals declined by 14 percent while the number of hospital beds declined by 11 percent.[4] The ratio of inpatient beds per 1,000 people declined from 6.2 in 1990 to 4.7 in 1997, the latter being much lower than the Organization for Economic Cooperation and Development (OECD) average of 7.4 beds.[5] More recently, the Canadian Institute for Health Information in its 2001 report, noted that over the last five years, more than 275 hospitals have been closed, merged, or converted to other types of care facilities.[6] In terms of actual consumption of hospital services, the rate at which Canadians were hospitalized reached an all-time low in 1997, with a discharge rate of 9,827.9 per 100,000 population, well below the peak of 16,802 in 1973.[7] Also, the average length of stay in a short-term hospital unit declined from 9.05 bed days in 1991–92 to 8.4 bed days in 1997.[8]

Despite the significant closures that have occurred, the process is still on-going. Ontario's Health Services Restructuring Commission (HSRC) (1996–2000) recommended the closure of thirty-one public hospitals, six private and six provincial psychiatric hospital sites.[9] In tandem with these recommendations, HSRC made recommendations for further public investment into home care and reform of primary care. More recently, in April 2001, the Fyke Commission on Medicare in Saskatchewan recommended that "dozens of small hospitals" be consolidated with six or seven "regional" hospitals into ten to fourteen "regional hospitals" and that "community care centres" replace hospitals in twenty-five to thirty communities.[10] These recommendations for hospital closures are premised on sweeping system reform and, in particular, a movement away from the solo fee-for-service model for physician practice and reimbursement.

In terms of sound health policy, it is difficult to quibble with the recommendations of either the HSRC or the Fyke Commission. There are safety gains associated with concentrating specialized surgical services into larger centres where higher volumes of the surgeries can be performed. The hospital closures in Ontario, however, preceded any fundamental reform of primary care or significant reinvestments in home care. The results have been saturation and chaos in emergency wards, with hospitals refusing to receive ambulances because of overcrowding. At least part of the problem seems to be that people are remaining in hospitals because of the absence of formal home care programs or a lack of nursing home beds and/or coordination between the hospital and home care providers and nursing homes.[11] People are also concerned about the burden being placed on patients and their families as patients are sent home from hospital while still needing various forms of medical care.

Public support for hospitals slated for closure or merger with others has been organized. In a series of cases in Ontario, hospitals such as Women's College Hospital challenged the HSRC's orders. To date, all these actions have been without success. In one case the court noted:[12]

> The court's role is very limited in these cases. The court has no power to inquire in the rights and wrongs of hospital restructuring laws or policies, the wisdom or folly of decisions to close particular hospitals, or decisions to direct particular hospital governance structures ...The only role of the court is to decide whether the Commission acted according to law in arriving at its decision.

While litigation has not been successful, political lobbying did force the HSRC to rethink its decision to close the francophone Montfort Hospital.[13] In general, however, there has been little resistance to the deinstitutionalization juggernaut. This lack of real resistance is in of itself an interesting phenomenon. Given widespread public concern and media coverage of hospital closures and growing waiting lists, this lack of resistance speaks to the strength of the forces that have converged to cause the shift from hospital to home care.

The Factors Fuelling Hospital Closures

There are at least five identifiable factors that underlie why hospitals are being closed and care shifted into the home. These factors, discussed further below, are developments in technology, changing demographics, an economic analysis of health insurance and health care service markets, government desire to reduce growth in public spending on health care and a shift to what is known as the "determinants of health" approach. In temporal terms, it is not apparent which factor, if any, arose first nor is it possible to say that each factor is wholly independent of the other four. What is clear, however, is that these factors have converged to create a very strong force to shift care away from hospitals and other institutions and into the home.

Technology

Technology has played an important role in the shift from hospital to home care. Advances in surgical techniques, combined with new and improved drugs, have enabled patients to recover faster than ever from surgical procedures and be in less need of intensive medical care in the recovery process. Examples include the use of computers to aid in surgery,[14] laparoscopy,[15] endoscopic surgery[16] and the use of new drugs and devices. New technologies have made it possible for home-based patients to receive treatments that previously required hospitalization. These include insulin pens, portable infusion pumps,[17] portable and stationary oxygen systems, and mechanical ventilators.[18] Advances in telecommunications technology have enabled the supply of various medical services at a distance[19] thus indirectly enabling further centralization of service providers into large hospitals in urban centres.

Advances in technology, however, also contribute to increased pressure on hospital budgets as new interventions, sometimes of questionable marginal benefit, are developed and introduced into the system. Often it seems that technology results in increased costs rather than savings. A survey of 50 leading US health economists in 1995 found that 82 percent agreed with the statement: "The primary reason for the increase in the health sector's share of GDP over the past thirty years is technological change in medicine."[20] Technology increases rather than lowering costs because technology is often developed with a view to improving quality of care or meeting new or previously unsatisfied health needs and not with a view to achieving the same outcome more cost effectively.[21]

Changing Demographics

The aging of the population is a factor bringing pressure to bear on the health care system and the shift to home care. This pressure is likely to continue for at least the next forty years as baby boomers age. In 1980, 9.4 percent of the population was aged over 65.[22] By 1998, 12.3 percent of the population was over 65, and this figure is estimated to reach 16 percent by 2016, 19 percent by 2020 and 22.6 percent by 2041.[23] Within the over-65 age group, the sharpest increase will be seen in the over-85 age group, which comprised 1.0 percent of the population in 1995 but which is projected to increase to 4.0 percent of the population by 2041.[24]

As the population greys, there will be an increasing proportion of people in transition from functional independence to functional dependence and in need of both medical and social services. This demographic trend will result in increasing pressure for more home care services. However, it is important to acknowledge that the magnitude of this pressure does not necessarily reflect a demand for home care rather than care in hospitals or other institutions. The received wisdom is that the elderly and others prefer to receive medical services and care in the home rather than in institutions.[25] *Prima facie*, this seems a reasonable assumption but closer examination reveals its limitations. A preference for care in the home as opposed to a hospital or other institution itself rests on the assumption that the quality of care will not be unacceptably diminished.

Clearly, the substitution of skilled health care professionals with untrained home care workers or family members must at least raise the question of the quality of resultant care. The prospects and costs of monitoring the quality of care delivered is diminished when care is shifted from a large institution into patients' homes. Home care patients may feel unable to voice complaints about the quality of care delivered by family members and may feel they are being a burden on their family or feel embarrassed that family members or friends are having to attend to their medical or personal care. Issues also arise as to liability for injury as a result of a family caregiver's negligence. Moreover, for some Canadians home may not be a warm, inviting, peaceful haven. Home may in fact be characterized by stress, overcrowding, a lack of proper heating, lack of adequate food, poverty,[26] loneliness[27] or even abuse.[28] So, while in the abstract most people would speak to the advantages of home care, this positive endorsement depends on a number of assumptions that may not hold in practice.

Presently there is very little evidence with regard to the quality of care received in institutions as opposed to the quality of care received in a home, whether formal services or supplied by family members. Research carried out has focussed on recovery times and the need for readmission as key outcome measures.[29] It is notoriously difficult, however, to measure the effectiveness of health care. Simply focussing on outcome measurements such as admission and readmission rates, mortality and morbidity misses significant aspects of quality that most people would consider important. These include minimization of pain and discomfort, caring kinds of health care services, respect for ones wishes and personal dignity.

Health Economics

An important factor that has fuelled hospital closures and the shift to home care is the impact of health economics. An economic approach is essential in order to design an efficient health care system. But there are problems if economy analysis is relied upon too heavily. As I discuss below, given its underlying utilitarian philosophy, economic analysis favours policies that maximize overall (population) health but is often not sensitive to the distribution of costs and benefits between citizens.

An economic analysis reveals two major problems with health insurance and health care service systems: moral hazard and information asymmetry.[30] Moral hazard is said to arise when an insured patient, after becoming ill, uses more health care than he or she would without insurance. Moral hazard occurs in private and public insurance systems—it doesn't matter where the insurance comes from. Insurance allows patients to not worry about the cost of care when they need it.[31] The other source of inefficiency in health care markets is what economists describe as an information asymmetry. What this means is that, in general, doctors know more than their patient about what is wrong with the patient and what health services will benefit the patient. Patients rely on doctors to tell them not only what is wrong with them (diagnosis) but also what is needed to fix the problem (treatment). So, although moral hazard is a problem, as discussed above, it is really a problem about doctor decisionmaking to the extent that patients rely on doctors to make decisions relating to their health. This leads to a phenomenon called "supplier-induced demand." This occurs when doctors, although facing fee restrictions, provide more services to patients in order to maintain their incomes.[32] Whether or not doctors do actually create demand for their own services is a matter of debate. But the most important issue is not whether doctors induce demand for their own services but that doctors have had little or no incentive to take into account the cost of things they prescribe or recommend.[33] While doctors are the gatekeepers to the rest of the system, historically they have not had to weigh the costs and benefits of their decisions. In fact, economists contend, many treatments recommended by doctors are of only marginal benefit or, indeed, ineffective.

Stoddart et al. note that the estimates of the cost of doctor-generated inappropriate use of health care services vary but are sometimes as large as 30 to 40 percent of all services, including hospital services and drugs.[34] Within Canada, variations between and within provinces with respect to the utilization of health care services that do not appear justified on the basis of differing health needs provide evidence for economists' arguments.[35] There are, for example, significant variations in the number of hysterectomies performed and no underlying objective clinical reason why there should be such wide variations.[36]

Alan Maynard is a well-known British health economist who often is invited to speak at Canadian health economics and policy conferences. He sums up what many health economists see as problems in health care systems:[37]

Due to third party payers, moral hazard and the reluctance of policy makers to design appropriate incentive structures to manipulate the behaviour of practitioners in efficiency and cost containing ways, physicians have been able to enhance demand for their services ... Government and insurers have been uncritical of the basis of this increased demand for health care. The rhetoric of "everything must be done for all patients" and "if it works, the intervention must be used" has been accepted uncritically in part because of the brilliant advocacy of provider agents and in part because of the ignorance of policy makers and society.

Thus, many health economists view the fact that doctors are not very sensitive to the cost of the varying services and treatments they supply or recommend as a key cause of cost escalation in health care systems. They emphasize that increased health care spending is not having a commensurate or, in some cases, any impact on health status.[38] They go on to argue that physicians resist having resources diverted away from the health care system to other areas (such as education, income support and tax reduction) as all money spent on the health care system, in one way or another, becomes income for physicians and other health care providers. They go on to conclude that, irrespective of real health needs, the more doctors and health care professionals there are in a system, the greater the total cost. Similarly, the more hospital beds, nursing staff and technology, the greater total costs. This is irrespective of real need since beds, staff and technology are simply resources used by physicians to supply more profitable services. Economists have advocated reductions in health care spending by cutting the number of hospital beds and cutting patients' length of stay in hospital, claiming that such reductions will not adversely impact on Canadians' "health."[39]

I have three criticisms to make of the assumption that cuts can be made to health care budgets without adversely affecting Canadians' health. First, focussing on health outcomes alone misses many aspects of the quality of care that people are concerned about. The difficulty is that health outcomes can presently only be measured by relatively crude outcome measures like mortality rates and morbidity rates. Relying on existing outcome measures alone fails to address what many consider important aspects of quality of care, including how long a patient is left in distress or in pain without assistance, how quickly a diagnosis and treatment is given so as to relieve anxiety and whether a patient is treated with dignity and respect and her or his wishes respected. Reliance on existing outcome measures means that the provision of "caring" services such as nursing, for which the quality and impact thereof are often difficult to measure, are seriously discounted by economists.[40] As a striking example of the economic perspective in this regard, Evans and Stoddart note:[41]

> Providers of care, particularly nurses, often emphasize their caring functions. The point here is not at all that caring is without importance or value, but rather that it is by no means the exclusive preserve of providers of health care. Furthermore, the "social contract" by which members of a particular community undertake collective (financial) responsibility for each other's health narrowly defined does not necessarily extend to responsibility for their happiness. "Caring" independently of any contemplated "curing" or at least prevention of deterioration, represents an extension of the "product line"—and sale revenue—of the health care system. If collective buyers of these services, public or private, have never in fact agreed to this extension, its ethical basis is rather shaky.

By contrast, philosophers and scholars in other disciplines do, however, argue that the priority of a health care system should, in fact, be caring rather than curing. Daniel Callahan writes:[42]

> Since medicine is a finite science and cures will eventually be ineffective, each person will, at some point, need caring. Therefore, the health care system's first premise should be that no one be abandoned, particularly those whom medicine cannot cure ...The highest priority should be that of care, displacing our present priorities in which cure is given the place of pride.

The second critique of the argument that health care resources can be cut without adversely affecting health is that this argument assumes that physicians, when faced with limited resources, will allocate resources optimally. However, physicians often lack good information about the cost-effectiveness and even effectiveness of many interventions. The Canadian "nonsystem" of solo fee-for-service practice also does not provide doctors with any incentive to prioritize different health care needs or factor cost into their treatment recommendations. In the face of restricted resources, rather than changing the way they practice medicine, doctors may find it easier to simply transfer costs to others through longer waiting times and lists. To be fair, most health economists recommend fundamental reform of the health care system, in particular primary care reform and a shift away from solo fee-for-service practice by doctors, in addition to hospital closures and consolidation. But the political economy has meant that while the economic analysis underpinning recommendations regarding hospital closures and consolidations are accepted and acted upon, the other, more difficult reform proposals are much more slowly, if ever, acted upon.

The third and final critique I have of the argument that health care resources can be cut without adversely affecting health is the assumption that the system should be oriented towards maximization of "health." This perspective speaks to the utilitarian philosophy that underlies economics. Although improving the overall health of the population (to the extent this can be measured) is undoubtedly important, the primary reason justifying government intervention in health care markets is an egalitarian one. In other words, the arguments in justice for government intervention in health care markets is that everyone should be entitled to *fair* share of health[43] or, as the next best proxy, health care services.[44] One can see the limitations of pursuing only the maximization of health of the population when considering the position of the dying, the disabled and the chronically ill. For these vulnerable populations, the provision of additional health care services may do little if anything to add to the population's "health."

The Determinants of Health

The focus on "health" outcomes rather than health care services supplied by physicians and the shift from institutional care to home and community care has also been supported by groups keen to see a shift away from the purely "medical model" to a more integrated, holistic approach. It has also converged with the rise in what is known as the "determinants of health literature."[45] Essentially, this literature argues that there are many other factors that contribute to health aside from the consumption of medical services, including nutrition, employment, socio-economic status, marital status and position at work. If the goal is the maximization of health, it may be better to transfer some of the spending resources for expensive hospital services to these other areas.

The difficulty with the determinants of health approach is that just as there is a paucity of evidence demonstrating the ultimate impact on health of curative health care services, so too is there a paucity of evidence about the impact of preventative measures. If the standard for public funding is conclusive evidence of an impact on health outcomes, then this justifies significant cuts to spending on the health care system without the transfer of savings to other areas of social spending. Yet the difficulties inherent in measuring the quality of health care are well documented.[46] The lack of evidence does not mean that health care services do not have an impact on health but that it is difficult to conclusively establish the magnitude of this effect. This suggests the need for further investment in monitoring and measuring the impact on health of various health care services, rather than retrenchment of health care spending in general.

Public Spending Retrenchment

In the 1990s, the views of health economists and advocates on the determinants of health approach dovetailed with the desire of governments (in many countries) to constrain the level of public spending on health care on fiscal and sometimes ideological grounds. In Canada throughout the 1990s, the key health reform initiative was to reduce the flow of resources into the system. The unstated assumption was that physicians and other health care providers, faced with limited resources, will direct resources to the greatest need and eliminate inefficiency and waste. Provincial governments focussed their cost-cutting efforts upon hospitals for two reasons. First, hospitals comprise the largest components of health care spending. Second, provincial government have significant control over hospital budgets compared to budgets for physicians (who are paid on a fee-for-service basis and, to some extent, can simply provide more services in response to fee reductions) and for drugs (where is there is a significant amount of private spending).

From the mid 1980s to the mid 1990s, Canada successfully pursued a policy of reducing growth in health care spending. Real total health care spending fell from $1,819.19 per capita in 1992 to $1,765.74 per capita in 1996.[47] The total spent on health care services as a percentage of GDP fell from 10.0 percent in 1992 to 9.2 percent in 1996.[48] Compared to other OECD countries, there was a sharp decline in Canada's public share of total health spending. Real per capita public spending began to decline in 1993 and continued to decline until 1997.[49] In 1990, Canadian public health expenditures per capita were 34 percent above the OECD mean; in 1997 Canada's public expenditures exceeded the OECD mean by 20 percent. However, the pace of spending has picked up again and the Canadian Institute for Health Information projects 4.4 percent and 4.8 percent increases in public sector spending for 1999 and 2000 respectively, adjusting for inflation and population growth.[50]

Cost-cutting and improving efficiency are often assumed to be one and the same. It is very important to make the simple but often overlooked point that cutting government spending is not the same as improving efficiency. Efficiency, from an economic perspective, takes into account all costs, wherever incurred in the public and private sector. Thus, cutting government spending will not be efficient if the result is that costs are simply shifted to the private sector. Despite the strong push towards moving care out of hospitals and into the home, there has been little evaluation of the cost-effectiveness of the delivery of different health care services in the home, whether provided by unpaid family members or by paid professionals. It is often simply assumed to be cost-effective because care by family members is "free." However, a true economic analysis would consider all the costs associated with shifting care away from institutions and into homes.

Some of the costs of the shift to home care were identified (although not quantified) in a study released in March 1997 by researchers in Alberta. They created a taxonomy of the hidden costs of informal elder care in the home which included emotional costs, physical and social well-being costs, labour costs, loss of employment opportunities, out-of-pocket costs for the caregiver, costs for the caregiver's employer arising from employees "accommodating their paid employment to their caregiving demands" (absenteeism, lower productivity) and costs associated with the "development and administration of family-friendly employee benefits."[51]

A report released in March 1998 by Saskatchewan's Health Care Services Utilization and Review Commission found that providing patients with home care where appropriate, instead of keeping them in the hospital, would save between $150 and $230 per day.[52] This research attempted to identify broader economic costs such as unpaid caregiver time but did so using as a proxy the hourly cost of hiring private home care services (estimated to be $15.00 per hour). The study did not quantify the *actual* employment costs of caregivers reducing their hours of work or giving up employment, foregone employment opportunities, foregone tax revenues, costs to employers or accommodating employees who need to engage in informal caregiving and costs associated with absenteeism, missed overtime, re-hiring and re-training. The unstated assumptions of this report are then that caregivers will rationally choose between giving up their own time and contracting out to private home care providers and that adequately trained home care providers are available in the private sector.

The Public/Private Mix
of Spending on Home Care

In conjunction with the closure of hospitals and reduction in hospital beds is an increasing emphasis on home care; however, it still comprises a relatively small component of total health care spending. Across Canada, on average, the percentage of total health care spending devoted to home care increased from 2.3 percent in 1990–91 to just under 4.0 percent in 1997–98.[53] Peter Coyte reports that, over the last decade, home care spending increased at a rate four times greater than other health care spending (9.0 percent vs. 2.2 percent).[54]

Although government spending on home care has, on average, nearly doubled in recent years as a percentage of total spending, the investments made in home care still pale in comparison to spending on hospitals. In 1996, 34.4 percent of total health care spending was on acute care. By 1999, this had fallen to 31.6 percent.[55] More importantly, increased government spending on home care does not reflect the magnitude of the cuts made to hospital spending. Between 1993 and 1996, total spending on hospital care fell by $1,205 million[56]

(I use the figures for total spending as there is very little private spending on hospital care in Canada because of prohibitions contained in the Canada Health Act). By comparison, between 1992–93 and 1995–96 public spending on home care only increased by $452.8 million.[57]

Canada does not have a national home care program, even though the National Forum on Health in 1997 recommended one be established.[58] Subsequently, the federal government promised in its "Red Book" to put in place a national home care program and a Pharmacare program. Towards this end, in 1998 the federal government hosted a national conference in Halifax with a view to formulating a national home care policy. Progress towards a national home care program has stalled, however, as the provinces have been very resistant to another cost-sharing national program. This is not surprising given that the federal government significantly reduced its financial contributions to the provinces for Medicare (covering hospital and physician services), while still expecting the provinces to maintain national standards as set out in the Canada Health Act.

Although Canada has no national home care program, all provinces and territories have some kind of publicly funded home care program. But across the country there are wide variations in terms of how home care quality is regulated[59] and what similarly situated patients are entitled to in terms of service delivery. There are significant differences across the country in terms of the percentage of total public health spending devoted to home care. In 1997–98, spending on home care as a percentage of total public health spending ranged from lows of 1.95 percent (PEI), 2.3 percent (Quebec) and 3 percent (Alberta and BC), to highs of 5.1 percent (Ontario and Newfoundland) and 5.8 percent (New Brunswick).[60] There are also variations between provinces and territories with regard to the range and volume of services and the use of means testing and user charges. An elderly person in Nova Scotia can receive home support services up to a limit of $4,000 a month, whereas a similarly situated person in Newfoundland can receive only up to $2,268 a month.[61]

In the absence of publicly funded services, home care must be bought in the private sector or provided by unpaid family members and friends. There are few empirical studies in Canada exploring the extent of private financing for home care services. Coyte estimates that 25 percent of spending on home care is privately financed (e.g., from out-of-pocket payments or from private insurance).[62] An indication of the burden of out-of-pocket costs for home care patients is given by a PriceWaterhouseCoopers study published in 1999. This study found 25 percent of home care clients reporting average out-of-pocket expenses of $407 per month on home care and $138 on prescription drugs.[63] Home care clients recently discharged from hospital spent approximately $200 per week on home care services. Apart from out-of-pocket costs, there are also the costs that unpaid family members incur in providing care. There is little empirical evidence of the extent of this, however some suggest that unpaid family members, friends and volunteers together provide about 80 percent of home-care services.[64]

What is Home Care?

Despite the rising importance of home care as a public policy issue there are remarkably few instances where "home care" is defined. While calling for a national home care program, even the National Forum did not define it. A 1990 Health Canada publication, *Report on Home Care* defines home care as:[65]

> an array of services enabling Canadians, incapacitated in whole or in part, to live at home, often with the effect of preventing, delaying, or substituting for long-term care or acute care alternatives.

What is lacking in this definition are details of the "array of services" to be provided and upon what basis Canadians should be entitled to have these services publicly funded.

The *Report on Home Care* suggests that home care can be defined narrowly as a post-hospital care service aimed at people with specific health problems or broadly as a province-wide program making no conceptual or administrative distinction among needs for medications, homemaking or income support.[66] "Home care," narrowly defined, includes services that have historically been provided in hospitals. For a number of reasons, these same medical needs are now being serviced outside of hospitals and in the home. The concern is that many services that, pursuant to the Canada Health Act, must be fully paid for by provincial governments if delivered in a hospital setting, do not have to be fully funded if provided in a home. Consequently, there is a risk that as provincial governments do not have to bear the full cost of the shift from hospital care to home care there will be a disproportionate emphasis on such a shift as a cost-saving device. Moreover, there is a justice concern that health care is being passively privatized and care will increasingly be given to those with the greatest capacity to pay as opposed to those in the greatest need.

The existence of relatively high levels of private financing for home care services stems from the fact that, pursuant to the constitutional division of powers, it has been interpreted that the provinces have the sole power to directly regulate health insurance and medical services.[67] As a consequence, the federal government is limited to using its spending power to encourage provinces to meet minimum standards in their provincial health care plans.[68] Thus the Canada Health Act is a mechanism by which the federal government attempts to achieve national standards by offering cash payments and tax points to those provinces that comply with the criteria set. It is important to realize that the Canada Health Act's five criteria of universality, portability, accessibility, nonprofit administration and comprehensiveness and the specific prohibition against user charges and extra billing *only* apply to hospital and physician services as defined in the Act. Thus there is nothing in the Canada Health Act which discourages provinces from allowing means testing or user charges to patients for drugs, medical equipment, nursing services, homemaking services and food services that are needed in the home. This would seem to be so even if these services are needed for the treatment of needs that would otherwise have to be treated in a hospital.[69]

"Home care," broadly defined, includes services that substitute for services provided by long-term care institutions for the elderly, disabled or chronically ill. Also included in a broader definition of home care would be preventative services that would forestall or delay admission into either a hospital or a long-term care institution. Services that fall within this broader definition of home care have not traditionally been fully publicly funded. Long-term care services have not been treated as a core component of Medicare and have not been fully publicly funded. In Nova Scotia, for example, an applicant for admission to a nursing home is means tested (considering income from all sources except his or her principal residence) to assess how much he or she can contribute to the costs of care.[70] Different provinces have different assessment criteria with some provinces, like Nova Scotia, setting fees according to income whereas in other provinces everyone pays a standard rate.[71]

The key difference between the narrow and broad definitions of home care is the time frame over which the services are required. In the narrow definition, home care services are generally required for a limited period during which an individual is restored to full capacity. In the broader definition, services are generally required over a much longer period as a person moves along a continuum from functional independence to total dependence. The array of services included in both the narrow and broad definition of home care is broad. The services needed may include those of a physician, registered nurse, nurse-aide, physiotherapist, occupational therapist and social worker as well as food preparation, general housekeeping and transportation services. Goods needed may include drugs, medical equipment (e.g., wheelchairs, lifts) and medical supplies (e.g., bandages, drips). Complementary services required are assessment and case management services.

The broad array of services that may be included in home care results in overlap by the traditional Medicare system and social service systems. Home care is unique in the health care system as the services required may include not only traditional medical services but also what may be thought of as community or social services such as social work and homemaking. However, the principles underlying Medicare are that services are allocated on the basis of medical need as opposed to ability to pay. Thus a millionaire and a homeless person are equally entitled to hospital and physician services without payment.

By contrast, Canada's social support system generally only provides assistance on a means-tested basis to those on low incomes. Thus, while there is universal entitlement to Medicare, there is none to housing or nutrition.

The fact that home care occurs at the intersection of the Medicare and social service systems, which are premised on different principles of access and entitlement, makes the question of how to design a home care system a complex one. The integrity of Medicare is maintained by essentially prohibiting private financing of hospital and physician services. The theory runs that by forcing nearly every Canadian into the publicly funded system, the quality of Medicare will be assured for rich and poor alike. As Weale notes, "The principle that services for poor people are poor services is about as well attested an observation as we are likely to find in social affairs."[72] However, with home care services, are we similarly persuaded that citizens should be prohibited from privately buying or have private insurance covering additional housekeeping, homemaking, and nursing service beyond that which is publicly funded? Should there be prohibitions on user charges and extra-billing for home care services just as there are for hospital and physician services? There may have different answers to these questions depending on whether home care services are viewed as a substitution for hospital services as opposed to long-term care needs.

In order to preserve the integrity of Medicare, there should be publicly funded home care covering services which, if they were not provided in the home, would otherwise require the patient to be admitted into hospital. This is necessary so that there is no resistance to the most cost-effective good or service being supplied in response to a particular health need. In other words, it is a misconceived system that forces or encourages patients to stay in hospital because they cannot afford the drugs or care they need at home. If it is expected or assumed that family or community members will supply services that are substitutes or complements to hospital services, then this raises questions of the quality of care delivered. Above and beyond safety and quality concerns, there must also be a public debate about the fairness of expecting family and community members to provide this kind of care. It is one thing to facilitate and encourage those family members who want to provide home care services. It is another thing again to require this of a patient's family or community, particularly where the family or community are reluctant to do so or are stretched to the breaking point.

With regard to home care services that are not substitutes for hospital services, we must, as a community, determine whether these services are of such significance and importance that justice demands that they too be publicly funded for everyone. In other words, should long-term care services be allocated on the basis of need as opposed to ability to pay? Or should responsibility for long-term care be something that is largely left to personal responsibility, with government assistance for the poor? Given that, barring premature death, old age and a decline in functional independence is predictable, it does not seem unjust to require individuals to take some degree of personal responsibility and save for the possibility of needing long-term care associated with aging. However, as long-term care can be very expensive, there is a need for a safety net for those on lower incomes.

In every province, home care is unique and distinct from other health care services as publicly funded home care services are viewed as a top-up to whatever can be provided in the community or by family members. The mission of Home Care Nova Scotia is to "deliver an array of services to assist Nova Scotians of all ages, who have assessed unmet needs, in order that they can achieve and maintain their maximum independence while living in the their own homes and communities." Unmet needs are defined as "needs which are not being met by existing formal services, or informal family or community supports."[73] Similarly, one of the objectives of the Saskatchewan home care program is to provide "supportive, palliative, and acute care that family, friends and neighbours cannot provide."[74] Thus, provincial home care programs are generally premised on the assumption that publicly funded services will only be provided when family and community are unable to provide the necessary care "for free."

In contrast to the Medicare system where entitlement depends solely upon an assessment of medical need, provincial home care programs like Home Care Nova Scotia take into consideration a person's entire circumstances by exploring physical, psychological, functional and social support needs. Thus, the assessment process for home care services is presently much more complicated than for Medicare services and has at least four components: determination of the nature and degree of disability or medical need; determination of the kinds of services needed to meet these needs; determination of whether the patient's home is a suitable place in which to supply the needed services; and determination of whether family members or others in the community are willing and able to provide the services needed.

The last element of the assessment process—determination of whether family members or others in the community are willing and able to provide the services needed—is fraught with the potential for stereotyping and bias. Stereotypical assumptions may be made about the ability of elderly men and elderly women to respectively care for themselves, about the ability of working daughters as opposed to working sons to care for elderly relatives, about the capacity of mothers to care for physically and/or mentally disabled children, and of the capacity and obligations of women with existing caring responsibilities.

The Distributional Implications
of Moving Medicare Home

In terms of distributional implications, there is the issue of the impact on people in rural areas, on people on low incomes and on family members. With regard to people in rural areas, the deinstitutionalization process has particularly focussed on closing small rural hospitals and consolidating hospitals in urban areas. It is true that there is evidence that some surgical procedures are more effectively and safely done in institutions that perform large volumes of procedures.[75] However, these better outcome rates must be balanced against the longer travelling times for rural people to hospitals, distance to emergency services, and the costs to patients, their families and their employers of having to take time off work to travel to urban centres. Because of both the distance from urban areas and the uneven distribution of publicly funded supports, the burden on family caregivers in rural areas is higher than in urban areas.[76]

The shift from caring in institutions to caring in homes creates additional burdens for those on lower incomes. Because the Canada Health Act only protects hospital and physician services, the shifting of care outside of hospital walls and into homes and communities has resulted in increased private costs for patients and their families in terms of drugs, medical equipment and the direct and indirect costs of informal or formal caregiving services. Private sector on health care has steadily increased over the last decade ($560.31 per capita in 1990 to $746.98 per capita in 1996).[77]

When considering the distributional implications of shifting costs away from the public sector and into the private sector, one has to be aware of the well-documented correlation between medical need and low socio-economic status.[78] To put it simply, the poorer a person is the more likely it is that he or she will need medical services. Thus, if the resources saved are not transferred to other social spending, privatizing care and shifting the cost of caring to patients and family members necessarily involves a net loss for the poor.

Poor women are particularly affected by the transition from institutional care to home care. First, they represent the majority of the elderly in need of care and assistance. Not only are there are a greater proportion of women who are elderly (as women live longer than men), but research indicates that a greater percentage of elderly women are in need of more assistance than their male peers with housework, meal preparation, shopping and moving around the house.[79] Elderly women are also more likely to live alone than any other group in the population. Statistics Canada reported that in 1996, 24 percent of the population was in one-person households.[80] Of these individuals, more than one-third (36 percent) were aged sixty-five and over.[81] Twenty-nine percent of people over the age of sixty-five lived alone,[82] and 58 percent of women aged eighty-five and over live alone.[83] Of all seniors, 58 percent are women, with the percentage increasing to 70 percent in the over-85 age group.[84] Thus, women as the receivers of care are disadvantaged by a move to home care as they may not have family members living with them to provide care or to provide supplemental care to whatever is publicly funded.

Women also bear a disproportionate share of the costs as caregivers. Although the figures vary from study to study, the general consensus is that women are not only significantly more likely to be caregivers but also supply significantly more hours of care.[85] According to Statistics Canada, 66 percent of informal caregivers are women, affecting approximately 14 percent of all Canadian women over the age of fifteen.[86] Female caregivers are also more likely to be called upon to provide the most stressful and intensely personal kinds of care: of those who are caring for dementia sufferers, 72 percent of informal caregivers are women.[87] Thus women, as caregivers, are more likely than men to incur the wider costs of home care such out-of-pocket costs for drugs and medical equipment and lost employment opportunities.

Conclusion

The mantra of nearly all policymakers is to focus more on health and less on access to health care services. This goal should not be uncritically accepted. It springs from an economic analysis of health care systems and economics and is grounded in a utilitarian philosophy. As such, it implicitly validates a goal of maximizing the aggregate production of health without regard for distributional considerations. Similarly, the "determinants of health" perspective is grounded in looking at "population" health or taking a public health perspective. The rhetoric of "health" may unwittingly result in the discounting of services for the vulnerable population, such as the terminally ill and the disabled, since providing extra resources for their health needs will contribute little to the overall healthiness of the population. What is clear is that better and more sophisticated measures of health than life expectancy and infant mortality are needed. Research is needed on the values Canadians place upon satisfying various health needs, and on the value of caring services like nursing, the quality and impact of which are intrinsically difficult to measure.

My second point is that any future home care program will not be able to be all things to all people. As a dwindling tax base supports an aging population, choices are going to have to be made between competing needs. When considering the future development of home care policy, the needs of the poor and particularly poor women must be addressed first since they are burdened with a disproportionate share of the costs in the shift from institutional care to care in the home. A key measure of any society's health care system is the degree to which it serves its most vulnerable members. In considering how best to design a national home care system, much can be learned from how other countries structure their entitlements to home care and long-term care, including the appropriate mix of public and private financing, the role of private insurance and the role of user charges. Canada may wish to closely examine the "exceptional medical expenses scheme" in the Netherlands. This program provides compulsory insurance for all citizens (funded by employer contributions) and covers long-term care and mental health services. Similarly, Germany and Japan have recently passed legislation providing for national long-term care programs.[88] These initiatives warrant close analysis.

My third point is that advocates of a national home care program must realize that to truly serve the poor and those on lower incomes, a home care program must include coverage for drugs and medical equipment. In its "Red Book" of election promises, the Liberal government promised to develop both national home care and Pharmacare programs. Federal Minister of Health Allan Rock has also said that he cannot envisage a satisfactory approach to home care that does not incorporate elements of Pharmacare.[89] The political momentum for a Pharmacare program has fallen away, partly because of opposition by drug companies, but also because many Canadians do not view it as a key issue. They may have drug coverage through their employer and the very poor and elderly are generally covered by a provincial plan. Many middle-class Canadians (and thus, many voters) do, however, consider home care a very big issue as they try to juggle work, family and caregiving commitments to elderly parents. Nonetheless, a full 14 percent of Canadians have no drug coverage. For these individuals, the financial burden of shifting from care in the hospital to care in the home can be very heavy. Also, serious consideration should be given to compensating individuals on low incomes for the time they spend in caregiving.

It is often difficult to measure the quality of health care and to draw linkages between the consumption of health care and health care outcomes. The shift to home care will increase the costs of monitoring quality since there are numerous sites of delivery (homes) rather than one central hospital or institution. Home care patients may be reluctant to complain or question the quality of care delivered by loved ones. Research into how to ensure the quality of care and the safety of home care patients must be carried out. Quality control should focus on the most vulnerable individuals. Assessors need to assess not only the willingness and capacity of family members to provide care but whether the home itself is suitable for the delivery of care.

My final point is that the assessment process (an assessor, generally either a nurse or social worker, is sent to the home to assess the ability of family members to provide needed care) will be key to ensuring women are not discriminated against. This assessment process is ripe with potential for stereotypical assumptions about the ability of men and women to care for themselves and for others, and about the importance and demands of other tasks men and women perform, in the workplace and at home. It is important to ensure that assessors do not assume that women, particularly women who are already at home with other caregiving responsibilities or are looking or training for work, are a free pool of labour to care for the elderly. When considering the capacity of women to provide home care to family members, clear central guidelines are required for the assessment process. The work women do, whether in or outside of the home, must be valued and taken into consideration.

NOTES

This research was funded by the Maritime Centre for Excellence in Women's Health. I would like to thank Fran Gregor, Kathy MacPherson, Fiona Bergin and Hope Beanlands for getting this project off the ground and for the all the insight and information I gained from the sessions we had discussing home care issues. Thanks also to Peter Coyte for his comments on an earlier version of this paper and to Martina Munden for her invaluable research assistance. All errors and omissions remain my sole responsibility.

1   For a recent collection of papers on home care in Canada, see *HealthcarePapers* (2000) 4:1.

2   "Insured health services" are defined in the Canada Health Act, 1986, c. C–6, to include all medically necessary hospital and physician services and surgical-dental services which need to be performed in a hospital.

3   Canadian Institute for Health Information, "Health Care in Canada 2000: A First Annual Report"; Table 9: "Where Health Care Dollars are Spent" (Ottawa: CIHI, 2000).

4   P. Tully and E. Saint-Pierre, "Downsizing Canada's Hospitals, 1986/87 to 1994/95" (1997) 8:4 Health Reports 33 at 35, 36 (Tables 2 and 3).

5   OECD, *OECD Health Data 2000: A Comparative Analysis of 29 Countries* (Paris: OECD, 2001) [hereinafter OECD Health Data 2000].

6   See Canadian Institute for Health Information, *Health Care in Canada 2001*, p. 27, online at http://www.cihi.ca.

7   OECD Health Data 2000.

8   Statistics Canada reports that the mean average length of stay (children and adults) for short-term units in 1991–92 was 9.05 bed days. The mean average length of stay fell to 8.79 in 1993–94. See *Statistics Canada, Hospital Indicators, 1991–92* (Statistics Canada: Ottawa, 1992), and *Hospital Indicators, 1993–94* (Statistics Canada: Ottawa, 1994). The 1997 figures are from the OECD Health Care Data 2000, *ibid.*

9   See the Health Services Restructuring Commission, *Looking Back, Looking Forward: The Ontario Health Services Restructuring Commission (1996–2000) A Legacy Report* (March 2000), online at http//www.hsrc.gov.on.ca.

10 The Commission on Medicare, *Caring for Medicare: Sustaining a Quality System*, April 2001 (Government of Saskatchewan: Regina, 2001), online at http://www.marketingden.com/medicare/Commission_on_Medicare-BW.pdf.

11   See, in the context of long-stay patients, C. DeCoster and A. Kozyrskyj, *Long-Stay Patients in Winnipeg Acute Care Hospital* (Winnipeg: Manitoba Centre for Health Policy and Evaluation, 2000).

12   *Pembroke Civic Hospital* v. *Ontario (Health Care Services Restructuring Commission)* [1997] O.J. No. 3142, No. 394/97 (at p. 10 of 35 in QL), Archie Campbell J.

13   J. Coutts, "Montfort Hospital to Remain Open," *The Globe and Mail* (14 August 1997) A4; J. Coutts, "Francophone Hospital to Get Partial Reprieve," *The Globe and Mail* (6 August 1997) A3.

14   See J. Fanta, "Video-Assisted Thoracic Surgery—Lobectomy, Penumonectomy" (1996) 75:8 *Rozhl-Chir.* 375–9.

15   See W.S. Geier, "An Overview of Consumer-Driven Ambulatory Surgery: Operative Laparoscopy," *Nurse Pract.* 20:36 (1995): 46.

16   P. Steffen, *et al.*, "Postoperative Analgesia After Endoscopic Abdominal Operations: A Randomized Double-Blind Study of Perioperative Effectiveness of Metamizole," *Chirug.* 68:8 (1997): 7806.

17   See D.S. Rich, "Evaluation of a Disposable, Elastomeric Infusion Device in the Home Environment," *Am. J. Hosp. Phar.* 49 (1992): 1712; P.B. New et al., "Ambulatory Antibiotic Infusion Pumps," *J. Pediatric Nurse* 6 (1991): 134; D.N. Williams et al., "Home Intravenous Antibiotic Therapy Using a Programmable Infusion Pump," *Arch. Intern Med.* (1989): 1157.

18   See T.L. Petty, "Lungs at Home," *Monaldi Arch. Chest Dis.* 51:1 (1996): 60.

19   See D.J. Wirthlin *et al.*, "Telemedicine in Vascular Surgery: Feasibility of Digital Imaging for Remote Management of Wounds" (1998) 27:6 J Vasc Surg 1089.

20   V. Fuchs, "Economics, Values and Health Care Reform" (1996) 86: 1 American Economic Review 1-24.

21   In part this has been due to the fact that insurance (whether public or private) has historically indemnified patients against all costs incurred or paid doctors for all services delivered. With the rise of managed care we are seeing much more active management of physician decision-making by both private and public insurers and efforts to control the influx of technology into health care systems.

22   CD-ROM: *1999 OECD Health Database* (Paris: OECD, 1999).

23   National Advisory Council on Aging, *1999 and Beyond: Challenges of an Aging Society* (Ottawa: National Advisory Council on Aging, 1999) at 3.

24   Statistics Canada, *A Portrait of Seniors in Canada*, 2nd. ed. (Ottawa: Statistics Canada, 1997), (Cat. No. 89–519–XPE).

25   N.L. McAllister and M.J. Hollander, "Seniors Perceptions of and Attitudes Toward the British Columbia Continuing Care System," *Health Reports* 5:4 (1993): 409 (Statistics Canada, Cat. No. 82–003); B. Samaroo, "Comfort Levels With The Dying," *Can. Nurse* 91:8 (1995): 53; W.C. McCormick et al., "Long-term Care Preferences of Hospitalized Persons With AIDS," *J. Gen. Intern Med.* 6:6 (1991): 524; D. Rich, "Physicians, Pharmacists and Home Infusion Antibiotic Therapy," *Am. J. Med.* 97:2 (1994): 3; T.R. McWhinney and M.A. Stewart, "Home Care of Dying Patient," *Canadian Family Physician* 40 (1994): 240. Also see the reference to a study by John Hopkins University referenced in M. MacAdam, "Home Care: It's Time for a Canadian Model," *HealthcarePapers* 1:4 (2000): 9 at 27, which found that 70 percent of consumers want to be cared for in their own homes, 11 percent in housing with supportive services, 10 percent in the homes of family members and 3 percent in nursing homes.

26 Statistics Canada reports that the percentage of the population classified as living on a low income after tax peaked was 12.2 percent in 1998, after peaking at 14.2 percent in 1996, online at http.www.statcan.ca/Daily/English/000612/d000612a.htm (accessed on 14 July 2000).

27 Statistics Canada reports that 35.6 percent of people over the age of sixty-five lived alone in 1996, online at http:www.statcan.ca/Daily/English/980609/d980609.htm#1996census (accessed on 14 July 2000).

28 Unfortunately, it seems that for many people, home is associated with violence. A 1997 study conducted by Statistics Canada found that 22,254 cases of spousal assault were reported to police stations. A 1993 national telephone survey conducted by Statistics Canada found that the rate of wife assault was 29 percent of ever-married women. People over the age of sixty-five were victims in 2 percent of all violent crimes reported to police, with 24 percent of these crimes being committed by a family member. Of the 2,313 assaults in the sample, 1,230 were committed against women (53.1 percent). Statistics Canada also reported that older women continued to be abused by their partners as they aged and that those older women who were abused were most often abused by a spouse (40 percent) or adult child (40 percent), online at http://www.statcan.ca/english/freepub/85-224-XIE/0009885-224-XIE.pdf).

29 See the studies done by the Health Care Services Utilization and Research Commission, *Hospital and Home Care Study, Summary Report No. 10* (Saskatchewan: Health Care Services Utilization and Research Commission, 1998) and M. Brownell, N.P. Roos and C. Burchill, *Monitoring the Winnipeg Hospital System: 1990–91 Through 1996–97* (Manitoba Centre for Health Policy and Evaluation, February 1999), online at http://www.cc.umanitoba. ca/centres/mchpe/1mchpe.htm.

30 For a full discussion see Colleen M. Flood, *International Health Care Reform: A Legal, Economic and Political Analysis* (London: Routledge, 2000), chap. 2.

31 How big a problem moral hazard is will depend on the kind of health service. Because of the very unpleasant side effects and risks associated with surgery, there are few people who would want more surgery than they are told they actually need or must have. With full insurance, however, a patient will likely be insensitive to the fact that one hospital is much more efficient at providing the needed surgery than another. Also, while people may not happily use more surgical services, they may use more home care services, massage therapy or psychotherapy services if they are offered.

32 One study showed that when doctor fees were frozen from 1971 to 1976 in Quebec, per capita service use grew at an annual rate of 9.6 percent. By 1976, per capita utilization was 58 percent higher than in 1971. See M.L. Barer, R.G. Evans and R.J. Labelle, "Fee Controls as Cost Control: Tales from the Frozen North," *The Milbank Quarterly* 66:1 (1988) 1.

33 For a discussion, see Colleen M. Flood, *International Health Care Reform: A Legal, Economic and Political Analysis* (London: Routledge, 2000), chap. 2.

34 See G.L. Stoddart, M.L. Barer, R.G. Evans and V. Bhatia, "Why Not User Charges? The Real Issues—A Discussion Paper" (Ontario: The Premier's Council on Health, Well-being and Social Justice, September 1993) at 6.

35 For a discussion, see National Forum on Health, "Creating a Culture of Evidence-Based Decision Making in Health" in *Canada Health Action: Building on the Legacy, Volume 11, Synthesis Reports and Issues Papers* (National Forum on Health, Ottawa, 1997) at 20.

36 See J. Coutts, "Too Many Hysterectomies Performed in Ontario Report Says," *The Globe and Mail* (26 February 1998) A4.

37 A. Maynard, "Health Care Reform: Don't Confuse Me With Facts Stupid!" in *Four Country Conference on Health Care Reform and Health Care Policies in the United States, Canada, Germany and the Netherlands, Conference Report* (Amsterdam and Rotterdam: Ministry of Health, Welfare and Sport, 1995) 47 at 54.

38 R.G. Evans and G. L. Stoddart, "Producing Health, Consuming Health Care" in R.G. Evans, M.L. Barer and T.R. Marmor, *Why are Some People Healthy and Other Not?: The Determinants of Health of Populations* (New York: Aldine De Gruyter, 1994) 27 at 38.

39 See D.E. Angus et al., *Sustainable Health Care for Canada, Synthesis Report* (Ottawa: University of Ottawa, 1995).

40 Colleen M. Flood, "Conflicts Between Professional Interests, The Public Interest, and Patients' Interest in an Era of Reform: Nova Scotia Registered Nurses," *Health Law Journal* (1997) 27.

41 See note 38, 27 at 61, fn. 8.

42 D. Callahan, "What is a Reasonable Demand on Health Care Resources: Designing a Basic Package of Benefits," *J. of Contemporary Health Law and Policy* 8 (1992): 1.

43 See N. Daniels, *Just Health Care* (Cambridge: Cambridge University Press, 1985). See also A. Wagstaff et al., "Equity in the Finance of Health Care: Some International Comparisons," *J. Health Econ.* 11:4 (1992): 361 at 363 and J.W. Hurst, "Reforming Health Care in Seven European Nations," *Health Affairs* (1991): 7. For a critique of the impact of economists on health policy values, see E.M. Melhado, "Economists, Public Provision and the Market: Changing Values in Policy Debate," *J. Health Polit. Policy Law* 23:2 (1998): 215.

44 G. Mooney, "What Does Equity in Health Mean?," *World Health Stat. Q.* 40 (1987): 196, as cited by R.A. Carr-Hill, "Efficiency and Equity Implications of the Health Care Reforms," *Soc. Sci. Med.* 39:9 (1994): 1189 at p. 1190.

45 See L.B. Lerer et al., "Health For All: Analyzing Health Status and Determinants," *World Health Stat. Q.* 51:1 (1998): 7; S. Birch, "As a Matter of Fact: Evidence-Based Decision-Making Unplugged," *Health Econ.* 6:6 (1997): 547; C.J. Frankish, C.D. Milligan and C. Reid, "A Review of Relationships Between Active Living and Determinants of Health," *Soc. Sci. Med.* 47:3 (1998): 287; L. Weinreb et al., "Determinants of Health and Service Use Patterns in Homeless and Low-Income Housed Children," *Pediatrics* 102 (3 Pt 1) (1998): 554; N.L. Chappell, "Maintaining and Enhancing Independence and Well-being in Old Age" in National Forum on Health, *Determinants of Health, Adults and Seniors* (Ottawa: National Forum on Health, 1997) at 90.

46 See D.M. Eddy, "Performance Measurement: Problems and Solutions," *Health Affairs* 17:4 (1998): 7 at 17.

47 See Canadian Institute for Health Information, *National Health Expenditures Database (NHEX): Total Health Expenditure by Source of Finance, Canada, 1975 to 2000-Current Dollars*, online at http://www.cihi.ca/facts/nhex 2000/table_A.2.3. shtml.

48 Idem.

49 C.H. Tuohy, Colleen M. Flood and M. Stabile, *How Does Private Finance Affect Public Health Care Systems? Marshalling the Evidence from OECD Nations* (Working paper submitted to the Journal of Health, Politics, Policy and Law.)

50 See Canadian Institute for Health Information, *Health Care in Canada 2001*, p. 72, online at http://www.cihi.ca.

51 J.E. Fast et al., *Conceptualizing and Operationalizing the Costs of Informal Elder Care, Final Technical Report to the National Health Research Development Program (NHRDP)*, 17 March 1997, at 4–11 and 12.

52 Health Care Services Utilization and Research Commission, *Hospital and Home Care Study, Summary Report No. 10* (Saskatchewan: Health Care Services Utilization and Research Commission, 1998).

53 Health Canada, *Public Home Care Expenditures in Canada 1975–76 to 1997–98: Fact Sheets* (Ottawa: Health Canada, 1998) at 3; Table 1, online at http://www.hc-sc.gc.ca/datapcb/datahesa/E_home.htm, and Peter Coyte, "Home Care in Canada: Passing the Buck" (National Leadership Roundtable on Health Reform, University of Toronto, 28 June 2000), online at http://www.utoronto.ca/hlthadmn/dhr/4.html.

54 P. Coyte, *ibid.* at p. 3.

55 See Canadian Institute for Health Information, *National Health Expenditures Database (NHEX): Total Health Expenditure by Source of Finance, Canada, 1975 to 2000-Current Dollars,* online at http://www.cihi.ca/facts/nhex 2000/table_A.2.3.shtml.

56 See Canadian Institute for Health Information, *National Health Expenditures Database (NHEX): Total Health Expenditure by Source of Finance, Canada, 1975 to 2000-Current Dollars,* online at http://www.cihi.ca/facts/nhex 2000/table_A.2.3.shtml.

57 In 1997–93, a total of $1,362.5 million in public monies were spent on home care; in 1995–96, the total was $1,815.3. See Health Canada, *Public Home Care Expenditures in Canada 1975–76 to 1997–98: Fact Sheets* (Ottawa: Health Canada, 1998) at 3.

58 National Forum on Health, *Canada Health Action: Building on the Legacy, Final Report of the National Forum on Health* (Ottawa: National Forum on Health, 1997) at 20.

59 See L. Soderstrom et al., "The Health and Cost Effects of Substituting Home Care for Inpatient Acute Care: A Review of the Evidence," *CMAJ* 160:8 (1999): 1151; J. Lavis et al., "Free-standing Health Care Facilities: Financial Arrangements, Quality Assurance and a Pilot Study," *CMAJ* 158:3 (1998): 359; K. Parr, Saskatchewan Health Services Utilization and Research Commission, *The Cost-Effectiveness of Home Care: A Rigorous Review of the Literature* (Saskatoon: HSURC, 1996). 60 P. Coyte, supra note 10.

61 M. Hollander, *The Identification and Analysis of Incentives and Disincentives and Cost-Effectiveness of Various Funding Approaches for Continuing Care* (Victoria, BC: Hollander Analytical Services).

62 P. Coyte, "Home Care in Canada: Passing the Buck" (unpublished working paper). This figure likely underestimates the true private cost of home care since it does not account for the cost of informal care by family members for which no actual monetary transactions occur.

63 PriceWaterhouseCoopers Health Care Group, *Health Insider: An Indepth Research Report on Consumer Health Issues* (Toronto: PriceWaterhouseCoopers, 1999).

64 E. Brody, "Women in the Middle and Family Help to Older People," *The Gerontologist* 21 (1981): 471 and E. Brody, "Parent Care as a Normative Family Stress," *The Gerontologist* 25:1 (1985): 19.

65 Health Canada, *Report on Home Care* (Ottawa: Health Canada, 1990) at 2.

66 *Ibid.* at 2.

67 See Justice Dickson in *Schneider* v. *The Queen*, [1982] 2 S.C.R. 112 at 137, who notes that "[t]he view that the general jurisdiction over health matters is provincial … has prevailed and is not seriously questioned." See also *Eldridge* v. *British Columbia (Attorney General)* (1997), 151 D.L.R. (4th) 577 at 595–6, per La Forest J.

68 For a discussion, see Colleen M. Flood, "The Structure and Dynamics of the Canadian Health Care System" in J. Downie and T. Caulfield (eds.), *Canadian Health Law and Policy* (Toronto: Butterworths, 1999) at 5–50.

69 This may be, however, the subject of negotiation between the federal and provincial governments. The federal government has, for example, strongly argued that the provisions of the Canada Health Act cover care delivered in out-patient clinics.

70 See Nova Scotia Department of Health, *Quick Facts—Nursing Homes/Homes for the Aged* (Halifax: Nova Scotia Department of Health, 1997).

71 National Advisory Council on Aging, *The NACA Position on the Privatization of Health Care* (Ottawa: National Advisory Council on Aging, 1997) at 28.

72 A. Weale, "Equality, Social Solidarity and the Welfare State," *Ethics* 100 (1992): 473 at 474.

73 "Home Care in Saskatchewan: A Portrait," working document prepared by the Canadian Home Care Association for the Health Transition Fund, Health Canada, 1998, pp. 1–2, 4.

74 *Ibid.*, at 3.

75 See K. Grumbach et al., "Regionalization of Cardiac Surgery in the United States and Canada: Geographic Access, Choice and Outcomes," *JAMA* 274:16 (1995): 1282. See also J. Coutts, "Larger Hospitals Safer, Study Maintains: Pancreatic-Cancer Sufferers Treated in Small Centres Twice as likely to Die After Surgery," *The Globe and Mail* (18 June 1998) A10.

76 See. J, Campbell, G. Bruhm and Susan Lilley, *Caregivers' Support Needs: Insights from the Experience of Women Providing Care in Rural Nova Scotia* (report presented to the Maritime Centre of Excellence for Women's Health, Halifax, November 1998).

77 See Canadian Institute for Health Information, *National Health Expenditures Database (NHEX): Total Health Expenditure by Source of Finance, Canada, 1975 to 2000-Current Dollars,* online at http://www.cihi.ca/facts/nhex 2000/table_A.2.3.shtml.

78 See R.G. Evans, M.L. Barer and T.R. Marmor, *Why Are Some People Healthy and Other Not?: The Determinants of Health of Populations* (New York: Aldine De Gruyter, 1994) and G.A. Kaplan, "People and Places: Contrasting Perspectives on the Association Between Social Class and Health," *Int. J. Health Services* 26:3 (1996): 507.

79 M.W. Rosenberger and E.G. Moore, "The Health of Canada's Elderly Population: Current Status and Future Implications," *Can. Med. Assoc. J.* 157:8 (1997): 1025.

80 Statistics Canada, *1996 Census: Private Households, Housing Costs and Social and Economic Characteristics of Families,* online at http://www.statcan.ca:80/Daily/English/980609/d980609.htm#1996CENSUS (accessed on 26 January 1999).

81 *Ibid.*

82 Health Canada, *Statistical Snapshot No. 5: Many Living Alone,* online at http://www.hc-sc.gc.ca/seniors-aines/pubs/factoids/en/no8.htm (accessed on 5 May 1999).

83 *Ibid.*

84 Health Canada, *Statistical Snapshot No. 5: More Women Than Men*, online at http://www.hc-sc.gc.ca/seniors-aines/pubs/factoids/en/no8.htm (accessed on 5 May 1999).

85 See E. Grunfeld et al., "Caring for Elderly People at Home: The Consequences to Caregivers," *Can. Med. Assoc. J.* 157:8 (1997): 1101.

86 Statistics Canada, *Who Cares? Caregiving in the 1990s* (General Social Survey, Ottawa, unpublished data, 1996), as quoted by J, Campbell, G. Bruhm and Susan Lilley in *Caregivers' Support Needs: Insights from the Experience of Women Providing Care in Rural Nova Scotia* (report presented to the Maritime Centre of Excellence for Women's Health, Halifax, November 1998) p. 9.

87 *Ibid.*

88 For a discussion, see M. MacAdam, "Home Care: It's Time for a Canadian Model," *HealthcarePapers* 1:4 (2000): 9 at 21.

89 See Allan Rock in his address to the conference on National Approaches to Pharmacare in K. Graham, *Proceedings of the Conference on National Approaches to Pharmacare* (Ottawa: Health Canada Publications, 1998).

5

HUMAN RIGHTS AND
HEALTH CARE REFORM
A CANADIAN PERSPECTIVE

BARBARA VON TIGERSTROM

Rights language is often used to make claims about health care, ranging from general claims that the public has a right to health or to health care, to specific claims to particular treatments or standards of treatment. Any agenda for health care reform needs to take account of such claims, in terms of both their political weight and their basis in law. Integrating human rights into the analytical framework for designing health care reform requires a clearer idea of the nature and validity of rights claims relating to health. The right to health has been receiving increased attention in the international legal community:[1] domestically, there have been a number of high-profile cases involving health care and the Canadian Charter of Rights and Freedoms[2] in recent years.[3] Although there is widespread—if not universal[4]—agreement that the right to health or health care should be protected as a human right, there is less consensus on what this means or what obligations it entails for governments. However, there is by now a substantial body of interpretation that can be used to define the content and scope of human rights relating to health.

The objective of this chapter is to examine this content and scope, and in particular to explore what it means for health care reform in Canada. While general claims of a "right to health care" or to "equity in health" have rhetorical force, they will be of limited use unless there is a clearer idea of how human rights need to be respected in health care and how reforms can be undertaken in a way that enhances, rather than undermines, respect for human rights. Specifically, this chapter will look at the relevance of human rights law in regards to two basic questions in health care reform: What health services should be provided, and how should they be provided? International and domestic human rights law relevant to health care will be reviewed, followed by implications for the structure of payment and delivery of health care, and the scope of health services to which access should be guaranteed.

The Right to Health in International Human Rights Law

The right to health is recognized in several major international human rights treaties to which Canada is a party. Article 12 of the International Covenant on Economic, Social and Cultural Rights (ICESCR)[5] provides:

1. The States Parties to the present Covenant recognize the right of everyone to the enjoyment of the highest attainable standard of physical and mental health.
2. The steps to be taken by the States Parties to the present Covenant to achieve the full realization of this right shall include those necessary for:

> (a) The provision for the reduction of the stillbirth rate and of infant mortality and for the healthy development of the child;
> (b) The improvement of all aspects of environmental and industrial hygiene;
> (c) The prevention, treatment and control of epidemic, endemic, occupational and other diseases;
> (d) The creation of conditions which would assure to all medical service and medical attention in the event of sickness.

The Convention on the Elimination of All Forms of Discrimination against Women (CEDAW) requires states to "eliminate discrimination against women in the field of health care in order to ensure, on a basis of equality between men and women, access to health care services" and in particular to ensure access to appropriate services in connection with pregnancy.[6] The Convention on the Rights of the Child (CRC) contains a very comprehensive provision, similar to that contained in the ICESCR but even more detailed. Specifically, it requires states to recognize "the right of the child to the enjoyment of the highest attainable standard of health and to facilities for the treatment of illness and rehabilitation of health," to "ensure that no child is deprived of his or her right of access to such health care services" and to take appropriate measures to "ensure the provision of necessary medical assistance and health care to all children with emphasis on the development of primary health care."[7]

The right to health does not, of course, oblige governments to guarantee that individuals will be healthy[8]—the reference to the "highest attainable" standard of health takes into account both individual variations and the availability of resources.[9] The Committee on Economic, Social and Cultural Rights (CESCR) has stated that "the right to health must be understood as a right to the enjoyment of a variety of facilities, goods, services and conditions necessary for the realization of the highest attainable standard of health."[10] This includes, but is not limited to, the right to health care.[11] Given the purpose of this chapter, health care is the focus. The right to health, however, also encompasses broader rights to health protection.

In determining the scope and content of a state's obligations under the right to health, it is necessary not only to look at the text of the provisions but also to consider general principles of international human rights law and interpretation of the relevant instruments, in particular the ICESCR. In relation to any right, states have obligations that have been classified into three types.[12] The obligation to respect rights means that the state must refrain from engaging in any conduct that would interfere with the enjoyment of the right to health, such as denying access to health care or causing harm to individuals' health through environmental damage. The obligation to protect rights requires states to prevent third parties from interfering with the right to health, for example by enforcing professional standards for medical professionals and ensuring that health care providers or insurers do not prevent access to health care. Finally, the obligation to fulfill the right to health requires governments to take positive steps toward the fulfilment of the right. These measures may include legislative recognition of the right to health, development and implementation of health protection policies and the provision of health facilities and services.

Other provisions in the ICESCR and their interpretation also help to identify the nature and scope of states' obligations with respect to the right to health. Article 2(1) requires each state party to "take steps, individually and through international assistance and co-operation, especially economic and technical, to the maximum of its available resources, with a view to achieving progressively the full realization of the rights recognized in the present Covenant by all appropriate means, including particularly the adoption of legislative measures." This has been interpreted to mean that states are not necessarily expected to achieve the full realization of the rights in the Covenant immediately, but must immediately begin to take steps toward their progressive realization, and continue moving expeditiously toward this goal.[13] These steps should include, but are not limited to, legislative measures; they should also include the provision of judicial remedies with respect to the rights in the Covenant.[14] Retrogressive measures "would require the most careful consideration and would need to be fully justified by reference to the totality of the rights provided for in the Covenant and in the context of the full use of the maximum available resources."[15] The Covenant does allow for some flexibility to take into account resource constraints, but a state is required to take steps "to the maximum of its available resources." This involves devoting sufficient resources to the fulfilment of economic, social and cultural rights, and also using those resources effectively and equitably.[16] For each right there are certain core obligations which must be fulfilled regardless of resource considerations.[17]

According to Article 2(2), the rights in the Covenant must be guaranteed to all without discrimination, and there is a specific provision (Article 3) requiring states to ensure the equal right of men and women to enjoy the rights. Although the obligations in the Covenant are generally progressive in nature, the requirement of nondiscrimination takes effect immediately.[18] States must "eliminate *de jure* discrimination by abolishing without delay any discriminatory laws, regulations and practices (including acts of omission as well as commission) affecting the enjoyment of economic, social and cultural rights," and must begin acting immediately to end *de facto* discrimination and discrimination by private persons.[19]

These general principles and provisions will assist in determining what specific obligations the right to health will entail. In sections III and IV below, the implications for how health care is funded and delivered, and what care must be provided, will be explored. Canada, as a party to the ICESCR and other treaties referred to above, must act in accordance with its obligations under these treaties. However, treaty obligations are not directly enforceable in Canadian domestic law; they must be implemented in legislation by the relevant level of government.[20] Even unimplemented provisions of international law may have an indirect impact on Canadian law, however, because they may be used by the courts in interpreting the Charter of Rights and Freedom or legislation.[21] The limited extent to which economic, social and cultural rights including the right to health are implemented in Canadian law has been a source of some concern to the Committee on Economic, Social and Cultural Rights.[22] One of the themes which will be explored below is the protection provided for the right to health in Canadian law, in particular the Charter. Another difficulty is that although Canada as a state is a party to these agreements and subject to their obligations, the provincial governments have primary responsibility in the area of health care. Therefore, although the federal government is responsible to the international community for its compliance with treaty obligations in this area, it has limited, and indirect, control over their fulfilment.

The Canadian Charter of Rights and Freedoms

There is no "right to health" explicitly recognized in the Canadian Charter of Rights and Freedoms. However, several sections of the Charter are relevant to health and have been used as the basis for claims in this context.

Section 7 of the Charter guarantees to everyone "the right to life, liberty and security of the person, and the right not to be deprived thereof except in accordance with fundamental justice." This section of the Charter requires a two-step analysis: first, it must be determined if there is an infringement of life, liberty or security of the person; second, if there is an infringement, it must be determined whether the infringement is contrary to the principles of fundamental justice. If so, there is a violation of section 7 and the analysis will proceed to the test for justification under section 1.

Security of the person has been held to include both physical and psychological integrity.[23] Since health is clearly linked to life and to security of the person, it seems reasonable that section 7 should protect a right to health, and convincing arguments have been made to this effect.[24] Such an interpretation would also be consistent with Canada's international obligations. However, existing jurisprudence suggests that the scope of section 7 is more limited, so that it may be applied to protect certain aspects of the right to health, but not the full scope of the right as recognized in the international instruments. For example, section 7 may prevent the state from interfering with an individual's physical and mental health through the threat of criminal sanctions in some cases,[25] but has not been successfully used to claim a right to certain treatment.[26]

The Charter's equality guarantees are also relevant to health and health care. Section 15(1) requires that individuals be guaranteed equality before and under the law and the equal protection and benefit of the law. A law or government action may infringe s. 15(1) without deliberately targeting or discriminating against a certain group, if it has an adverse effect on that group. However, not every distinction or instance of differential treatment or effect will constitute discrimination. The Supreme Court of Canada has recently stated the following test to determine if there is a violation of s. 15(1):[27]

(A) Does the impugned law (a) draw a formal distinction between the claimant and others on the basis of one or more personal characteristics, or (b) fail to take into account the claimant's already disadvantaged position within Canadian society resulting in substantively differential treatment between the claimant and others on the basis of one or more personal characteristics?

(B) Is the claimant subject to differential treatment based on one or more of the enumerated and analogous grounds?

and

(C) Does the differential treatment discriminate, by imposing a burden upon or withholding a benefit from the claimant in a manner which reflects the stereotypical application of presumed group or personal characteristics, or which otherwise has the effect of perpetuating or promoting the view that the individual is less capable or worthy of recognition or value as a human being or as a member of Canadian society, equally deserving of concern, respect, and consideration?

This three-step test is not a strict test or formula but summarizes the central issues to be addressed.[28] The third component requires that the differential treatment be "discriminatory in a substantive sense," which means that it violates the fundamental purpose of s. 15(1). This purpose is "to prevent the violation of essential human dignity and freedom through the imposition of disadvantage, stereotyping, or political or social prejudice, and to promote a society in which all persons enjoy equal recognition at law as human beings or as members of Canadian society, equally capable and equally deserving of concern, respect and consideration."[29]

This inquiry is to be undertaken using a comparative approach[30] and taking account of contextual factors including pre-existing disadvantage, the relationship between the grounds and the claimant's characteristics or circumstances, the ameliorative purpose or effects of the impugned provision and the nature of the interest affected.[31] The claimant must show that the purpose of s. 15 has been infringed by the impugned law.

Even where a violation of a right protected by the Charter is established, it is open to the government to attempt to justify the violation under section 1, which provides that the rights and freedoms in the Charter are guaranteed "subject only to such reasonable limits prescribed by law as can be demonstrably justified in a free and democratic society." The courts have developed a framework for analyzing this test, which requires the government to show the objective of the legislation or other action is pressing and substantial, that the infringement is rationally connected to this objective, that it impairs rights as little as possible and that the effect of the infringement is proportional to the objective.[32]

Finally, it is important to bear in mind that not all conduct within the health care system will be subject to the Charter. The Charter applies to the acts of government,[33] which most obviously includes legislation but also extends to other official government actions. It does not apply to private actors unless their actions can be attributed to government.[34] In order to determine whether the Charter applies in a given situation, it is necessary to look at both the actor involved and the nature of the action. For example, in *Stoffman* v. *Vancouver General Hospital*, the Court held that the Charter did not apply to a hospital in respect of its adoption and administration of a regulation on hospital privileges. The hospital was not part of government and "the provision of a public service, even if it is one as important as health care, is not the kind of function which qualifies as a government function" for the purposes of the

Charter.[35] However, where a hospital or other actor in the health care system is implementing a specific government policy or program, rather than merely providing services, the Charter will apply. Therefore, in *Eldridge* v. *British Columbia (Attorney General)*, it was held that hospitals carry out a specific government objective in providing medically necessary services under the Hospital Insurance Act and conduct related to this will therefore be subject to the Charter. Similarly, the Medical Services Commission, in determining whether a service is a benefit under the Medical and Health Care Services Act, clearly acts in a governmental capacity and is subject to the Charter.[36] Finally, although this discussion will focus on the Charter, it should also be remembered that in cases where the Charter does not apply, the conduct of private actors may be subject to similar restrictions, for example the obligation not to discriminate, under human rights legislation.

Structure of Payment and Delivery of Health Care

One of the important questions in health care reform is what roles the public and private sectors should play in the payment and delivery of health care. There is a wide variety of options available within a framework of four rough classifications, depending on whether financing and provision of services, respectively, are predominantly private or public.[37] Canada's system is generally categorized as having public financing and private delivery, although there is in fact a significant and growing proportion of private financing.[38] Privatization of health care, which has been defined as "a *process* in which nongovernment actors become increasingly involved in the financing and/or provision of health care services,"[39] is often part of cost-containment and efficiency strategies in health care reform.[40] In Canada, efforts to privatize financing or delivery of services have been the cause of substantial concern and controversy, as witnessed by the public debates regarding Bill 11, the Health Care Protection Act, in Alberta.[41] Human rights language and the right to health care are sometimes invoked in this context, reflecting concerns that privatization may have a negative impact on equitable access to health care. Human rights law does not provide any set formula for the public/private mix in health care, but provides some limits and criteria for policy choices in this area.

Generally speaking, a state's obligations with regard to economic, social and cultural rights, including the right to health, do not require the adoption of any particular political or economic system, and states have a wide margin of discretion as to how they choose to fulfill their obligations. The ICESCR is neutral in this regard and does not compel the adoption of any particular approach, so long as it respects rights (those contained in the Covenant as well as human rights generally).[42] The specific obligation in the ICESCR with respect to health care is "the creation of conditions which would assure to all medical service and medical attention in the event of sickness"; the CRC requires states to "ensure the provision of necessary medical assistance and health care to all children." CEDAW requires states to ensure equal access to health care services by men and women, and to ensure appropriate pregnancy-related services, "granting free services where necessary." Apart from this provision in CEDAW, which states that free services must be provided where necessary, international instruments do not require health care to be provided free of charge.[43] However, "health facilities, goods and services must be affordable for all. Payment for health care services ... have to be based on the principles of equity ensuring that these services, whether privately or publicly provided, are affordable for all, including socially disadvantaged groups."[44]

Therefore, it will be a question of fact in each case whether the approach taken by Canada or another state party is fulfilling its obligations under these agreements—hence the crucial importance of monitoring and reporting procedures.[45] In making policy decisions about health care, states should be required to take into account the available evidence in order to gauge the likely impact of any reforms. For example, the World Health Organization (WHO) has formulated a number of "key design features" for universal access to health care, and notes that there is increasing international consensus on these features.[46] If a government chooses policies which, on the best available evidence, seem likely to undermine the fulfilment of its obligations rather than progressively realize the right to health, or if monitoring and reporting reveal that recent reforms have had a retrogressive effect, that government must be prepared to meet a strict burden of justification: "As with all rights in the Covenant, there is a strong presumption that retrogressive measures taken in relation to the right to health are impermissible. If any deliberately retrogressive measures are taken, the State party has the burden of proving that they have been introduced after the most careful consideration of all alternatives and that they are duly justified by reference to the totality of the rights provided for in the Covenant in the context of the full use of the State party's maximum available resources."[47]

It is also clear that a state cannot avoid its obligations under the ICESCR or other international treaties by privatizing services.[48] Even if services are privately financed and/or provided, the state still remains ultimately responsible for ensuring that its obligations are being met, in this case that there is universal and equal access to adequate health care. States are specifically required to "ensure that privatization of the health sector does not constitute a threat to the availability, accessibility, acceptability and quality of health facilities, goods and services" as part of their obligation to protect the right to health.[49] Serious concerns have been raised regarding the potential detrimental effect on equitable access of increasing privatization in health care.[50] Therefore, if governments choose to privatize, they will be required to justify this choice and/or to implement measures to prevent the potential harms.

A related question is whether individuals would be able to claim that they have a right to health services which are funded or delivered in a certain way, for example to privately insured health care. As one author has suggested:[51]

> [P]articularly in light of the accessibility and comprehensiveness of the current public system, it is unlikely that a right to health care would be read so expansively as to entitle an individual to demand unlimited freedom of access to services or to choice of providers, free from any restrictions. In other words, it is unlikely that section 7 [of the Charter] could be successfully invoked to challenge existing provisions of the Canada Health Act, or to challenge further restrictions on access to private health care services, on the grounds that such restrictions amount to a deprivation of the right to health care.

This was tested in a recent Quebec case, *Chaoulli v. Québec (Procureure générale)*.[52] Dr. Chaoulli and Mr. Zéliotis brought an action challenging the provisions in Quebec legislation which prohibit payment by private insurance for services which are insured under the provincial health insurance plan.[53] The plaintiffs claimed that this prohibition infringed their rights under section 7 of the Charter, and that they should be permitted to take out private insurance to cover medical and hospital services provided by physicians who had opted out of the public system. The motivation for this challenge was summed up thus in Dr. Chaoulli's testimony: "If I fall gravely ill ... I want to be able to spend my money on saving my life rather than paying for my funeral."[54]

The plaintiffs claimed that given the limits on access in the public system, the prohibition of parallel private insurance constituted a violation of life and security of the person; in addition, it interfered with an important personal decision and therefore infringed their liberty.[55] In considering these claims, the Court first examined the scope of section 7. The section does not protect purely economic rights, but may protect rights which are intimately related to life, liberty and security of the person but have an incidental economic component. Justice Piché accepted that section 7 protects a right to health care, but not that it protects the right of physicians to practice without restriction in the private sector. As long as the public health care system provides access to the services required, the prohibition on private insurance does not infringe section 7 rights. However, the evidence of numerous physicians and surgeons, experts in health policy and administration, and other individuals heard by the Court indicated that there were serious problems with access in certain sectors. To the extent that sufficient access is not available in the public system, the prohibition may constitute an infringement.

However, the plaintiffs failed to establish that this potential infringement was contrary to the principles of fundamental justice. Justice Piché found that the adoption of these sections "was motivated by considerations of equality and human dignity and, thus, it is clear that there is no conflict with the general values promoted by the Canadian Charter."[56] The evidence heard by the Court showed that allowing a parallel private system would affect the rights of the rest of the population. It would threaten the integrity, functioning and viability of the public system. The purpose of the impugned provisions is to prevent these effects and guarantee the existence of a high-quality public health care system in Quebec.[57] As a result, it was concluded that the infringement of life, liberty and security of the person was in accordance with the principles of fundamental justice, and there was no violation of section 7. The Court also dismissed arguments under sections 12 (cruel and unusual treatment or punishment) and 15 of the Charter.

From this case and the earlier discussion it is evident that a human rights analysis using the Charter or international human rights law instruments will not direct governments to adopt any particular structure for the provision of health services in every case, or require them to allow private provision and/ or payment of services. What human rights law will provide is a framework for evaluating existing structures or policies, or any proposed reforms. It should help to guide policy development toward the goals of quality, access and equity in health care.

Scope of Coverage

In the previous section, the fact that states are obliged to ensure access to health care for all, regardless of how health services are financed or provided, was discussed. This raises the obvious question: To what, exactly, must access be ensured? There is near-unanimous realization that no system can provide all services that might be needed or desired by every individual. The WHO refers to the "new universalism": "Universal coverage means coverage for all, not coverage of everything."[58] However, the question of what must be covered is an extremely difficult one which has defied satisfactory resolution despite the huge volume of writing devoted to it.

International materials provide some indications of what must be assured to all under the right to health. Specific requirements are contained in some instruments: for example, the CEDAW requires the provision of pregnancy-related care, and the CRC also specifically refers to pre- and postnatal care, as well as measures to diminish infant and child mortality, primary health care and preventive health care. This, of course, still leaves open large questions about the scope of such services to be provided (e.g., what is the scope of primary or preventive care?). Attempts have also been made at the international level to define the minimum core content of economic, social and cultural rights, including the right to health. This core content includes the minimum obligations which states are required to satisfy unless they can demonstrate that this is impossible, even using all available resources for this purpose as a matter of priority.[59] The recent General Comment by the CESCR on the right to health defines the core obligations as including, *inter alia*: essential primary health care; ensuring the "right of access to health facilities, goods and services on a nondiscriminatory basis, especially for vulnerable or marginalized groups"; providing "essential drugs, as from time to time defined by WHO's Action Programme on Essential Drugs"; and ensuring equitable distribution of health facilities, goods and services.[60]

A wealthy country like Canada would be expected to satisfy these core obligations and to treat them as a minimum, while working toward the progressive realization of the right to health through all appropriate measures and to the maximum of available resources. As a result, this core content, even if it were more fully defined, does not exhaust the range of health care to which access must be ensured in Canada. Some of the discussion in American literature regarding "basic standards" or "decent minimum" health care is similarly of limited usefulness.[61] A developing body of jurisprudence under the Charter of Rights and Freedoms has attempted to define the limits of individuals' entitlements under the right to health care in the Canadian context.

As noted above, some have suggested that section 7 of the Charter, which recognizes the right to "life, liberty and security, and the right not to be deprived thereof except in accordance with the principles of fundamental justice," includes a right to health care.[62] The jurisprudence on this subject is not encouraging, however. For example, in *Brown v. British Columbia (Minister of Health)*,[63] the plaintiff challenged the British Columbia government's decision to place AZT under the provincial Pharmacare Plan, so that all persons with HIV/AIDS, except those on social assistance or in long-term care facilities, would have to pay part of the cost of the very expensive drug. The plaintiff's argument, based on section 7 of the Charter of Rights and Freedoms, was rejected, in part because the Court held that the impact of the law itself was merely the economic hardship and reduction in the standard of living that would be suffered by those who have to pay for the drug, which is not within the protection given by section 7.[64] The Court also held that any deprivation of life, liberty or security of the person was caused by the disease itself, not the law.[65]

Reliance on section 7 in other cases has similarly been unsuccessful. In *Ontario Nursing Home Association v. Ontario*, a claim by a nursing home resident was rejected because, although "with greater funding he might receive more care," there was no evidence that the care provided was inadequate. Section 7 "does not deal with property rights and as such does not deal with additional benefits which might enhance life, liberty or security of the person."[66] In *Fernandes v. Manitoba (Director of Social Services, Winnipeg Central)*, Mr. Fernandes was denied an allowance to provide for a caregiver in his home. He required an attendant for sixteen hours a day and, without assistance for home care, would have to live in a hospital. Therefore, he argued that the denial of assistance would infringe his rights to liberty and security of the person by effectively confining him to hospital. The Manitoba Court of Appeal disagreed, stating that the "desire to live in a particular setting does not constitute a right protected under s. 7 of the Charter."[67] More recently, the appellants in the *Cameron* case, discussed below, sought to rely on section 7 as well as section 15 at trial, but their arguments on section 7 were summarily dismissed by the trial judge and were not pursued on appeal.[68]

The usefulness of section 7 in this context may be restricted by the limited scope of application of the section. This is not necessarily, as some have suggested,[69] because section 7 recognizes only "negative" rights to be free from government interference. The distinction between positive and negative rights is problematic in any case, and in the recent case of *New Brunswick (Minister of Health and Social Services) v. G. (J.)*[70] the Supreme Court of Canada held that section 7 may require the government to provide funding for legal counsel in certain types of proceedings, which suggests that a court may be willing to require the government to provide funding or take other measures to comply with section 7. Furthermore, while this decision does not explicitly discuss the issue, its decision implies that section 7 can protect a right which has an economic aspect. At issue in the case was not whether the appellant was permitted to be represented by counsel, but whether she was entitled to public funding for counsel if she could not afford to pay. The British Columbia Supreme Court's characterization of the complaint in *Brown* as merely one of economic deprivation not addressed by section 7 is questionable in light of this decision. The recent decision of the Quebec Superior Court in *Chaoulli* not only accepted that section 7 includes a right to health care[71] but also found, following earlier statements by the Supreme Court and other courts, that section 7 could protect rights that have an incidental economic aspect but are intimately related to life, liberty or security of the person.[72]

However, the *New Brunswick* decision also suggested, as have previous decisions of the Supreme Court, that the application of section 7 is limited to situations where the complainant's rights have allegedly been infringed "as a result of an individual's interaction with the justice system and its administration."[73] If the application of section 7 is limited to this context, this would reduce its usefulness in claiming a right to health care in many situations.

Given these limitations, it may be difficult to use section 7 to effectively enforce a government's obligation to fulfill the right to health by ensuring access to health care.[74] However, in Canada there is already a commitment, through the Canada Health Act and the establishment of provincial health care plans, to the provision of health care. In this context, the obligation of nondiscrimination comes to the forefront. The international instruments require the right to health to be guaranteed to all persons without discrimination:[75]

> By virtue of articles 2(2) and 3, the Covenant proscribes any discrimination in access to health care and underlying determinants of health, as well as to means and entitlements for their procurement, on the grounds of race, colour, sex, language, religion, political or other opinion, national or social origin, property, birth, physical or mental disability, health status (including HIV/AIDS), sexual orientation and civil, political, social or other status, which has the intention or effect of nullifying or impairing the equal enjoyment or exercise of the right to health.

States must guarantee equality of access to health care and health services, including provision of health insurance and facilities where required, prevention of discrimination in the provision of health care and health services, and ensuring equitable distribution of resources.[76]

In Canadian law, the actions of government in the area of health care are subject to the Charter's equality guarantees in section 15(1). The Supreme Court "has repeatedly held that once the state does provide a benefit, it is obliged to do so in a nondiscriminatory manner."[77] There have been a number of decided cases in Canada in which claimants have alleged violations of s. 15(1) in relation to health services, although to date only a few of these cases have been successful.

In *J.C. v. Forensic Psychiatric Service Commissioner*,[78] the complainant J.C. had been committed to a psychiatric institution in which there were a number of different units for patients at different stages of recovery. J.C. wished to move into a part of the facility (the "Cottages") which was used as a "stepping stone" before release into the community, with a home-like environment and considerable freedom. Professional assessments indicated that this would be appropriate for her; however, the request was denied because of the institution's policy, based on budget considerations, not to allow female residents to be placed in this part of the facility. No alternative was available for female residents. The BC Supreme Court found that the policy excluding women from this program did constitute discrimination, stating: "J.C. by most accounts needs the benefit of the Cottage program to make the transition into the community. She has been denied that program because of her gender and for no other reason."[79] This violation of her equality rights could not be justified under section 1 since, in the opinion of the Court, the need to operate within current budget restrictions was not a sufficiently important objective to warrant the limitation of a constitutional right.[80] Furthermore, the rational connection with the infringement was weak, since "no one has suggested additional funds could not be made available or that changes could not be made to existing programs to accommodate the requested transfer," and the extinguishment of J.C.'s right to equal treatment outweighed any competing interests.[81]

A section 15(1) claim was also successful in another BC case, *Eldridge v. British Columbia (Attorney General)*. In this case, the plaintiffs challenged the province's refusal to fund medical interpretation services for deaf persons as insured health services. The claim was unsuccessful in the BC Supreme Court and Court of Appeal. However, the Supreme Court of Canada found that there was a violation of section 15(1), not in the legislation itself which set up the schemes for insured medical and hospital services, but in the decisions under those statutes not to fund sign-language interpretation. The lack of funding for this service had an adverse effect on deaf persons because it deprived them of the ability to benefit equally from the provincial health care system. Given the importance of effective communication to the provision of medical services, the failure to ensure that deaf patients could communicate with health professionals meant they would not receive the same level of care. The Court found, furthermore, that "[i]f we accept the concept of adverse effects discrimination, it seems inevitable, at least at the s. 15(1) stage of the analysis, that the government will be required to take special measures to ensure that disadvantaged groups are able to benefit equally from government services."[82] In this case an attempt at justification under section 1 based on budgetary constraints was also rejected. The Court found that to deny the claimants "equal access to services that are available to all" could not be described as a "minimal impairment" of their equality rights, especially given that the total estimated cost of providing the interpretation services was only $150,000, or approximately 0.0025 per cent of the total provincial health care budget.[83]

Both of these cases involve situations where the claimant is denied equal access to services which are generally available to others, based on a personal characteristic (gender in *J.C.* and disability in *Eldridge*). In other cases, there have been claims of discrimination where the government refuses to fund a specific treatment which is required by or relevant to particular groups of individuals, for example those with a certain disease or condition. The case of *Brown v. British Columbia*,[84] referred to above in relation to section 7, concerned the refusal to fully fund AZT, a drug for persons with HIV/AIDS;

Cameron v. *Nova Scotia*[85] was a challenge to the provincial government's refusal to fund *in vitro* fertilization (IVF) and intra-cytoplasmic sperm injection (ICSI), used by infertile couples attempting to conceive a child. Both of these claims failed; however, a s. 15(1) challenge succeeded in the recent case of *Auton* v. *British Columbia*,[86] in which it was claimed that the refusal to fund intensive early behavioural intervention for autistic children was discriminatory.

These two general categories of cases correspond to two ways of rationing services: by individual ("by patient") or by service. "Rationing by patient occurs when a particular medical service is available, but not to everyone who might benefit from it."[87] So, for example, in *J.C.*, a certain type of program was available for psychiatric patients, but not to J.C. because of her gender; in *Eldridge*, insured medical and hospital services were available to all residents of the province but deaf persons were effectively denied equal access because of the lack of services to allow them to communicate with their health care providers.[88] Rationing by service, on the other hand, "occurs when only certain medical services are covered."[89] In the case of *Brown*, many services and certain types of medications were fully funded by the province (cancer drugs and immunal suppression drugs for transplant patients), but not AZT. In *Cameron*, the province funded many hospital and medical services, including some for infertility, but not *in vitro* fertilization (IVF) or intra-cytoplasmic sperm injection (ICSI). The provincial health insurance plans in Canada employ both types of rationing:[90] some services are simply not covered, others are generally available but are not provided to certain individuals either as a matter of explicit policy (through conditions placed on the coverage of services) or as a result of less explicit rationing at various levels in the health care system. Either type of rationing may potentially be discriminatory, but the analysis plays out somewhat differently in each case.

In many respects, claims of discrimination involving rationing by service are more difficult to resolve. Decisions not to fund a certain medical good or service may be based on a number of different factors, including effectiveness, safety, cost and ethical or social concerns. In *Brown*, the Court accepted that the distinction between drugs that were fully funded and AZT, which was not, was based on "clinically relevant grounds."[91] It may often be difficult for a court to adequately assess such grounds and determine whether they are legitimate. Decisions involving medical judgement have long been considered the exclusive domain of medical professionals—so much so that some courts have taken the position that anti-discrimination law was not meant to apply to medical judgements as opposed to other kinds of judgements.[92] However, decisions to fund or provide certain services ostensibly based on clinical grounds may in fact conceal discriminatory intent or effect. For example, in the *Auton* case, the Court noted, "The absence of treatment program for autistic children must consciously or unconsciously be based on the premise that one cannot effectively treat autistic children. The extensive evidence in this case shows that assumption to be a misconceived stereotype."[93] Even legitimate clinical grounds may reflect systemic discrimination or at least a social structure which makes the funding decision discriminatory in its effect. For example, "the greater the improvement in quality or length of life from a treatment, the more likely it is that the treatment will be funded. Social organization may act on this relationship between quality of life and likelihood of funding to the detriment of persons with disabilities" because social organization may exacerbate the impact of disability on an individual's life, causing individuals with disabilities to receive a smaller improvement in quality of life, which in turn makes it less likely that a treatment will be funded.[94] In addition, social conditions may influence the availability of treatments, because of priorities for medical research and treatment, and the cost of treatments. As a result, "just as considerations of medical benefit are not 'neutral' measures for allocation decisions, neither are considerations of cost."[95]

How then, can it be determined whether a denial of funding or access for a particular service is discriminatory? "It cannot be the case ... that whenever funding is denied for a treatment or procedure that is specifically relevant to or required by persons with a particular medical condition or disability, the mere fact of the denial will be sufficient for a finding of discrimination."[96] However, the possibility that it may well be discriminatory in certain cases must be acknowledged. Distinguishing between these types of cases is likely to be difficult, but the structure of analysis that developed for sections 15(1) and 1 of the Charter, to determine whether there is discrimination and whether that discrimination can be justified, can be used.

A "synthesis" of the guidelines for determining whether section 15(1) has been infringed has been set out by the Supreme Court of Canada in recent cases:[97]

> First, does the impugned law (a) draw a formal distinction between the claimant and others on the basis of one or more personal charac-teristics, or (b) fail to take into account the claimant's already disad-vantaged position within Canadian society resulting in substantively differential treatment between the claimant and others on the basis of one or more personal characteristics? If so, there is differential treat-ment for the purpose of s. 15(1). Second, was the claimant subject to differential treatment on the basis of one or more of the enumerated and analogous grounds? And third, does the differential treatment discriminate in a substantive sense, bringing into play the *purpose* of s. 15(1) of the Charter in remedying such ills as prejudice, stereotyping, and historical disadvantage? The second and third inquiries are con-cerned with whether the differential treatment constitutes discrimi-nation in the substantive sense intended by s. 15(1).

The first part of this test, which requires the claimant to establish a distinction, will often not present much of an obstacle in these cases. Where access is denied to a medical good or service that has particular relevance to a specific group, for example those with a certain disease or condition, there will likely be differential treatment based on a personal characteristic (the disease or condition, and in some cases associated personal characteristics as well—for example in *Brown*, at the relevant time 90 per cent of the identifiable group, HIV-positive individuals, were homosexual or bisexual males, which gave rise to a claim based on sexual orientation as well as disability[98]). If a specific funding decision cannot be characterized as a direct, formal distinction, the funding policy (schedule of benefits under the provincial health insurance plan) or legislative structure can be said to have an adverse effect on the relevant group. However, it is possible that in some cases the nature of the good or service will be such that its exclusion cannot be shown to have a differential impact on any identifiable group.

The next stage is to determine whether the personal characteristic(s) on which the distinction is based can be characterized as an enumerated or analogous ground. As just noted, in some cases there may be an enumerated or analogous ground such as gender, sexual orientation or age, which is shared by the group needing the service. Otherwise, the question will be whether the disease or condition for which the service is required can be considered a mental or physical disability, or an analogous ground. In some cases, the answer to this question may seem straightforward; in others it may be more difficult. In *Cameron*, the members of the Nova Scotia Court of Appeal disagreed as to whether infertility is a disability.[99] "The question might be asked whether everybody requiring medical services is disabled, mentally or physically."[100] Courts in Canada and elsewhere have struggled with the definition of "disability" and the outcome of this consideration can assist in determining whether an individual's need for medical services means that she is disabled.[101] For the purposes of this article,[102]

> an important factor in determining whether a particular condition amounts to a disability is the principle that Charter guarantees should be given a broad and liberal construction, and not be interpreted in an unduly technical, contorted or restrictive manner. Thus, if a court is in doubt as to whether a particular condition counts as a physical disability, it should resolve its doubt in the plaintiff's favour. Having done so, the court ought to turn to the core question under section 15, namely, whether the Charter plaintiff was denied equality rights on account of his or her physical disability.

While there may be some cases in which the relevant conditions do not amount to a disability, claims should not be shut down at this stage unless this is quite clear.

The most difficult part of the section 15 analysis, then, will likely be the third stage of the *Law* test which requires a claimant to establish that the differential treatment on the basis of an enumerated or analogous ground constitutes discrimination. As the Court stated in *Brown*, "[I]t is true that the funding policy affects an identifiable group. That can be said, for example, of those taking insulin, drugs for tuberculosis, or cystic fibrosis. But can it be said that the special funding programs for cancer and transplant patients (and not those drugs or AZT) constitutes an inequality which is discriminatory, for that is what s. 15 of the Charter prevents."[103] According to *Law*, differential treatment will be discriminatory if it is contrary to the purpose of the Charter, in that it has "the effect of perpetuating or promoting the view that the individual is less capable or worthy of recognition or value as a human being or as a member of Canadian society, equally deserving of concern, respect, and consideration." This is to be assessed contextually on a case-by-case basis, and the Court suggested a number of factors which will be relevant.

First, although pre-existing disadvantage is not necessary or sufficient in itself to establish discrimination,[104] "probably the most compelling factor favouring a conclusion that differential treatment imposed by legislation is truly discriminatory will be, where it exists, pre-existing disadvantage, vulnerability, stereotyping, or prejudice experienced by the individual or group."[105] This will depend on the nature of the disability or other personal characteristic, and the extent to which individuals with that characteristic have been subject to disadvantage independent of the government action being challenged. For example, in *Brown* the trial judge acknowledged the fact that individuals who are gay and/or HIV positive had historically been, and were at the time of trial, the targets of discrimination and persecution.[106] This should have been relevant to the analysis of whether the exclusion of coverage for AZT was discriminatory. Although the majority judgement in *Cameron* accepted that infertile couples were subject to pre-existing disadvantage, it recognized that they "do not appear to suffer consequences of their disability to the same extent" as other disabled persons.[107] The extent to which pre-existing disadvantage can be used as an indicium of discrimination will clearly be a matter of degree, depending on the nature of the disability or other characteristic, the social context and other factors.

Another contextual factor is the relationship between the grounds upon which the distinction is made and the claimant's characteristics or circumstances: "[I]t will be easier to establish discrimination to the extent that impugned legislation fails to take into account a claimant's actual situation, and more difficult to establish discrimination to the extent that legislation properly accommodates the claimant's needs, capacities, and circumstances."[108] Also relevant is the "ameliorative purpose or effects of impugned legislation or other state action upon a more disadvantaged person or group in society."[109] It could be argued, for example, that exclusion of a certain treatment is necessary because its prohibitive cost would deprive others of important benefits, or because it could be harmful to some other group for another reason (perhaps ethical considerations, for example). The existence of an ameliorative purpose or effect does not necessarily mean that the law or policy does not discriminate, however, and it may still require justification under s. 1 or the operation of s. 15(2).[110] Finally, the nature and scope of the interest affected may be relevant.[111]

It has been quite rightly pointed out that these factors include matters that are normally considered at the stage of the section 1 analysis, when the government is required to justify a violation, and that this raises concerns that too much of the burden is being shifted onto the claimant under this third part of the *Law* test.[112] It has always been accepted that not every distinction on enumerated or analogous grounds constitutes discrimination. It is not yet clear, however, whether the test as stated in *Law* will impose an additional burden on claimants as compared to earlier formulations of the s. 15 analysis.[113] The claimant will not necessarily be required to adduce "data, or other social science evidence not generally available, in order to show a violation of the claimant's dignity or freedom"; this may be clear merely on the basis of judicial notice and logical reasoning by the court.[114] However, a court "must be satisfied that the claimant's assertion that differential treatment imposed by the legislation demeans his or her dignity is supported by an objective assessment of the situation."[115] While this may be clear in principle, it will likely often be difficult in application. For example, in *Cameron* the Court found that, looked at objectively, "[t]he impact of the denial of these procedures to the infertile perpetuates the view that they are less worthy of recognition or value. It touches their essential dignity and self-worth. I agree with the appellants that this denial sends a powerful message to the infertile."[116] By contrast, the Court in *Brown* was of the opinion that "[i]f the plaintiffs have suffered stigma, loss of esteem and perception of discrimination" because of the decision to fund cancer and transplant drugs and not AZT, "they have suffered unreasonably."[117] These findings, placed side-by-side and viewed in their respective contexts, seem difficult to reconcile, highlighting the difficulty inherent in judging whether a perception of diminished dignity and self-worth is "unreasonable."

The most difficult distinctions, among cases concerning denial of coverage under section 15(1), will likely be drawn at this third step of the analysis. If a claimant can successfully establish all three elements of the *Law* framework of analysis, then further distinctions may be drawn at the stage of justification under section 1. If there is a section 15(1) violation, the government has the opportunity to demonstrate that the violation is nevertheless a "reasonable limit" which "can be demonstrably justified in a free and democratic society."

The first stage of the section 1 test requires the government to show that it has a "pressing and substantial objective" for the legislation or other action that infringes the claimant's rights. In some cases the government may be able to show that there are factors such as safety or effectiveness concerns which justify excluding services from coverage.[118] However, the motivation will likely often be partly—and sometimes exclusively—the desire to minimize costs in the health care system. Therefore, a key question here will be the extent to which the government will be permitted to use budgetary considerations and the need to limit expenditures as a pressing and substantial objective. Although it has been stated that financial considerations alone cannot justify an infringement of the Charter,[119] the Court has also stated that "governments must be afforded wide latitude to determine the proper distribution of resources in society," particularly when they must make choices among disadvantaged groups in providing benefits.[120] Two recent cases came to conflicting conclusions on this issue: in *Cameron*, the majority accepted budgetary pressures in the Nova Scotia health care system as an objective justifying denial of coverage, while in *Auton*, the objective of making "'judicious use' of limited health care resources" could not justify the violation of s. 15(1) rights.[121]

Assuming that financial considerations can be relied on in at least some cases as an objective justifying infringements, whether the attempt at justification is ultimately successful will depend on the government meeting the other elements of the test under section 1. It is not sufficient merely to plead lack of funds. The government must meet the "proportionality test," i.e., it must show that the measure is rationally connected to the objective, that it impairs rights as little as reasonably possible (minimal impairment) and that its harmful effects are proportional to its objective. Where the government seeks to rely on financial constraints as an objective for infringing constitutional rights, the courts should be vigilant to ensure that these remaining elements of the test are met. Whether it is legitimate to deny access to a medical good or service needed by an identifiable group may depend on a number of factors, including the cost of the good or service relative to the overall budget,[122] whether the government is devoting maximum available resources to health as required by international commitments and whether the government's priorities for funding are rationally designed to maximize health and equitable access to health care. The advice of international authorities (such as the WHO) on the allocation of priorities to realize the right to health may be helpful in making this type of assessment. While it may not be appropriate for the courts to scrutinize budgetary policies in detail, it is reasonable to require a government which seeks to rely on financial constraints to show that it has made reasonable efforts to allocate its budget in a rational and "rights-friendly" manner. Some of these factors can be addressed through the proportionality analysis under section 1.

Comments made by the Supreme Court in the *Eldridge* decision suggest that the minimal impairment analysis may be crucial to determining whether denial of coverage may be justified. The Court distinguished the situation in which deaf persons were essentially being denied "equal access to services that are available to all" from a case where claimants might "demand that the government provide them with a discrete service or product, such as hearing aids, that will help alleviate their general disadvantage."[123] The former situation was described as one which did not minimally impair the claimants rights, but the implication is that the latter, which is more like both *Cameron* and *Brown*, might be a minimal impairment. However, whether this is the case will surely depend on the nature of the service which is excluded and its importance to the members of the group at issue.[124]

In the rational-connection analysis, assessments of long-term cost-effectiveness may have an important role. The Court's decision in *Auton* may have been affected by the recognition that "[i]n a broad sense, it is apparent that the costs incurred in paying for effective treatment of autism may well be more than offset by the savings achieved by assisting autistic children to develop their educational and societal potential rather than dooming them to a life of isolation and institutionalization."[125] If providing a treatment or preventive measure will be cost-effective in the long run, exclusion of funding is not rationally connected to the objective of saving money.

The application of sections 15(1) and 1 of the Charter will not provide any easy answers to questions about the scope of coverage in health care. However, they do provide a framework of analysis with which there can be an attempt to separate legitimate and reasonable decisions from those which have a discriminatory purpose or effect and cannot be justified as reasonable limits on rights. These distinctions will be inextricably tied up with considerations about medical judgment, effectiveness, cost and other factors, but the analysis requires careful scrutiny of these factors through the lens of equality and human rights concerns.

Implications for Health Reform

This discussion has focussed on several prominent questions in health care reform and suggested some ways in which human rights law can make a contribution to the analysis of these questions. There are also many other implications for the health care system which can be drawn from human rights law in the domestic and international spheres. For example, the importance of monitoring the impact of existing arrangements and reforms on the enjoyment of the right to health has already been mentioned.[126] In addition, the existence of effective mechanisms for public accountability and the availability of remedies for violations is essential.[127] This has implications for the legal system as well as for health care, since remedies for violations, to be effective, must be provided for in law as well as internal procedures, and the existence of adequate remedies will depend on the extent to which the right to health is recognized and implemented in Canadian law.

Realization of the right to health will have important implications beyond the health care system *per se*, including the legal system, social services and other government functions. Access to information has an important role in health protection.[128] Finally, attention to other areas of human rights, such as privacy and the rights of indigenous peoples,[129] should also have a significant impact on health reform and health policy development.

When people think of human rights and health care they may think of a narrow range of issues, in particular claims regarding entitlements to particular health services. Human rights law can certainly assist in analyzing these types of claims. It also has far-reaching implications for health care and health care reform in a variety of areas, including the scope of coverage, the public/private mix in payment and provision of services, regulation of health service providers, and the allocation of resources and budgetary priorities. A human rights analysis will not necessarily provide a single blueprint for any of these areas of policy, but it can help to identify the goals and parameters, and provide a framework of analysis for assessing whether the existing or proposed system is acceptable.

NOTES

1   See Committee on Economic, Social and Cultural Rights, CESCR General Comment 14: The Right to the Highest Attainable Standard of Health, 22nd Sess., UN Doc. E/C.12/2000/4 (2000) [hereinafter General Comment 14]; B.C.A. Toebes, *The Right to Health as a Human Right in International Law* (Antwerp: Intersentia, 1999).

2   Part I of the Constitution Act, 1982, being Schedule B to the Canada Act, 1982 (UK), 1982, c.11 [hereinafter Charter].

3   Recent cases include *Cameron v. Nova Scotia (Attorney General)* (1999), 177 D.L.R. (4th) 611, [1999] N.S.J. No. 297 (N.S.C.A.) (QL), leave to appeal to S.C.C. refused [1999] S.C.C.A. No. 531, aff'g (1999), 172 N.S.R. (2d) 227, [1999] N.S.J. No. 33 (N.S. S.C.) (QL) [hereinafter *Cameron*]; *Chaoulli v. Quebec (Procureure générale)*, [2000] J.Q. No. 479 (QL) and *Auton (Guardian ad litem of) v. British Columbia (Minister of Health)*, [2000] B.C.J. No. 1547 (B.C.S.C.)(QL).

4   For a critical view of the right to health, see R.A. Epstein, *Mortal Peril: Our Inalienable Right to Health Care?* (Reading, MA: Addison-Wesley, 1997). This book provoked numerous rebuttals, including the following symposium: "Is America's health care system in mortal peril?" (1998) 3 *U. Illinois L. Rev.* 683.

5   16 December 1966, 993 U.N.T.S. 3; Can.T.S. 1976 No. 46 [hereinafter ICESCR].

6   18 December 1979, 1249 U.N.T.S. 13 Can.T.S. 1982 No.31 [hereinafter CEDAW], article 12.

7   20 November 1989, UN G.A. Res. 44/25, 29 I.L.M. 1340 (1990), Can.T.S. 1992 No.3 [hereinafter CRC], article 24.

8   General Comment 14, *supra* note 1 at paras. 8–9.

9   *Ibid.* at para. 9.

10   *Ibid.*

11   There has been a great deal of discussion as to whether the rights under the ICESCR are properly referred to as the "right to health" or the "right to health care," "right to health protection," or some other phrase. The consensus seems to be that the "right to health" is preferable since it is more inclusive and thus better reflects the content of the rights recognized in the Covenant. See V.A. Leary, "Implications of a Right to Health" in K.E. Mahoney and P. Mahoney, eds., *Human Rights in the Twenty-first Century* (Dordrecht: Martinus Nijhoff, 1993) 481 at 484–6; Toebes, *supra* note 1 at 16–24.

12   On the origins of the tripartite typology of obligations, see Toebes, *supra* note 1 at 307–11. For discussions of the application of these three types of obligations to the right to health, see Toebes, *supra* note 1 at 311ff; General Comment 14, *supra* note 1 at paras. 34–7; P. Hunt, *Reclaiming Social Rights: International and Comparative Perspectives* (Aldershot, England: Dartmouth, 1996 at 130–3.

13   The Limburg Principles on the Implementation of the International Covenant on Economic, Social and Cultural Rights, UN Doc. E/CN.4/1987/17, Annex, reprinted in (1987) 9 *Hum. Rts. Q.* 122 [hereinafter Limburg Principles] at paras. 16, 21; Committee on Economic, Social and Cultural Rights, CESCR General Comment 3: The Nature of States Parties Obligations, 5th Sess. (1990) [hereinafter General Comment 3], paras. 2, 9.

14   Limburg Principles, *ibid.*, at paras. 18, 19; General Comment 3, *ibid.* at paras. 3–7; Committee on Economic, Social and Cultural Rights, CESCR General Comment 9: The Domestic Application of the Covenant, 19th Sess. (1998), UN Doc. E/C.12/1998/24.

15   General Comment 3, *supra* note 13 at para. 9.

16   Limburg Principles, *supra* note 13 at paras. 27–8.

17   Limburg Principles, *supra* note 13 at para. 25; *General Comment 3, supra* note 13 at paras. 10–11.

18   Limburg Principles, *supra* note 13 at para. 35.

19   Limburg Principles, *supra* note 13 at paras. 38, 40.

20   *Baker v. Canada (Minister of Citizenship and Immigration)*, [1999] 2 S.C.R. 817; *Francis v. The Queen*, [1956] S.C.R. 618; *Capital Cities Communications Inc. v. Canadian Radio-Television Commission*, [1978] 2 S.C.R. 141.

21   *Baker, ibid.* at para. 70. The Court was divided on this point in *Baker*, but the majority found that it was permissible to refer to unimplemented obligations in international law to interpret the Immigration Act. See also *R. v. Keegstra*, [1990] 3 S.C.R. 697; W.A. Schabas, *International Human Rights Law and the Canadian Charter* (Scarborough, ON: Carswell, 1996).

22   Committee on Economic, Social and Cultural Rights, Concluding Observations of the Committee on Economic, Social and Cultural Rights: Canada, 19th Sess., UN Doc. E/C.12/1/Add.31 [hereinafter Concluding Observations].

23 R. v. *Morgentaler (No. 2)*, [1988] 1 S.C.R. 30 [hereinafter *Morgentaler*]; *Singh* v. *Minister of Employment and Immigration*, [1985] 1 S.C.R. 177; *Rodriguez* v. *British Columbia (Attorney General)*, [1993] 3 S.C.R. 519.

24 M. Jackman, "The Regulation of Private Health Care under the Canada Health Act and the Canadian Charter" (1995) 6:2 *Constitutional Forum* 54 at 56; M. Jackman, "The Right to Participate in Health Care and Health Resource Allocation Decisions Under Section 7 of the Canadian Charter" (1995/96) 4:2 *Health L. Rev.* 3 at 3–5. On the right to life and health see Leary, "Implications of a Right to Health," *supra* note 11 at 486–7; Toebes, *supra* note 1 at 260–4; D. O'Sullivan, "The allocation of scarce resources and the right to life under the European Convention on Human Rights" (1998) *Public L.* 389.

25 See *Morgentaler*, *supra* note 23: "'Security of the person' must include a right of access to medical treatment for a condition representing a danger to life or health without fear of criminal sanction" (at 90 per Beetz J.). *Morgentaler* struck down the Criminal Code provisions on abortion as contrary to section 7 of the *Charter*. *R.* v. *Parker*, [2000] O.J. No. 2787 (Ont. C.A.) involved a section 7 challenge to the prohibition of marijuana under the Narcotic Control Act, R.S.C. 1985, c. N–1 and the Controlled Drugs and Substances Act, S.C. 1996, c. 19. The legislation was found to infringe the appellant's section 7 rights because it did not adequately provide for medical use which was required by the appellant. "Preventing Parker from using marijuana to treat his condition by threat of criminal prosecution constitutes an interference with his physical and psychological integrity" and therefore violates his rights to liberty and security of the person. The violation is not in accordance with the principles of fundamental justice and could not be justified under section 1.

26 See *infra* notes 63–8 and accompanying text.

27 *Law* v. *Canada (Minister of Employment and Immigration)*, [1999] 1 S.C.R. 497 [hereinafter *Law*] at para. 88. These guidelines were subsequently reaffirmed and applied in *Granovsky* v. *Canada (Minister of Employment and Immigration)*, [2000] 1 S.C.R. 703 [hereinafter *Granovsky*].

28 *Law*, *ibid.*; *Winko* v. *British Columbia (Forensic Psychiatric Institute)*, [1999] 2 S.C.R. 625 at para. 76.

29 *Law*, *supra* note 27 at para. 51.

30 *Ibid.* at paras. 55–8.

31 *Ibid.* at paras. 62ff.

32 This test was first set out in the case of *R.* v. *Oakes*, [1986] 1 S.C.R. 103 and later summarized in *Egan* v. *Canada*, [1995] 2 S.C.R. 513 at para. 182. Depending on the nature of the alleged infringement, at the first stage of the test it may be appropriate to examine the objective of the legislation generally, or of the specific impugned provision, omission or other action, or both: *Vriend* v. *Alberta*, [1998] 1 S.C.R. 493 at paras. 109–11.

33 *Charter*, *supra* note 2, s. 32.

34 *McKinney* v. *University of Guelph*, [1990] 3 S.C.R. 229 at 273–4.

35 [1990] 3 S.C.R. 483 at 516.

36 [1997] 3 S.C.R. 624 at paras. 49–52.

37 A. Stewart, "Cost-containment and Privatization: An International Analysis" in D. Drache and T. Sullivan, eds., *Market Limits in Health Reform: Public Success, Private Failure* (London: Routledge, 1999) 65 at 66.

38. See C. Flood, "The Structure and Dynamics of Canada's Health Care System" in J. Downie and T. Caulfield, eds., *Canadian Health Law and Policy* (Toronto: Butterworths, 1999) 5 at 29–30.

39 J. Muschell, *Privatization in Health* (Geneva: World Health Organization, 1995), quoted in Stewart, *supra* note 37 at 66.

40 Stewart, *supra* note 37 at 65.

41 Health Care Protection Act, S.A. 2000, c. H–3.3. The Act was introduced as Bill 11 in the 4th Session of the 24th Legislature on 2 March 2000 and passed in May; it was proclaimed in force on 28 September 2000.

42 General Comment 3, *supra* note 13 at para. 8.

43 Toebes, *supra* note 1 at 249.

44 General Comment 14, *supra* note 1 at para. 12.

45 Committee on Economic, Social and Cultural Rights, CESCR General Comment 1: Reporting by States Parties, 3rd Sess. (1989); on monitoring see General Comment 14, *supra* note 1 at para. 57; A.R. Chapman, "Monitoring Women's Right to Health under the International Covenant on Economic, Social and Cultural Rights" (1995) 44 *Am. U.L. Rev.* 1157; T.B. Jabine, "Indicators for Monitoring Access to Basic Health Care as a Human Right" in A.R. Chapman, ed., *Health Care Reform: A Human Rights Approach* (Washington: Georgetown University Press, 1994) 233.

46 World Health Organization, *World Health Report 1999: Making a Difference* (Geneva: World Health Organization, 1999) at 43–4.

47 General Comment 14, *supra* note 1 at para. 32.

48 Toebes, *supra* note 1 at 249. See also Committee on the Elimination of Discrimination against Women, CEDAW General Recommendation 24: Women and Health, 20th Sess. (1999) at para. 17: "The Committee is concerned at the growing evidence that States are relinquishing these obligations as they transfer State health functions to private agencies. States parties cannot absolve themselves of responsibility in these areas by delegating or transferring these powers to private sector agencies. States parties should therefore report on what they have done to organize governmental processes and all structures through which public power is exercised to promote and protect women's health. They should include ... the measure they have taken to ensure the provision of such services."

49 General Comment 14, *supra* note 1 at para. 35.

50 See D. Wikler, "Privatization and Human Rights in Health Care: Notes from the American Experience" in Mahoney and Mahoney, eds., *supra* note 11, 495.

51 Jackman, "The Regulation of Private Health Care," *supra* note 24 at 57.

52 *Supra* note 3.

53 *Loi sur l'assurance-maladie*, L.R.Q., c. A–29, s. 15; *Loi sur l'assurance-hospitalisation*, L.R.Q., c. A–28, s. 11. Some, but not all, other provinces have similar provisions in their provincial health insurance legislation: e.g., Alberta Health Care Insurance Act, R.S.A. 1980, c. A–24, s. 17; Medicare Protection Act, R.S.B.C., c. 286, s. 45; Health Insurance Act, R.S.O. c. H.6, s. 14.

54 *Chaoulli, supra* note 3 at para. 38 [translated by author].

55 *Ibid.* at para. 94–5.

56 *Ibid.* at para. 260.

57 *Ibid.* at para. 263.

58   *World Health Report 1999, supra* note 46 at 43.

59   General Comment 3, *supra* note 13 at para. 10.

60   General Comment 14, *supra* note 1 at para. 43. See also Maastricht Guidelines on Violations of Economic, Social and Cultural Rights, reprinted in (1998) 20 *Hum. Rts. Q.* 691, at para. 9. For more information on essential drugs, see World Health Organization, Essential Drugs and Medicines Policy, online at www.who.int/medicines (accessed on 17 July 2000).

61   See M.A. Baily, "Defining the Decent Minimum" in Chapman, ed., *supra* note 45, 167.

62   See *supra* note 24.

63   (1990), 66 D.L.R. (4th) 444 (B.C.S.C.).

64   *Ibid.* at 467.

65   *Ibid.* at 466–7.

66   (1990), 74 O.R. (2d) 365 (Ont. H.C.J.) at 378.

67   (1992), 78 Man. R. (2d) 172 at 182–3.

68   *Cameron* v. *Nova Scotia (Attorney General)* (1999), 172 N.S.R. (2d) 227 (N.S.S.C.) at 250. In *Auton, supra* note 3 at para. 111, the BC Supreme Court found that it was it was unnecessary to consider the arguments relating to section 7 and decided the case on the basis of section 15(1).

69   Canadian Bar Association Task Force on Health Care, *What's Law Got to do with it? Health Care Reform in Canada* (Ottawa: Canadian Bar Association, 1994) at 25–6.

70   [1999] 3 S.C.R. 46.

71   *Supra* note 3 at para. 223.

72   *Ibid.* at para. 221.

73   *Supra* note 70 at para. 65. This is not necessarily limited to criminal matters; *ibid.* This was recently confirmed in the Supreme Court's decision in *Blencoe* v. *British Columbia (Human Rights Commission)*, 2000 SCC 44 at para. 45–6. See also *Reference re ss. 193 and 195.1(1)(c) of the Criminal Code*, [1990] 1 S.C.R. 1123; *B. (R.)* v. *Children's Aid Society of Metropolitan Toronto*, [1995] 1 S.C.R. 315.

74   Section 7 may be more effective in enforcing the government's obligation to respect (refrain from interfering with) the right to health; see *supra* note 25 and accompanying text.

75   *General Comment 14, supra* note 1 at para. 18.

76   *Ibid.*, paras. 19, 43.

77   *Eldridge, supra* note 36 at para. 73, citing *Tétrault-Gadoury* v. *Canada (Employment and Immigration Commission)*, [1991] 2 S.C.R. 22, *Haig* v. *Canada (Chief Electoral Officer)*, [1993] 2 S.C.R. 995, at pp. 1041–2, *Native Women's Assn. of Canada* v. *Canada*, [1994] 3 S.C.R. 627, at p. 655, *Miron* v. *Trudel*, [1995] 2 S.C.R. 418.

78   (1992), 65 B.C.L.R. (2d) 386.

79   *Ibid.* at 397.

80   *Ibid.* at 398.

81   *Ibid.* at 399.

82   *Eldridge, supra* note 36 at para. 77.

83   *Ibid.* at paras. 87, 92, 94.

84 *Supra* note 63.

85 *Supra* note 3.

86 *Supra* note 3.

87 D. Orentlicher, "Destructuring Disability: Rationing of Health Care and Unfair Discrimination Against the Sick" (1996) 31 *Harv. C.R.-C.L. L. Rev.* 49 at 53.

88 *Eldridge* at first glance may appear to be more like *Cameron* and *Brown* in that it involved a claim for specific services required by deaf persons. However, interpretation services were auxiliary services required in order to allow deaf persons to benefit equally from the whole range of other insured services, not specific services for the amelioration of their condition (see *Eldridge, supra* note 36 at para. 92). Therefore, the claim was really for equal access to health services generally.

89 Orentlicher, *supra* note 87 at 53.

90 Some authors distinguish between "rationing," which occurs at an individual level, and "resource allocation," which refers to decisions made at a macro or policy level. See M.B. Kapp, "De Facto Health-Care Rationing by Age: The Law has no Remedy" (1998) 19 *J. Legal Med.* 323 at 323, n. 1. This distinction is not relevant for the purposes of this article. The level at which the decision is made will, however, likely affect whether the Charter applies or not.

91 *Supra* note 63 at 462–3.

92 See Orentlicher, *supra* note 87 at 59, citing *United States* v. *University Hospital,* 729 F.2d 144 (2d Cir. 1984). This may apply especially in the context of individual clinical treatment decisions; see Kapp, *supra* note 90 at 346.

93 *Supra* note 3 at para. 127.

94 Orentlicher, *supra* note 87 at 68.

95 *Ibid.* at 69–71 (passage quoted is at 71).

96 B. von Tigerstrom, "Equality Rights and the Allocation of Scarce Resources in Health Care: A Comment on *Cameron* v. *Nova Scotia*" (1999) 11:1 *Constitutional Forum* 30 at 38.

97 *Law, supra* note 27 at para. 39; the three steps are also set out at para. 88, see *supra* note 27 and accompanying text. The test has been applied in subsequent cases, for example, *Granovsky, supra* note 27 at para. 41ff.

99 The majority judgment stated that "I do not think it can be seriously disputed that a person unable to have a child has a physical disability": *Cameron, supra* note 3 at para. 145; see also at para. 175. The minority judgment, in contrast, stated that while in "some contexts this dysfunction would be viewed as a 'disability'" it did not fall within the meaning of disability for the purposes of section 15, "[n]or can a realistic argument be advanced that infertility, if not within the enumerated ground of 'disability', constitutes an analogous ground." *Ibid.* at paras. 265–6.

100 *Cameron, supra* note 3 at para. 173.

101 For discussions of some of this jurisprudence, see von Tigerstrom, *supra* note 96 at 35–7; R.W. Zinn and P.P. Brethour, *The Law of Human Rights in Canada: Practice and Procedure,* looseleaf (Aurora, ON: Canada Law Book, 1996) at 5–9ff; M.D. Lepofsky and J.E. Bickenbach, "Equality Rights and the Physically Handicapped" in A.F. Bayefsky and M. Eberts, *Equality Rights and the Canadian Charter of Rights and Freedoms* (Toronto: Carswell, 1985) 323 at 343–6. The decision of the Supreme

Court of Canada in *Granovsky, supra* note 27, contains an extensive and useful discussion of the ground of disability at paras. 31ff.

102 Lepofsky and Bickenbach, *ibid.* at 345.

103 *Brown, supra* note 63 at 462.

104 *Law, supra* note 27 at paras. 65, 67.

105 *Ibid.* at para. 63.

106 *Brown, supra* note 63 at 457.

107 *Cameron, supra* note 3 at para. 192.

108 *Law, supra* note 27 at para. 70.

109 *Ibid.* at para. 72.

110 *Ibid.* at para. 73. Section 15(2) provides: "Subsection (1) does not preclude any law, program or activity that has as its object the amelioration of conditions of disadvantaged individuals or groups including those that are disadvantaged because of race, national or ethnic origin, colour, religion, sex, age or mental or physical disability."

111 *Ibid.* at para. 74.

112 J. Ross, "*Law v. Canada*: A Convergence of Ways or a New and Uncharted Path?" (Legal Education Society of Alberta Constitutional Cases Seminar, Faculty of Law, University of Alberta, 17 May 2000) [forthcoming in *Constitutional Forum*].

113 See *ibid.*

114 *Law, supra* note 27 at para. 77.

115 *Ibid.* at para. 60.

116 *Cameron, supra* note 3 at para. 202.

117 *Brown, supra* note 63 at 463–4.

118 E.g., *Cameron, supra* note 3.

119 *Schachter* v. *Canada*, [1992] S.C.R. 679 at 709.

120 *Eldridge, supra* note 36 at para. 85, citing *McKinney, supra* note 34, *Egan, supra* note 32.

121 *Supra* note 3 at para. 151.

122 This was a factor in *Eldridge*; see *supra* note 36 at para. 87.

123 *Eldridge, supra* note 36 at para. 92.

124 In *Auton, supra* note 3, the BC Supreme Court found that the denial of funding for treatment for autistic treatment could not be classified as a minimal impairment (at para. 151). The Court characterized it as "the exclusion of effective treatment for autistic children" (at para. 151) and stated that the province "provides no effective treatment for the medical disability of autism" (para. 154). This suggests that if the treatment denied is perceived as being the only or most effective treatment for a particular condition, its exclusion is less likely to be considered a minimal impairment.

125 *Ibid.* at para. 147. It is not clear that the Court in that case considered cost-effectiveness as part of the rational connection test; it is addressed in the context of assessing the government's objective.

126 *Supra* note 45 and accompanying text. The federal government has recently pledged to increase its monitoring of compliance with the Canada Health Act in response to the passage of Bill 11, the Health Care Protection Act, in Alberta.

Health Canada, News Release 2000–46, "Health Minister responds to Bill 11" (11 May 2000). On supervisory mechanisms and the Canada Health Act, see the chapter by Sujit Choudhry in this volume.

127 See *General Comment 14, supra* note 1 at para. 59; *Concluding Observations, supra* note 22 at para. 12; Virginia A. Leary, "Justiciability and Beyond; Complaint Procedures and the Right to Health" (1995) 55 *I.C.J. Rev.* 105. Concerns have been raised in the past about complaints resolution in health care in Alberta, highlighting problems of fragmentation, lack of public awareness, backlog and inconsistency; D. Anderson, *Fractured Voices: A Report on the Fairness Business in Alberta* (Edmonton, AB: Canadian Mental Health Association, Alberta Division, 1995). Since that time, efforts have been made to reform and improve complaints resolution in the Alberta health care system. See Provincial Health Council of Alberta, *Appeal Mechanisms Review: Final Report* (Edmonton, AB: Provincial Health Council of Alberta, 1996); Alberta Health, *Achieving Accountability in Alberta's Health Care System* (Edmonton, AB: Alberta Health, 1998).

128 See, for example, J. Welsh, "Freedom of Expression and the Healthy Society" (1998) 3 *Health & Hum. Rts.* 67.

129 See *General Comment 14, supra* note 1 at para. 27. As part of the efforts of indigenous peoples in Canada to reclaim control over their communities, there has been an ongoing process of transferring control of health programs from the federal government to First Nations and Inuit communities: Health Canada, *A Second Diagnostic on the Health of First Nations and Inuit People in Canada* (November, 1999) at 29–30, online at http://www.hc-sc.gc.ca/msb/fnihp/pdf1/diag2_e.pdf.

6

A NEW DIRECTION IN
MENTAL HEALTH LAW
BRIAN'S LAW AND THE PROBLEMATIC IMPLICATIONS
OF COMMUNITY TREATMENT ORDERS

PETER CARVER

In June 2000 the Ontario Legislature passed Brian's Law,[1] a series of significant amendments to that province's Mental Health Act.[2] The amendment which received most public attention introduced "community treatment orders" into law.[3] Ontario thereby joined Saskatchewan[4] as the only two provinces to employ this mechanism for requiring persons with serious mental illness living in the community to comply with proposed psychiatric treatment. This article seeks to apply a legal analysis to the provisions of Brian's Law for the purpose of examining certain implications of introducing legal "coercion" into community mental health services. In particular, the analysis seeks to provide context to the two principal critiques which have been made of compulsory community treatment laws: (1) that they do not work as intended; (2) that they compromise important individual rights which, in Canada, are guaranteed by the Canadian Charter of Rights and Freedoms.

This Ontario initiative is the most dramatic example to date of a new direction in Canadian mental health law reform. The distinctive feature of mental health statutes is their coercive nature: they provide authority for the compulsory delivery of medical treatment to persons who have not sought and may actively not wish to receive treatment. This coercion has traditionally been achieved through involuntary hospitalization, combined with authority to provide treatment in the absence of the patient's consent. In the latter third of the twentieth century, reform in mental health law meant ameliorating the coercive aspects of the law, by expanding procedural and substantive legal rights of mental patients. In Canada, such reforms included narrowing the criteria for civil commitment, increasing access to information on legal rights and representation, and facilitating administrative tribunal review of physicians' decisions to detain and treat. Reforms in the law coincided with "de-institutionalization," the significant downsizing of large psychiatric hospital facilities with long-term patient populations, and a consequent emphasis on community-based services.

In recent years, criticism of law reform directed at "patients' rights" and of the de-institutionalization of the mental health system has grown. Many people associate these developments with abandoning care for persons with serious mental illness, and hold them partly responsible for the problem of homelessness in Canada's urban centres. An increasingly strong voice expressing concerns of this kind comes from organizations which represent family members of the seriously mentally ill. Groups like the Schizophrenia Society have joined forces with members of the psychiatric profession to raise important questions about gaps in the mental health service system, including difficulties in obtaining intervention and treatment for relatives living in the community. One of the major concerns of this constituency is that of treatment noncompliance, which is viewed as a significant contributor to the "revolving door" phenomenon in mental health service delivery: persons are hospitalized at a point of acute mental illness, when their symptoms are stabilized through the use of anti-psychotic medications; once stabilized and no longer committable, they are discharged back into the community; no longer under legal constraint, they stop taking medications, resulting in deterioration to the point of again requiring hospitalization. Legislative reforms, perceived and actual, which have expanded patients' rights, have come in for a large share of the blame for problems of this kind:[5]

> The Mental Health Act [of Ontario] is a practical and moral failure. It hinders the provision of better mental health care to the people who most require it, thus holding back mental health reform. It prevents us from acting compassionately towards people who are suffering, sometimes horribly, from the effects of untreated mental illness. It denies incapable people access to necessary care and treatment. It deprives people of liberty who could be treated in the community, subject to some legal constraints, but who must instead be held in a hospital. And it threatens public safety by hindering the provision of care that might prevent people from becoming so ill they pose a threat of harm to others.

One goal of this constituency has been to broaden the grounds for civil commitment to allow for intervention before a person's illness reaches the point of causing imminent physical harm to self or others. A second goal has been to extend a degree of control over the ongoing treatment of persons with mental illness living in the community, outside psychiatric hospital facilities.[6]

The community treatment order appears to be a straightforward response to the second objective. It invokes the law to require compliance with psychiatric treatment. By complying, persons with chronic mental illness have a better chance of controlling their symptoms. The vicious cycle of repeat hospitalizations can be broken. The intentions are humane and laudable. The difficulty is that law is often a blunt instrument to bring to bear on complex public health issues. Laws intended to control behaviour viewed by others as self-destructive rarely work as intended. At worst, they may come to stigmatize an underlying illness rather than the behaviour it causes. At best, they may simply be ineffective.

Ontario and Saskatchewan are not the first jurisdictions to legislate compulsory community treatment. Forms of community treatment orders have existed for several years in the laws of most American states.[7] The term used in the US is "outpatient committal," or OPC. These statutory provisions have given rise to a considerable literature, both in the fields of legal scholarship,[8] and in psychology and psychiatry.[9] A striking feature of the literature is the degree to which scepticism and doubt exist about the efficacy of outpatient committal. While a detailed survey of this literature is beyond the scope of this article, a few comments about it may help frame the discussion to follow.

Legal writers have noted that the term "OPC" covers a considerable range in the nature of legislative schemes directed at requiring persons with mental illness living in the community to comply with treatment plans. Several have sought to distinguish between the different schemes:[10]

1. Conditional discharge: a person already involuntarily hospitalized is released into the community, on terms and conditions devised by the hospital treatment team, while remaining under the original commitment order;

2. Diversion: a person who would otherwise be committed to a psychiatric hospital is instead allowed to remain in the community, on terms and conditions related to following psychiatric treatment;

3. Preventive commitment: a person who would not otherwise meet criteria for involuntary hospitalization is nevertheless ordered to follow terms and conditions of a treatment plan, in order to prevent their deteriorating to the point of hospitalization.

In Canadian terms, "conditional discharge" provisions already exist in all provincial mental health statutes, usually under the rubric of "leave of absence." The CTO schemes in Ontario and Saskatchewan are not leave-of-absence provisions. A question addressed toward the end of this article is whether they more closely resemble the diversion or the preventive commitment model.

Commonly noted problems with OPC laws include the wide range of utilization among states, with many states making rare use of the law;[11] the difficulty in enforcing OPC orders, and the absence of enforcement mechanisms in many states;[12] the "limited positive outcomes," understood in such terms as reduced hospital re-admission rates, reported by many empirical studies, and the difficulty of measuring outcomes.[13] One study describes the latter as a difficulty in separating the effects of intensive community treatment from effects resulting specifically from the order to comply with an intensive treatment program.[14] It concludes:[15]

> It is clear that legislation authorizing outpatient commitment is not in itself sufficient to establish an effective outpatient commitment program. The legislation must also specifically address issues such as liability [of physicians], fiscal support, and fiscal incentives and establish clear consequences for noncompliance. Many of the outpatient laws now in effect amount to nothing more than paper tigers without teeth.

The complex statutory provisions enacted in Ontario to create the community treatment order scheme give rise to similar doubts. As a legal measure intended to produce health results, CTOs warrant legal analysis. As a coercive measure which restricts personal choice and liberty, that analysis necessarily involves consideration of the Charter of Rights and Freedoms. The Charter is a significant part of the legal context in which CTOs will be implemented. The argument below suggests that this context properly limits the ways in which community treatment orders can be enforced. If enforcement is illusory, the effectiveness of a law intended to make people comply with medical treatment they do not want, for whatever reason including illness itself, is thrown very much into question.[16]

I. The Community Treatment Order: Legislative Context

Community treatment orders need to be understood in the context of mental health law and, in particular, the context provided by the traditional areas in which coercion has long existed: (1) civil commitment, or involuntary hospitalization; and (2) treatment without consent. Following a review of these two areas of legal coercion, including their status under the Charter, the amendments introduced in Ontario by Brian's Law will be summarized. This section of the paper concludes by setting out certain dilemmas involved in the design of CTO provisions.

A. The Context of Mental Health Law

Mental health law in Canada is a matter of provincial jurisdiction. Consequently, there is considerable variety from province to province in the language and operational details of mental health law. The general structure of the provincial statutes tends, however, to be common. Given its subject matter, this article refers mostly to legislation in Ontario. Where helpful to illustrate a particular point or anomaly, reference will be made to the legislation of other provinces.

1. Involuntary Hospitalization: Civil commitment has a substantive and a procedural dimension. The substantive goes to the criteria for committal. Gerald Robertson has identified three criteria for committal to hospital commonly found in provincial mental health statutes: (a) a diagnosis of mental illness or mental disorder; (b) "dangerousness," in the sense that a causal link must be identified between the mental disorder and the person's posing a danger, or risk, to his or her own or others' safety; (c) that the person require treatment in a psychiatric facility, and not be suitable for admission to hospital on a voluntary basis.[17] Each of these three criteria is found in the pre-amendment Ontario Mental Health Act in the following form:

> 20. (1) The attending physician, after observing and examining a person who is the subject of an application for assessment under section 15 or who is the subject of an order under section 32, ...
>
> (c) shall admit the person as an involuntary patient by completing and filing with the officer in charge a certificate of involuntary admission if the attending physician is of the opinion both that the person is suffering from mental disorder of a nature or quality that likely will result in,
>
> (i) serious bodily harm to the person,
>
> (ii) serious bodily harm to another person, or
>
> (iii) imminent and serious physical impairment of the person,
>
> unless the person remains in the custody of a psychiatric facility and that the person is not suitable for admission as an informal or voluntary patient.

The general procedural scheme for civil commitment in Canada has three principal stages: (1) intervention in the community; (2) examination by one or two physicians or psychiatrists for purpose of identifying whether the person meets commitment criteria; and (3), review of a committal by an administrative tribunal, on application by the involuntary patient.[18] In Ontario, such reviews are conducted by the Consent and Capacity Board.

The traditional coercive measures of involuntary hospitalization and treatment without consent implicate individual rights protected in the Charter, most particularly sections 7 and 9:[19]

7. Everyone has the right to life, liberty and security of the person and the right not to be deprived thereof except in accordance with the principles of fundamental justice.

9. Everyone has the right not to be arbitrarily detained.

Given that the interference with these rights represented by mental health laws is premised, in large part, on a person's having a mental disability, they should also fall under the scrutiny of equality rights analysis under section 15(1):

15. (1) Every individual is equal before and under the law and has the right to the equal protection and equal benefit of the law without discrimination based on race, national or ethnic origin, colour, religion, sex, age or mental or physical disability.

As several commentators have pointed out, however, the impact of the Charter on Canada's mental health laws has been relatively limited to date.[20] This is more true of the issue of civil committal, or involuntary hospitalization, than it is of committal under the Criminal Code, and of the right to refuse treatment. Most challenges to involuntary hospitalization have dealt with the procedures employed in committal. A relative handful have addressed the substantive committal criteria. In only one case was the challenge successful. In *Thwaites*,[21] the Manitoba Court of Appeal struck down the existing criteria in that province's Mental Health Act. The Court ruled the criteria permitted arbitrary detention by not setting objective standards related to mental condition and risk of harm, but merely authorized committal where in the opinion of a physician a person "should be confined as a patient at a psychiatric facility." The Court rejected the argument that it was appropriate for the legislature to essentially delegate the issue of when a person's liberty could be restricted on the grounds of mental illness entirely to the professional judgement of individual medical practitioners. Philp J.A. stated: "I do not think it can be said that, in the absence of a dangerousness or like standard, the provisions impair as little as possible the right of a person 'not to be arbitrarily detained.'"[22]

The committal criteria in BC's Mental Health Act were challenged in 1993 in *McCorkell*.[23] The plaintiff argued that section 20 of the Act violated sections 7 and 9 of the Charter by authorizing committal where two physicians certified that the person examined "requires care, supervision and control in a Provincial mental health facility for his own protection or for the protection of others." The plaintiff's position was that the provision was unconstitutional for vagueness, and that only criteria based strictly on dangerousness could meet the standard for civil restriction of an individual's liberty. Further, it was argued, measures for involuntarily hospitalizing a person in his or her own interests, as opposed to the protection of public safety, should appropriately proceed by way of guardianship law, requiring court order, with all the procedural protections afforded by the judicial process. Donald J. rejected these arguments. In particular, he rejected the plaintiff's attempt to draw an analogy between criminal law, in which the state's power to restrict liberty is circumscribed by extensive substantive and procedural protections for accused persons, and mental health law: "Statutes dealing with criminal law are penal in nature; incarceration is a punishment of culpable individuals and serves the objectives of public safety and denunciation of crime. The Mental Health Act involuntarily detains people only for the purpose of treatment; the punitive element is wholly absent."[24]

No Canadian court has yet found that "dangerousness" to self and others is the minimum basis for involuntary committal required by the Constitution.[25] Isabel Grant writes that judges have repeatedly justified civil commitment laws under the state's *parens patriae* power—i.e., the state's responsibility to protect vulnerable persons who are unable to protect themselves.[26] Grant posits that because they emphasize the therapeutic purpose of mental health legislation, Canadian judges refuse to analogize civil commitment to detention under the criminal law, with all its protections for the liberty interests of accused persons.

This idea is reflected in an emerging doctrine in Supreme Court equality rights jurisprudence: that government programs which are intended to ameliorate the "factual" disadvantages imposed by disability do not constitute discrimination. In *Eaton*,[27] the Supreme Court rejected a challenge to an education appeal board's decision to place a child with cerebral palsy in a segregated class placement, in large part because the Court viewed the placement as an effort by school officials to accommodate the child's special educational needs resulting from her disability. In *Law*, Iacobucci J. described the *Eaton* decision in these terms:[28]

> Another possibly important factor will be the ameliorative purpose or effects of impugned legislation or other state action upon a more disadvantaged person or group in society. As stated by Sopinka J. in *Eaton*, supra, at para. 66: "the purpose of s. 15(1) of the Charter is not only to prevent discrimination by the attribution of stereotypical characteristics to individuals, but also to ameliorate the position of groups within Canadian society who have suffered disadvantage by exclusion from mainstream society."

A similar analysis appears in *Winko*,[29] a case dealing with criminal committal of persons found "not criminally responsible by reason of mental disorder" ("NCRMD") under the Criminal Code. The plaintiff alleged that the failure of Parliament to "cap" the period for committal of NCRMD accused at the maximum sentence for the offence giving rise to committal reflected the discriminatory nature of the Code provisions. The Court rejected the argument, finding the individualized assessment called for by the Code to be the "very antithesis of discrimination":[30]

> It does not disadvantage or treat unequally the NCR accused, but rather recognizes the NCR accused's disability, incapacity and particular personal situation, and based upon that recognition, creates a system of individualized assessment and treatment that deliberately undermines the invidious stereotype of the mentally ill as dangerous.

2. Treatment Without Consent: The issue of consent to treatment is one of the most vexed issues in mental health law. The starting place for an analysis of consent is the common law principle that every person has the right to be free from interference with his or her physical integrity.[31] In the absence of the person's consent, any such interference, including medical treatment, constitutes the tort of battery. To be valid, consent must be given by a person who is competent to consent. Competence to consent to medical treatment is the ability to understand the nature and consequences of the treatment, and of not receiving the treatment.[32]

A person who is incapable of giving consent to treatment is at risk of not receiving medical treatment. One of the more significant areas of legislative reform in Canada in recent years has been the proliferation of provincial guardianship and health consent statutes which seek, among other things, to fill this "gap" by providing mechanisms through which "substitute decision-makers" (SDMs), usually close family members, can be recognized for the purposes of making health decisions for those unable to do so on their own behalf.[33] Those statutes have generally also instructed SDMs to follow the wishes respecting medical treatment expressed by a person before becoming incapable. This allows for pre-planning one's own medical treatment in anticipation of later incapacity.

For a long time, Canadian mental health statutes authorized directors or physicians of psychiatric hospitals to provide treatment to involuntarily committed patients without obtaining their consent to treatment. It was assumed that serious mental illness rendered a person incapable of giving consent to treatment. Two legal developments have challenged this assumption. The first is a new understanding of decisionmaking capacity, which treats each area of decision-making in a person's life as a distinct area of competency. That is, "global incompetence" should not be assumed on the basis of an incompetence in one area of activity, nor on the basis of a particular mental disability.[34]

Second, section 7 of the Charter makes the right to consent to treatment a constitutionally protected right to "security of the person." Legislation that purports to deny the right of a capable person to refuse medical treatment may constitute a violation of section 7, subject to its being found in accordance with the principles of fundamental justice, or to be saved pursuant to section 1.

Due to the often episodic nature of mental illness, recognition of the right to refuse treatment has particular importance with respect to wishes expressed at a time of treatment competence. This was the issue in *Fleming* v. *Reid*.[35] Statutory provisions then in existence in Ontario recognized that psychiatric treatment for an incapable person committed under the Mental Health Act could be permitted if consent was obtained from the authorized substitute decision-maker. That person, however, was obliged to act on the treatment wishes of the person expressed at a time of competence. *Fleming* concerned two patients, each of whom expressed wishes at a time when they were competent that they did not wish the treatment that psychiatrists later proposed. The substitute decision-makers, acting under statutory obligation, refused treatment. The psychiatrists applied to the Review Board to override the refusal, pursuant to then s. 35 of the Mental Health Act, which authorized an override "in the best interests" of the patient. The Ontario Court of Appeal struck down this provision of the Mental Health Act. The Court ruled that by authorizing treatment in the face of a competent refusal, the provision violated section 7. As the statute provided this could be done without a hearing into whether the patient's competent wishes should be honoured, the violation was not in accord with the principles of fundamental justice, nor could it be saved under section 1.

Ontario law has since incorporated the *Fleming* principle.[36] The Consent and Capacity Board does not have the authority to override a competent treatment refusal. At most, a party may apply to the board to challenge whether a patient's refusal of treatment was expressed at a time of competence. The situation in other provinces varies greatly. At the opposite end from Ontario (and Nova Scotia) is British Columbia, which has retained in its Mental Health Act a long-standing provision that the authorization of treatment for an involuntary patient by the director of a psychiatric facility is deemed to be given with the consent of the patient.[37] In the middle are provinces like Alberta and Manitoba, which recognize an involuntary patient's right to refuse treatment, but authorize review boards, on application, to override a competent refusal in the patient's best interests. Those statutory provisions are vulnerable to Charter challenge on the basis of the principles developed in *Fleming*.[38]

Saskatchewan is the lone province to make it part of the substantive criteria for involuntary hospitalization that an individual be incapable of giving or withholding consent to treatment. This helps to avoid the dilemma which presently exists in Ontario—i.e., the possibility of committing a person to hospital who may be found competent to refuse psychiatric treatment.

B. The CTO Provisions in Brian's Law

Brian's Law makes a number of changes to Ontario's mental health legislation, and to associated provisions in the province's Health Care Consent Act, 1996.[39] One amendment removes the word "imminent" in section 20(1)(c)(iii), presumably to permit intervention at an earlier point in the anticipation of a person's serious physical impairment.

This paper is concerned more with two amendments that create a statutory regime targeted specifically at "revolving-door clients" of the mental health system. The first sets out new grounds for involuntary hospitalization which operate in addition to the existing harm criteria. The second series of amendments deals with the provisions of the new community treatment order. These two areas of legislative amendment are closely linked, and to some extent the implementation of each appears dependent on the other. The new involuntary committal criteria appear in section 20.1:

(1.1) The attending physician shall complete a certificate of involuntary admission or a certificate of renewal if, after examining the patient, he or she is of the opinion that the patient,

(a) has previously received treatment for mental disorder of an ongoing or recurring nature that, when not treated, is of a nature or quality that likely will result in serious bodily harm to the person or to another person or substantial mental or physical deterioration of the person or serious physical impairment of the person;

(b) has shown clinical improvement as a result of the treatment;

(c) is suffering from the same mental disorder as the one for which he or she previously received treatment or from a mental disorder that is similar to the previous one;

(d) given the person's history of mental disorder and current mental or physical condition, is likely to cause serious bodily harm to himself or herself or to another person or is likely to suffer substantial mental or physical deterioration or serious physical impairment;

(e) has been found incapable, within the meaning of the Health Care Consent Act, 1996, of consenting to his or her treatment in a psychiatric facility and the consent of his or her substitute decision-maker has been obtained; and

(f) is not suitable for admission or continuation as an informal or voluntary patient.

This provision creates a new class of persons subject to civil commitment in Ontario that might be termed the "treatable, chronically mentally ill." For members of this class, the history of their mental disorder, and of its treatment, serves as a significant predictor of harm. This largely replaces the need for the observation of present behaviour and conduct on which to base the prediction. Other matters to note: the previous treatment is not described as having been provided in a psychiatric hospital so may refer to treatment in the community, including that provided under a community treatment order. Second, a person is only committable under this provision if he or she has already been determined to be incompetent to consent to treatment, and consent has been obtained from a substitute decision-maker. This appears to eliminate the possibility of committing a person to hospital who could then not be treated because of a valid treatment refusal. Potentially difficult questions, such as how to identify a record of past successful treatment, or what "a mental disorder that is similar to the previous one" means in practice, await physicians relying on this section.

The overall import of section 20.1 is nevertheless clear: it provides a means of hospitalizing individuals who are known to the mental health system, in circumstances in which their condition and behaviour might not result in committal under the harm criteria set out in section 20.

The community treatment order provisions in Brian's Law are extensive. Most are incorporated into a new section 33.1 of the Mental Health Act. The criteria for issuing a CTO are set out in ss. 33.1(4):

> (4) A physician may issue or renew a community treatment order under this section if,
>> (a) during the previous three-year period, the person,
>>> (i) has been a patient in a psychiatric facility on two or more separate occasions or for a cumulative period of 30 days or more during that three-year period, or
>>> (ii) has been the subject of a previous community treatment order under this section;
>> (b) the person or his or her substitute decisionmaker, the physician who is considering issuing or renewing the community treatment order and any other health practitioner or person involved in the person's treatment or care and supervision have developed a community treatment plan for the person;
>> (c) within the 72-hour period before entering into the community treatment plan, the physician has examined the person and is of the opinion, based on the examination and any other relevant facts communicated to the physician, that,
>>> (i) the person is suffering from mental disorder such that he or she needs continuing treatment or care and continuing supervision while living in the community,
>>> (ii) the person meets the criteria for the completion of an application for psychiatric assessment under subsection 15 (1) or (1.1) where the person is not currently a patient in a psychiatric facility,

> (iii) if the person does not receive continuing treatment or care and continuing supervision while living in the community, he or she is likely, because of mental disorder, to cause serious bodily harm to himself or herself or to another person or to suffer substantial mental or physical deterioration of the person or serious physical impairment of the person,
>
> (iv) the person is able to comply with the community treatment plan contained in the community treatment order, and
>
> (v) the treatment or care and supervision required under the terms of the community treatment order are available in the community;
>
> (d) the physician has consulted with the health practitioners or other persons proposed to be named in the community treatment plan;
>
> (e) subject to subsection (5), the physician is satisfied that the person subject to the order and his or her substitute decision-maker, if any, have consulted with a rights adviser and have been advised of their legal rights; and
>
> (f) the person or his or her substitute decision-maker consents to the community treatment plan in accordance with the rules for consent under the Health Care Consent Act, 1996.

The target group for CTOs is, again, the "revolving-door client." The definition here is more specific, in that to be subject to a CTO a person must have been hospitalized on at least two occasions or for thirty days or more within the previous three years. The legislation does not limit the previous hospitalizations to involuntary committals. Therefore, individuals who voluntarily admit themselves to psychiatric facilities can thereby become eligible for CTO committal.

The necessary components of the "community treatment plan," to be incorporated in the CTO, are set out in section 33.7:

> 33.7 A community treatment plan shall contain at least the following:
>
> 1. A plan of treatment for the person subject to the community treatment order.
>
> 2. Any conditions relating to the treatment or care and supervision of the person.
>
> 3. The obligations of the person subject to the community treatment order.
>
> 4. The obligations of the substitute decision-maker, if any.
>
> 5. The name of the physician, if any, who has agreed to accept respon-

sibility for the general supervision and management of the community treatment order under subsection 33.5 (2).

6. The names of all persons or organizations who have agreed to provide treatment or care and supervision under the community treatment plan and their obligations under the plan.

The CTO expires after six months unless it is renewed (s. 33.1(11) and (12)). Express obligations are placed on the person subject to the CTO (hereafter, the "CTO subject") to comply with the community treatment plan, or on the SDM to make "best efforts" to obtain the subject's compliance (ss. 33.1 (6)(d) and 33.1(9)). Should the CTO subject fail to comply with the terms of the CTO, or should he or she or the substitute decision-maker withdraw consent to the community treatment plan, the attending physician may issue an "order for examination" which serves as a thirty-day authority for police officers to apprehend the person and bring him or her to the physician for an examination (ss. 33.3 and 33.4). The provisions dealing with compliance are discussed in greater detail below. Finally, the Act includes a mechanism to ensure that the implementation of community treatment orders in Ontario is subject to early and periodic review by the Minister of Health.[40]

The Saskatchewan scheme differs from that in Ontario in the following pertinent respects. A person is liable to being made subject to a CTO if he or she has been hospitalized in a psychiatric hospital on three occasions, or for a cumulative total of sixty days, in the previous two years. Only persons who are incompetent to consent to treatment can be the subject of a CTO, and no provision is made for a requirement to obtain the consent of a substitute decision-maker. To be effective, a CTO must be "validated" by a second physician. The CTO remains in effect for three months and is renewable. The other significant difference between the Ontario and Saskatchewan mental health statutes is that the latter does not contain involuntary hospitalization criteria for the "treatable, chronically mentally ill" class.[41]

C. Dilemmas of Design

The community treatment order provision in the Ontario Mental Health Act is introduced by a statement of purpose which seems unusual in its detail. It was added following committee hearings, and may well represent the drafters' attempt to pin down the elusive nature of the Legislature's creation:

33.1(3) The purpose of a community treatment order is to provide a person who suffers from a serious mental disorder with a comprehensive plan of community-based treatment or care and supervision that is less restrictive than being detained in a psychiatric facility. Without limiting the generality of the foregoing, a purpose is to provide such a plan for a person who, as a result of his or her serious mental disorder, experiences this pattern: The person is admitted to a psychiatric facility where his or her condition is usually stabilized; after being released from the facility, the person often stops the treatment or care and supervision; the person's condition changes and, as a result, the person must be re-admitted to a psychiatric facility.

The statement of purpose contains within it two arguable propositions. These go to the heart of what the CTO seeks to accomplish. First, is an "order" necessary to the provision of a comprehensive plan of community-based treatment or care and supervision? Surely such a plan could be provided in the absence of an order. This could be done in the context of a voluntary therapeutic relationship. The purpose of the CTO is therefore not to provide a treatment plan, but to produce *compliance* with the treatment plan. The community treatment order is justified to the extent, and only to the extent, that it produces compliance where this previously did not occur. A significant problem is how it is conceived as doing this. A legal provision is usually thought to produce compliance with a specified course of conduct by imposing sanctions on noncompliance. The sanction is the legal consequence of failing to comply with the legal obligation and, as such, is exterior to the mandated course of conduct. In the case of the CTO, however, imposing a separate sanction for failure to comply with a treatment plan would have connotations of punishing a person because of his or her illness. This means that any sanctions for noncompliance with a CTO must make sense both in medical and legal terms. How can this be achieved?

The second dilemma is captured by the question: In what way is a CTO a "less restrictive" alternative to hospitalization? In order to be so, it would seem to need to be an alternative to hospitalization that is available. This is somewhat inconsistent if the purpose of the legislation is to require treatment in the community at a point earlier than when detention in hospital is considered necessary. If committal criteria are relaxed in order to make hospital and community true alternatives, does this represent an expansion of the coerciveness of mental health laws, as opposed to creating a less restrictive alternative to hospitalization?

These two dilemmas, in the context of Brian's Law, are further explored below.

II. The Dilemma of Coercing Treatment Compliance

Section 33.1(3) of the Ontario Mental Health Act states that community treatment orders are intended to provide a "comprehensive plan of community-based treatment or care and supervision." This phrase implies that a CTO not intended to be used to support a bare treatment plan that merely calls for a person to appear for appointments to receive medications. It implies that the CTO will support plans that involve intensive interaction between the CTO subject and a treatment team. This should include the "assertive community treatment" (ACT) method for providing services to persons with serious chronic mental illness. The Ontario government's major initiative in mental health prior to introducing Brian's Law involved funding fifty-one ACT teams throughout the province. Assertive community treatment is a recognized approach to supporting persons with serious and chronic mental illness living in the community.[42] It views the provision of anti-psychotic medications as only a part of the interaction with the client. Psychiatric nurses, occupational therapists and social workers deliver other parts of the program which are intended to support the client in developing and maintaining daily living and vocational skills. Providing these services by outreach visits to the client, rather than by meeting the client in office appointments, is an important feature of ACT programs. The main drawback to these programs is their expense, given the low ratio of professionals to clients. Assertive community treatment programs and other forms of comprehensive community mental health service address themselves to several of the very problems which can be seen as giving rise to noncompliance with treatment. They do this through outreach, intensive interaction, ongoing discussion of events in the client's life, maintaining housing and employment or other vocational activity. To the extent that CTOs are issued in conjunction with comprehensive programs of this kind, it may be difficult to separate the effects on compliance of the CTO from that of the program itself. If the precise purpose of the CTO is to enhance compliance with treatment, it is crucial to understand how it may, or may not, accomplish this goal.

This may seem an odd question to ask. The CTO is a statutory "order," issued by a physician or physicians, which expressly calls for compliance. In other words, it looks like any other lawful order. One does not usually ask in what way an order is compulsory. The expectation is that a mandatory order will be obeyed. Sanctions for breaching a mandatory provision of the law are generally of secondary interest.

The question has relevance, however, given the particular problem the CTO is intended to address, and the nature of the activity—medical treatment—which it seeks to mandate. The CTO is directed at a perceived problem of treatment noncompliance. The target population is one that presumably exhibits discontent or difficulty in maintaining a proposed treatment regimen. Since noncompliance is the very problem at which the CTO is directed, the means with which the legislation seeks to obtain compliance with its terms has special significance. To state this issue in another way, why should a CTO produce greater compliance with psychiatric treatment in the community than the offer of treatment in the first place? The answer involves considering two matters: (1) the role of consent in a community treatment plan; (2) sanctions for noncompliance with a CTO. Following that, a further possible source of compliance is examined: the statutory obligations imposed on treatment providers.

A. The Issue of Consent

In Ontario, *Fleming* v. *Reid* and the Health Care Consent Act enacted following that decision have resulted in a situation in which a competent refusal of treatment cannot be overridden. Brian's Law deals with this situation by providing that a person who is competent to consent to treatment can only be made subject to a CTO if he or she *consents* to the community treatment plan which is incorporated in the order. The implications of this approach are intriguing. In essence, it means that any person who is treatment-competent must consent to be ordered to comply with a treatment plan. For these individuals, in what way can it be said that a CTO is an "order," or has coercive authority? After all, the coercive power of the state is not generally imposed only with the agreement of the individual on whom it is to be imposed.

Some might argue that a consensual CTO scheme allows willing individuals to bind themselves or contract to follow a certain course of conduct, with sanctions or penalties should they fail to do so. Consent to health care is not, however, conceived as creating a contractual relationship. Consent to treatment can be freely withdrawn—i.e., withdrawn without sanction—at any point prior to the provision of treatment's becoming physically irreversible.[43] The Ontario legislation in fact allows a treatment-competent person to withdraw his or her consent to a CTO at any time. It does, however, impose a statutory sanction on such a withdrawal: on being notified of withdrawal from the CTO, the attending physician may issue a CTO warrant to apprehend the person for an examination.

One is left to ask whether this scheme justifies the use of a coercive approach. A valid consent to treatment is understood as one that is given freely, not under threat or pressure. If a person is perfectly content to consent to a CTO, why is the CTO even necessary? The person and the treatment provider(s) might just as well, and perhaps more easily, enter into the "usual" consensual arrangement for receiving treatment. This leaves one uncomfortable implication: the benefit of the CTO for treatment-competent persons is the unspoken idea that consent will be pressured by an express or implied threat of involuntary hospitalization if the individual does not agree to a CTO. Consent given under pressure, however, may not be valid. It also may have implications for Charter rights, a matter discussed in section III.

Under the Saskatchewan legislation, a CTO is made available only with respect to persons who are incompetent to give or withhold consent to treatment.[44] This is consistent with that province's criteria for civil commitment, which apply only to incompetent persons. It should be noted, however, that a degree of mental competence must exist if CTOs are to provide any benefit whatsoever. That is, it must be assumed that a CTO subject is competent to understand that he or she is being placed under an order to comply, and what compliance requires in the particular case. Otherwise, it is not "compliance" that is being sought, but simply an order authorizing certain things to be done to a person who is unable to understand what they are or why they are being done. Indeed, both the Ontario and Saskatchewan statutes make it a requirement for issuing a CTO that the physician find the person able to comply with the CTO. It has been suggested that this demands a refined series of assessments that may be difficult to operationalize.[45]

In Ontario, the CTO provisions state that where a person is incompetent to consent to treatment, consent to the community treatment plan in a CTO may be given by a substitute decision-maker. This appears consistent with the scheme set out in that province's Health Care Consent Act. It is not clear, however, whether the latter statute authorizes a SDM to consent to "care and supervision," which might be contemplated as part of a community treatment plan, but which would appear to be beyond what is meant by "treatment" in a strict sense. The role of a SDM in consenting on a person's behalf to a "comprehensive plan of treatment or care and supervision" suggests an ongoing role and responsibility for that person, unlike the more precise, time-limited intervention generally contemplated by guardianship legislation. This is reinforced by the obligation on the SDM to make "best efforts" to obtain the CTO subject's compliance. The later provision appears to make the SDM, likely to be a close family member, not just a giver of consent, but an enforcer of the CTO. This may create a conflict of interest for the SDM who, in the absence of previously expressed competent wishes, is directed by the Health Care Consent Act to make decisions in the person's best interests, first taking into account the person's values and beliefs.[46]

B. The Issue of Enforcement

Quite apart from the issue of consent, how is the CTO is understood to be enforceable? The simplest answer also goes to voluntariness: people are generally law-abiding, and willingly comply with lawful orders. People with mental illness should be considered no less likely to comply with legal obligations than anyone else. This should not be discounted as a possible basis for success of certain CTO orders. Persons who might otherwise drift away from treatment could well continue with it if they are legally required to do so.

However, if compliance with psychiatric treatment is as significant a problem as the passage of Brian's Law would suggest, voluntariness seems a thin reed on which to rely. Most laws require sanctions to be effective in the long run. This would seem at least as likely to be the case where dealing with "noncompliant" behaviour is the objective of the law. Certainly, ambiguity over enforcement mechanisms for OPC provisions has been cited as a reason for their relative disuse, and possibly for their ineffectiveness, in some American states.[47]

What sanctions exist to enforce CTOs in Ontario and Saskatchewan? The first point to make is the obvious one that the usual means of enforcing an "order," the contempt power of the superior courts, is not available. First, CTOs are issued by physicians, not by courts. Neither province has purported to make the CTO an order that can be filed in court and have the force of a court order. The penal nature of a contempt recourse would, in any event, seem wholly inappropriate to a therapeutic measure like the CTO.

This latter point is crucial. It would also apply, it is submitted, with respect to any thought of making involuntary hospitalization the "automatic" consequence of a person's breaching the terms of a CTO. The conceptual and constitutional foundation for civil commitment in Canadian law does not permit committal to hospital for other than a person's meeting statutory criteria related to therapeutic need. This would certainly exclude committal for noncompliance with the terms of a CTO.

The Saskatchewan and Ontario statutes do not, in fact, make committal the consequence of noncompliance with the terms of a CTO. Rather, they provide that, in the event of perceived noncompliance, the attending physician may issue an order authorizing the apprehension of the CTO subject for the purpose of bringing him or her to the physician for an examination.[48] The Ontario provision reads as follows:

> 33.3(1) If a physician who issued or renewed a community treatment order has reasonable cause to believe that the person subject to the order has failed to comply with his or her obligations under subsection 33.1 (9), the physician may, subject to subsection (2), issue an order for examination of the person in the prescribed form.
>
> (2) The physician shall not issue an order for examination under subsection (1) unless,
>
> (a) he or she has reasonable cause to believe that the criteria set out in subclauses 33.1 (4) (c) (i), (ii) and (iii) continue to be met; and
>
> (b) reasonable efforts have been made to,
>
> > (i) locate the person,
> >
> > (ii) inform the person of the failure to comply or, if the person is incapable within the meaning of the Health Care Consent Act, 1996, inform the person's substitute decision-maker of the failure,
> >
> > (iii) inform the person or the substitute decision-maker of the possibility that the physician may issue an order for examination and of the possible consequences; and

(iv) provide assistance to the person to comply with the terms
of the order.

(3) An order for examination issued under subsection (1) is sufficient
authority, for 30 days after it is issued, for a police officer to take the
person named in it into custody and then promptly to the physician
who issued the order.

(4) The physician shall promptly examine the person to determine
whether,

    (a) the physician should make an application for a psychiatric
assessment of the person under section 15;

    (b) the physician should issue another community treatment
order where the person, or his or her substitute decision-maker,
consents to the community treatment plan;

or

    (c) the person should be released without being subject to a com-
munity treatment order.

This power to issue a form of warrant for the noncomplying CTO subject
is the sole mechanism enforcing compliance in the two statues. While
involuntary committal might well result from an examination by the attending
physician, this is not necessarily the outcome. It would ensue only if the
noncompliant CTO subject was assessed as meeting the criteria for committal
that apply generally, irrespective of the existence of a CTO. In fact, in the
Ontario statute, the examination cannot itself result in a person's being
certified, but only to an application for the further procedural step of a
psychiatric assessment.

The possibility that in Ontario the noncompliant CTO subject will, on
examination, be found committable to hospital is increased by two factors: first,
a physician is required to form an opinion that the subject is likely
committable before issuing an order for examination (hereafter, the "CTO
warrant"). The Saskatchewan legislation differs in this respect, in that
noncompliance alone is sufficient basis for the order for apprehension. Second,
the new section 20.1 of the Ontario Mental Health Act—the "treatable,
chronically mental ill" provision—has added grounds for committal which are
similar to the grounds for issuing a CTO. If a person was made subject to a
CTO, that person likely fulfills several of the criteria set out in s. 20.1.

The fact, common to both jurisdictions, that the sole enforcement
mechanism for noncompliance is the CTO warrant, a form of expedited
process for authorizing police officers to convey a person for a mental
examination, is not insignificant. Certainly, one of the consistent complaints of
family members of chronically mental ill persons is the difficulty they
encounter in obtaining help, including from police, to get their unwilling
relative to a physician or to hospital when symptoms of acute illness appear.

The question with which this discussion began must nevertheless be asked again: in what way does this scheme enhance community treatment? The success of the CTO warrant process in producing either better treatment compliance, or at least earlier intervention with persons whose condition may be deteriorating in the community, seems itself likely to depend on several factors linked to program design. These include the responsiveness of police officials to acting promptly on CTO warrants; the degree to which physicians are able to distinguish noncompliance from "slip-ups" arising from a host of factors, many of which are endemic to poverty—missed transportation connections, loss of housing, missed telephone communication, etc.—and the ease with which noncompliant CTO subjects can be physically located. What most of these factors relate to is the close monitoring involved in an intensive treatment program. Only if the treatment plan keeps the treatment team in active and frequent communication with the CTO subject is the CTO warrant process likely to function well.

A treatment team providing services to a person without benefit of a CTO would seem as likely to become aware of deterioration in a person's mental or physical condition requiring hospitalization as a team operating under a CTO. Having the person on a CTO might permit an easier apprehension for the purpose of obtaining an examination and assessment; the difference may well be marginal.

C. Treatment Provider Obligations: A Right to Treatment?

Brian's Law provides one further mechanism by which the CTO may enhance treatment compliance: the imposition of legal obligations on treatment providers. The attending physician assumes the following responsibilities in addition to those related to assessment and treatment of the CTO subject:

- to develop a community treatment plan (s. 33.1(2)(b));
- to ensure, before issuing the CTO, that the "treatment or care and supervision" set out in the plan are, in fact, available in the community (s. 33.1(2) (c)(v));
- to consult with any other health practitioners to be named in the plan (33.1(2)(d));
- to ensure that the CTO subject has consulted with a rights adviser (s. 33.1(2)(e));
- to ensure that copies of the order get to appropriate parties, including any health practitioners named in the plan (s. 33.1(7));

In addition, s. 33.5(1) makes the physician responsible for monitoring the plan's progress:[49]

33.5(1) A physician who issues or renews a community treatment order ... is responsible for the general supervision and management of the order.

American commentators have noted that the success of OPC programs seems at least as much related to the "commitment" made to them by service providers, as to the subject's willingness to cooperate.[50]

Persons with serious mental illness and their families have long complained that it is difficult to obtain services and the ongoing involvement in their lives of physicians and service providers in the community. The foregoing provisions of Brian's Law may imply a form of "right to treatment" for CTO subjects that has not hitherto had a strong foundation in Canadian law.[51] It seems unlikely, however, that the individual client will be in a position to enforce this "right." Compliance with these obligations will largely be a matter of professional ethics and program management.

To the degree that CTO provisions are seen as creating added administrative responsibility on treatment providers, as well as exposure to increased risk of liability, they may have built-in disincentives to their use. The obligations imposed on attending physicians, particularly of supervision and management of the community treatment plan, will place a premium on CTO services being offered out of well-resourced mental health facilities. This is as it should be. These provisions make manifest the inappropriateness of a family physician responding to a request to issue a CTO for a relative with mental illness, while not having the ability or even the intention to remain involved in its progress and management.

The obligations on treatment providers appear to be a statutory *quid pro quo* for the authority to place a person under the terms of a community treatment order. Indeed, the CTO provisions in Brian's Law could be viewed as a form of informal contract.[52] An informal contract describes the nature of the relationship involved in the delivery of any comprehensive treatment program. The Ontario legislation adds little by way of practical enforceability to this ordinary relationship between treatment provider and client.

III. Dilemma of a Less Restrictive Alternative to Involuntary Hospitalization

It could be argued that whether or not community treatment orders increase compliance, their role and function is in any event not intrusive with respect to personal autonomy. Whatever benefit they provide should easily outweigh any cost to individual rights.

The purpose clause in the Ontario legislation describes community treatment orders as "less restrictive" than involuntary hospitalization. The "least restrictive alternative" principle developed in US constitutional law from the idea that when government limits personal liberties in the pursuit of legitimate state interests, it should do so in the least restrictive manner. The same principle forms part of the balancing test performed in applying section 1 of the Charter to impugned legislation.[53] Kaiser argues that it is an important principle to be applied wherever state authority is brought to bear on persons with mental disabilities for therapeutic purposes.[54] He notes that the principle can apply with respect to decisions about whether providing care in an institutional setting is necessary, as well as to more and less intrusive modalities of medical treatment.

The reference to "less restrictive" in s. 33.1(3) of Ontario's Mental Health Act does not appear to be so much a guide to decision-making as a description of what community treatment orders are intended to provide. As such, is it an accurate description? There are two lines of argument, one legal, the other more theoretical, for suggesting that it is not.

A. Hospitalization and Community Treatment as Mutually Exclusive Courses of Action

It seems indisputable that the difference between being physically confined in a hospital setting and living in the community represents a difference between a "greater" and a "lesser" restriction of liberty. Whether a community treatment order is a "less restrictive" *alternative* to hospital commitment, however, is not so straightforward. The answer depends on the method of analysis. It might be argued, for instance, that imposing a CTO is less restrictive because, as a result of its effectiveness, the CTO subject is less likely to be hospitalized in the future. This consequentialist argument could be used to justify any number of measures which would be extraordinarily intrusive in the short term, so long as the ultimate therapeutic effects were thought to be beneficial. It does not seem helpful. What is "less restrictive" is better identified in terms of the immediate impact on the degree of liberty experienced by the individual.

One way to address this question is to ask whether the CTO, in the same circumstances, is an available alternative to the more restrictive recourse of involuntary hospitalization. This issue has been the subject of extensive discussion in American literature on outpatient committal. There, the distinction has been made between OPC provisions which constitute "preventive commitment," as opposed to those which operate as alternatives to involuntary hospitalization. Conditional discharge provisions (in Canada, "leaves of absence") are classified in the latter group. "Preventive commitment" refers to committal to a community order for treatment that is available *before* a person becomes committable to hospital, on criteria that are lower than those for involuntary hospitalization. Such provisions are viewed as being relatively uncommon in the US.[55]

Do the Ontario CTO provisions operate as preventive commitment, or as an alternative to hospitalization? The former appears to be the better description. For one thing, when the assessing physician identifies the criteria for involuntary hospitalization in a patient's condition, he or she has no discretion. The Mental Health Act says the physician "shall" admit the person as an involuntary patient.[56] Second, the criteria for hospital committal and CTO committal have been drawn in mutually exclusive terms. The criteria for involuntary hospitalization under section 20(5) of the Mental Health Act include that the person will cause or suffer harm unless he or she "remains in the custody of a psychiatric facility," and is "not suitable for admission ... as an informal or voluntary patient." Saskatchewan has a similar provision. Such criteria embody the least restrictive principle. It could be argued that the CTO creates a new alternative, such that the person need not be hospitalized in order to avoid harm. The new alternative, of course, is not community treatment, but the prospect of compliance with community treatment. For reasons given in Part II, those prospects seem uncertain.

In a more substantive sense, the criteria for committal to a community treatment order do not meet the harm criteria for involuntary hospitalization. The former include the person's history of recent repeat hospitalizations. In addition, a physician is required to find that this history shows that if the person does not receive psychiatric treatment in the community, he or she is likely to meet the harm criteria. This only makes sense if it is given a future connotation—i.e., that the person *will* meet those criteria if treatment is not received. In other words, a person is committable to a CTO at an earlier stage than to involuntary hospitalization.

Brian's Law added s. 20.1 to the legislation in Ontario. In effect, this section tracks the CTO provisions by making a person subject to involuntary hospitalization on the basis of a history of previous hospitalizations, combined with observation of present physical or mental condition:

> 20(1.1) (d) given the person's history of mental disorder and current mental or physical condition, is likely to cause serious bodily harm to himself or herself or to another person or is likely to suffer substantial mental or physical deterioration or serious physical impairment ...

These criteria bring the standard for involuntary hospitalization closer to that for the CTO and, indeed, closer to a form of preventive commitment.

This raises a further question of method: should the measure of "less restrictive alternative" be whether hospital committal was an alternative to the

CTO under the old legislation, or under the new amended legislation? In the latter case, the CTO may appear to be less restrictive only in the sense that the threshold for hospital committal has been lowered as part of the scheme for introducing the CTO itself. That too seems like a somewhat impoverished meaning for the term "less restrictive alternative." Exaggerating to make the point, it would be like saying that a reform in criminal law which changed the maximum sentence for robbery from fourteen years in prison to a choice between life in prison without parole or the death penalty, had created the life sentence as a less restrictive alternative.

This discussion of whether, in fact, the CTO is a less restrictive alternative to hospitalization is not a mere technicality. Among other things, it will affect the way community treatment orders are experienced by those subject to them. A "less restrictive alternative" offers an option to what would otherwise be the severe intrusion into liberty represented by detention in hospital. "Preventive commitment," however, involves the extension of coercion into the community, where it did not previously exist.

As American literature suggests, leave-of-absence provisions would not be viewed as preventive commitment. As a form of phased discharge from hospital, they represent a reducing of restrictions. Leave provisions occur within the context of an existing involuntary commitment. Should a person on leave fail to adhere to the conditions, or suffer decompensation, the leave is revocable and the person can be returned to hospital under the authority of the original committal. In the recent amendments to the BC Mental Health Act, the Legislature opted to enhance their leave provisions rather than go to a CTO model.[57] There are reasons to think that the CTO approach might operate best at the discharge from hospital stage, but the provisions in Saskatchewan and Ontario clearly are not limited in that way.

B. The Community as a Sphere of Freedom from Constraint

The second argument against seeing community treatment orders as less restrictive than involuntary hospitalization is more theoretical. This could be considered the "strong" argument for rejecting the idea of community committal as a less restrictive alternative. The argument goes to a fundamental question about the relationship between "coercion" and "community." Schwartz and Costanzo argue that the significant distinction for purposes of a least restrictive approach is that between coercion and no coercion, rather than that between "community" and "hospital." Does "community"—a term defined neither in the Saskatchewan nor Ontario legislation—merely connote living outside the walls of a designated psychiatric facility, or does it inherently refer to a sphere of liberty that is qualitatively different from the experience of "coercion," or legal constraint? How far can terms of a community treatment plan go before there is no appreciable difference between involuntary hospitalization and CTO committal? Terms of "care or supervision" that restricted a person to living at a particular residential location would raise this issue most forcefully.

IV. Community Treatment Orders and the Charter of Rights and Freedoms

The status of the existing coercive aspects of provincial mental health laws was examined briefly in Part I. The community treatment order, as a further measure of coercion, also seems likely to engage sections 7 and 9 of the Charter which deal with rights of liberty and security of the person. It also raises issues of equality rights under section 15(1) of the Charter. Interests giving rise to Charter issues would include the following:

(1) Security of the person: The community treatment order is a measure which seeks to enforce compliance with a course of psychiatric treatment. To the extent that it does so, with respect to a person who does not wish to comply, it violates that person's physical integrity.

(2) Liberty: The community treatment order by definition does not involve detention in a psychiatric hospital. However, "liberty interests" in section 7 are not limited to issues of the physical freedom to move. The Supreme Court has stated that "liberty" also goes to the personal autonomy necessary to the making of significant choices in life.[58] Community treatment plans incorporated into the terms of CTOs can go beyond "treatment," to "care and supervision." Should care and supervision include such matters as maintaining a residence, engaging in regularly scheduled activities and personal care and grooming, the CTO would implicate interests of personal autonomy. Moreover, if terms of care and supervision went so far as to require the CTO subject to live in a particular residence, it is arguable that it is no longer dealing with "community" treatment at all. It is restricting the CTO subject to living in a "facility," however small or integrated into a surrounding neighbourhood.

(3) Equality rights: A person is made subject to a community treatment order, which denies the benefits of "liberty" enjoyed by other persons living in the community, on the basis of mental disability, in fact largely on the basis of a history of mental disability. Recent Supreme Court jurisprudence has made it clear that a distinction in law based on an enumerated ground such as disability is not enough to establish discrimination

under section 15(1); the distinction must harm the dignity interests of members of the affected group, such as by stigmatizing them in the eyes of society, or evidencing society's lesser respect for them as equals.[59] In the case of CTOs, the argument would be made that being subject to such an order is stigmatizing, that it singles persons out as being less capable and deserving of exercising autonomy. The CTO provisions have the potential of making persons indefinitely subject to renewable CTOs, creating a virtual permanent class[60] of persons unable to exercise rights equally with others in the community.

It is beyond the scope of this article to look in detail at the arguments available with respect to potential Charter claims. The substantive criteria supporting issuance of community treatment orders in Ontario and Saskatchewan are narrowly drawn to capture only persons who have a demonstrated recent need for therapeutic intervention. This, combined with the relative lack of success of past Charter challenges to the substantive criteria for involuntary hospitalization discussed in Part I, suggest the statutory regimes for CTOs may well pass Charter scrutiny. Plaintiffs would encounter two particular hurdles: (1) the consent requirement in Ontario; (2) the argument that CTOs are "less restrictive" than the alternative of involuntary hospitalization. These arguments relate to earlier discussions and deserve further attention here.

A. Consent

The requirement in Ontario for consent by competent persons to a treatment plan may well dispense with section 7 arguments that the CTO is a deprivation of security of the person. The issue in *Fleming* concerned a statutory override of a competent refusal. In Part II it was suggested that the consensual nature of community treatment orders for competent persons may mean that they simply are not coercive. To the extent this is true, the CTO may be viewed as an insignificant intrusion on individual rights.

One caveat with respect to the requirement for consent is that Brian's Law provides a form of sanction to the withdrawal of consent by a CTO subject: the attending physician is authorized to issue an order for examination, the "CTO warrant." Still, this authority is to be exercised only where the physician believes the person is otherwise committable. It seems unlikely that the warrant is such a constraint on the giving of consent in the first place that it supports a claim that the CTO violates "security of the person." Of greater concern are informal pressures which may be brought to bear on an individual at the point of giving consent. There may well be a tendency among treatment providers and concerned family members to imply that a failure to consent to a CTO will result in involuntary hospitalization. Since criteria for hospital committal and CTO committal are described in mutually exclusive terms, this is not the case. To the degree that a person consents to a treatment plan under a "threat" of this nature, the consent could be vitiated, possibly giving rise to liability in tort. Should the "threat" emanate from someone viewed as a government actor, a remedy for breach of Charter rights might be sought under section 24 of the Charter.[61]

A last point concerning the provision of treatment under a CTO is that the statutory provisions do not appear to give sufficient authority for using physical force to provide medical treatment. Here, there is a distinction between "coerced" and "forced" treatment. The former refers to coercion by law. The CTO provisions are coercive only in this sense. Express statutory authority would be needed to permit treatment providers to restrain and force medication on an unwilling client.[62] Such express authorization of the use of force could not be saved by consent provisions, and might well breach the right to security of the person guaranteed by section 7 of the Charter.

B. Less Restrictive Alternative

A second conceptual barrier to a Charter challenge is the argument that the CTO is, in purpose and effect, less restrictive of personal liberty than the alternative of involuntary hospitalization. This issue is important both in section 7 and section 15 analysis. Under section 7, an important part of the legal analysis involves measuring the nature and extent of the deprivation of "liberty" interests against the importance of the policy objective being pursued in the legislation. To the extent a community treatment order appears less restrictive of individual liberty than the alternative of hospitalization, it is more likely to be upheld under section 7.

Similarly, a claim of discrimination under section 15 starts with identifying appropriate comparator groups. The individual or group claiming it has been discriminated against needs to show "in comparison to whom." Recent Supreme Court jurisprudence has underlined the importance of this step.[63] A section 15 claim against Brian's Law would likely turn on whether a court found the comparison between CTO subjects and involuntarily committed hospital patients pertinent. A court could choose to compare CTO subjects with all other persons living in the community not subject to the constraints of a treatment order. The discussion in Part IV was intended to show that the latter position has some merit. This is far from suggesting that a section 15 challenge to Brian's Law would succeed. It indicates the nature of the argument which would need to be developed to underpin any such litigation.

Conclusion

The discussions in Parts II and III of this article both speak to the value of considerable caution being exercised in the implementation and use of continuing treatment orders. Part II examined the problem of how the CTO is expected to produce compliance with psychiatric treatment. While a full appreciation of this issue would require a detailed understanding of the sources of noncompliance, the legal design of the CTO itself suggests the difficulty: an absence of meaningful enforcement. Those people who exhibit the strongest will not to comply with treatment may, if competent, refuse to consent. If a CTO subject is noncompliant, the recourse is apprehension for an examination of mental condition. Only if a person is then assessed to be committable would involuntary hospitalization follow. In this way, the community treatment order seems to add little to what a treatment provider might well say to a person when negotiating a voluntary course of community treatment: "If you don't follow up with this plan, you may well become ill again and have to return to hospital." The best subject for a CTO may be an individual who does not pose a significant problem of noncompliance, but who needs the occasional reminder or inducement to maintain treatment and contact with program staff, and for whom the CTO can serve that purpose. In this light, it seems CTOs should not be issued for the hardest cases, but should be issued selectively and in accordance with available resources for intensive interaction. The consequence of operating in any other way may well be a descending spiral of CTOs not being monitored, not being "enforced," and falling into greater disrespect and disuse.

A further consequence of the indiscriminate use of CTOs could be a significant infringement of individual rights. The analysis in Part III was intended to suggest that even if making out a Charter case against the statutory regime for compulsory community treatment may prove difficult, there is a serious argument to be made for the position that CTOs do not have as benign an impact on lives as the phrase "less restrictive" might suggest. If it is indeed the case that CTOs can be issued in circumstances which would not previously, or presently, result in involuntary hospitalization, then a constraint on liberty has been extended where none existed before.

The legal analysis presented in this paper suggests that the benefits of CTOs are likely to be limited at best. The essential task remains to improve the quality and availability of therapeutic and support services in the community. This is important to the success of CTOs. The irony is that improved community services would encourage voluntary compliance with treatment programs and make CTOs largely unnecessary.

NOTES

1   S.O. 2000, c. 9. The full name of the statute is An Act, in memory of Brian Smith, to amend the Mental Health Act and the Health Care Consent Act, 1996, to come into force on 1 December 2000 (section 49). Brian Smith was an Ottawa sports broadcaster who was shot and killed in 1995, outside the television station where he worked. He was killed by a man previously diagnosed and treated for paranoid schizophrenia.

2   RSO 1990, c. M 7.

3   The issue was highly controversial. A useful way of following the controversy is to review the submissions made to the hearings of the Legislative Committee on General Government dealing with Bill 68 (Brian's Law) between its announcement in April 2000 and passage on 21 June 2000. The website is www.ontla.on.ca/committees/committeesindex.htm. Two of the leading organizations taking opposing sides in this debate are the Ontario chapters of the Schizophrenia Society and the Canadian Mental Health Association. I am indebted to both for providing me with various materials produced by their respective head offices.

4   The Mental Health Services Act, SS 1984 85–86, c. M–13.1, as amended to introduce community treatment orders by the Mental Health Services Amendment Act, 1993, S.S. 1993, c. 59. The amendments were proclaimed in 1995. These provisions of the Act were further amended by the Mental Health Services Amendment Act, 1996, S.S. 1996, c.17.

5   "Enough is Enough: The Case for Reforming Ontario's Mental Health Act," the Schizophrenia Society of Ontario, 11 May 1999, online at www.schizophrenia.on.ca/enough.htm (accessed on 22 November 2000).

6   Brian's Law responds to these two objectives with respect to Ontario's mental health legislation. Recent reform initiatives in Saskatchewan and BC have also addressed these objectives. Mental Health Amendment Act, 1998, S.B.C. 1998 c. 35–1, proclaimed into law 15 November 1999; amending Mental Health Act, R.S.B.C. 1996, c. 288. See Saskatchewan amending statutes, *supra*, note 4.

The first objective of expanding committal criteria has been met in part by adding the phrase "substantial mental or physical deterioration" to those criteria, in each jurisdiction. As serious physical deterioration resulting from mental disorder likely justified committal under existing criteria, the real effect of this phrase would appear to be with respect to illness at the point it is causing "substantial mental deterioration" alone. Committal on this basis does not appear to have yet been the subject of judicial consideration in Canada.

In BC, the second objective was met by more clearly authorizing leaves of absence from involuntary hospitalization. Two further changes to the BC legislation are noteworthy. Review panels, to which involuntary patients may apply for review of their committal, are expressly directed to take into consideration a number of factors going to whether the patient, if discharged to the community, may experience a deterioration in his or her condition. In addition, the Legislature provided to involuntary patients the right to obtain a second psychiatric opinion with respect to treatment proposed by the attending hospital psychiatrist. This latter provision is unique in Canada.

7   Israel has introduced similar statutory provisions. See A. Kanter and U. Aviram, "Israel's Involuntary Outpatient Commitment Law: Lessons from the American Experience" (1995) 29 *Israel L. Rev.* 565.

8   Listed here are only those articles which were found of particular assistance in this study: J.T. Hinds, "Involuntary Outpatient Commitment for the Chronically Mentally Ill" (1990) 69 *Nebraska L. Rev.* 346; Charles W. Lidz, "Coercion in Psychiatric Care: What Have We Learned from Research?" (1998) 26 *Journal of the American Academy of Psychiatry and the Law* 631; S.J. Schwartz and C.E. Costanzo, "Compelling Treatment in the Community: Distorted Doctrines and Violated Values" (1987) 20 *Loyola of Los Angeles L. Rev.* 1329; E.D. Furlong, "Coercion in the Community: The Application of *Rogers* Guardianship to Outpatient Commitment" (1995) 1 *New England J. of Criminal and Civil Confinement* 485; Erika F. King, "Outpatient Committal in North Carolina: Constitutional and Policy Concerns" (1995) 58 *L. & Contemp. Probs.* 251.

9   E. Fuller Torrey and J.D. Kaplan, "A National Survey of the Use of Outpatient Commitment" (1995) 46 *Psychiatric Services* 778, is a useful overview. The Ontario division of the Canadian Mental Health Association produced a comprehensive listing in "Community Treatment Orders: a Survey of Recent Literature," January 2000, online at www.ontario.cmha.ca/mhic/CtoEvid.pdf (accessed on 22 November 2000).

10 King, *supra* note 8.

11 Torrey and Kaplan, *supra*, note 9. It should be noted that, unlike King, *ibid.*, Torrey and Kaplan distinguish between OPC, as a court-ordered treatment applying to persons living in the community, and "conditional release," as a discharge from hospital on condition that a person continue with treatment. They note the greater use and perceived advantages of conditional release in states where both mechanisms are available.

12 Hinds, *supra* note 8.

13 M.S. Swartz *et al.*, "New Directions in Research on Involuntary Outpatient Commitment" (1995) 46 *Psychiatric Services* 381. The authors criticize the studies that were most favourable to OPC for failing to account for selection criteria for research subjects that made it likely the subjects would show improvement.

14 *Ibid.* at 383.

15 *Ibid.* at 783.

16 The Saskatchewan Ministry of Health is in the process of producing its first evaluative report on community treatment orders. Preliminary quantitative material made available by the Ministry shows that 180 CTOs were issued between the start of the program in July 1995 and December 1998. This may represent about sixty different individuals, given that eighty-five CTOs specifically tracked related to twenty-eight subjects (who were subject on average to two renewals). Memo from the Community Care Branch, Saskatchewan Health (10 May 2000).

17 G.B. Robertson, *Mental Disability and the Law in Canada* (Scarborough, ON: Carswell, 1994) at 384–96.

18 The Canadian model of procedure for civil commitment differs from than that employed in the US. There, committal is a matter of court order, rather than medical certification. A court hearing prior to committal supplants the role of the after-the-fact administrative review. A consequence for OPC laws is that it is often courts which are involved in exploring this alternative, rather than physicians as in Canada.

19 The rights set out in sections 7, 9 and 15 are subject to the limits described in section 1 of the Charter: "The Canadian Charter of Rights and Freedoms guarantees the rights and freedoms set out in it subject only to such reasonable limits prescribed by law as can be demonstrably justified in a free and democratic society."

20 See Robertson, *supra*, note 17; I. Grant, "Mental Health Law and the Courts" (1991) 29 *Osgoode Hall L. J.* 747; H.A. Kaiser, "Mental Disability Law" in J. Downie and T. Caulfield, eds., *Canadian Health Law and Policy* (Toronto: Butterworths, 1999) 217 at 259–64.

21 *Thwaites* v. *Health Sciences Centre Psychiatric Facility* (1988) 40 C.R.R. 326 (Man. C.A.).

22 *Ibid.* at 332. The Court may have been comforted in coming to this decision by knowing that new mental health legislation setting out objective criteria for committal, including "substantial mental or physical deterioration," had been enacted by the Manitoba Legislature, but not yet proclaimed. The committal criteria in the amended legislation were subsequently upheld in *Bobbie* v. *Health Sciences Centre* (1989) 49 C.R.R. 376 (Man. Q.B.).

23 *McCorkell* v. *Riverview Hospital* [1993] B.C.J. No. 1518 (S.C.).

24 *Ibid.*, para. 45.

25 The issue of whether "dangerousness" is the necessary basis for committal under the Criminal Code of Canada provisions governing the disposition of cases involving persons found "not criminally responsible by reason of mental disorder" (NCRMD) arose in *Winko* v. *Forensic Psychiatric Services* [1999] 2 SCR 625. Winko argued that his Charter s. 7 rights were infringed by his facing an onus to establish that he did not constitute a danger to society in order to obtain an absolute discharge. The Court majority concluded that read properly, section 654.72 of the Code did not impose an onus on the NCRMD accused. Rather, it found an onus on the Court or review board to make a positive finding that the NCRMD accused poses a risk to society in order to justify restricting that person's liberty, either by involuntary hospitalization or a discharge from hospital on conditions. Thus, dangerousness to society provides the only basis under which a person's liberty can be limited under the criminal law. Whatever risk an ongoing mental disorder might create for the NCRMD accused's own safety could not justify his continued involuntary hospitalization, nor even the placing of conditions on his release into the community. In other words, there is no *parens patriae* basis for state intervention via the criminal law into the lives of NCRMD accused.

This does not mean that danger to society is the standard for civil commitment. The Supreme Court was only dealing with the power of the criminal law to detain or impose conditions on an NCRMD accused. It seems fair to ask, however, whether the meaning of "liberty" in section of the Charter could mean such different things for persons in each system. Whether a person is committed criminally or civilly is often a result of capricious events and decisions. The individual experience is often very much the same.

26 *Supra* note 20.

27 *Eaton* v. *Brant County Board of Education* [1997] 1 SCR 241.

28 *Law* v. *Canada (Minister of Employment and Immigration)* [1999] 1 SCR 497, at para. 72.

29 *Supra* note 25.

30 *Ibid.* at para. 90, per McLachlin J.

31 See, for discussion of the issue of consent in medical treatment, E. Picard and G.B. Robertson, *Legal Liability of Doctors and Hospitals in Canada* (Scarborough, ON: Carswell, 1996) at 39–86. For a specific legal statement on the right of a competent person to refuse life-saving treatment, see *Malette* v. *Shulman* (1987) 63 O.R. (2d) 243, aff'd 72 O.R. (2d) 417 (C.A.). This decision was relied on in *Fleming* v. *Reid, infra* note 35.

32 Picard and Robertson, *ibid.*, at 61–2.

33 See generally R. Gordon and S. Verdun-Jones, *Adult Guardianship Law in Canada* (Scarborough, ON: Carswell, 1992). Examples of recently introduced substitute decisionmaker legislation include, in Ontario, the Substitute Decisions Act, 1992, S.O. 1992, c. 30, as amended, and the Health Care Consent Act, 1996, S.O. 1996, c. 2, Schedule A, and in BC, the Adult Guardianship Act, R.S.B.C. 1996, c. 6, proclaimed 28 February 2000 by B.C. Reg 12/00.

34 See, for example, *Canadian Disability Rights Council* v. *Canada* [1988] 3 F.C. 622 (F.C.T.D.), in which a provision of the federal election law which made persons involuntarily committed to hospital ineligible to vote was found to violate section 3 of the Charter of Rights and Freedoms. Reed J. ruled that it was inappropriate to equate the mental disability required for committal with competence to vote.

35 *Fleming* v. *Reid* (1991) 82 D.L.R. (4th) 298 (Ont. C.A.).

36 Provisions on consent, the obligations of substitute decision-makers with respect to consent, and the applications which can be made to the Consent and Capacity Board are now found in the Health Care Consent Act, *supra* note 33.

37 R.S.B.C. 1996, c. 288, s. 31(1).

38 That such challenges have not been made is reflective of the inherent difficulty of bringing such cases forward. Quite apart from the usual issues of expense and legal resources, issues of "mootness" frequently defeat these attempts. That is, hospital stays often end well before cases get to court, raising a basic issue of whether it is useful for them to proceed. In *Rogerson* v. *Alberta Hospital* [A.J. No. 870] (20 July 1999), the Alberta Surrogate Court ruled that it would deal with a challenge to s. 29 of the Act despite a mootness objection; the plaintiff's personal circumstances nevertheless had changed, and the case did not proceed.

39 S.O. 1996, c. 2, Schedule A.

40 S. 33.9(1) The Minister shall establish a process to review the following matters:

1. The reasons that community treatment orders were or were not used during the review period.

2. The effectiveness of community treatment orders during the review period.

3. Methods used to evaluate the outcome of any treatment used under community treatment orders.

(2) The first review must be undertaken during the third year after the date on which subsection 33.1 (1) comes into force.

(3) A review must be completed every five years after the first review is completed.

(4) The Minister shall make available to the public for inspection the written report of the person conducting each review.

41 Civil commitment in Saskatchewan continues to take place under the "harm" criteria, set out in section 24(2)(a), as follows:

> (i) the person is suffering from a mental disorder as a result of which he is in need of treatment or care and supervision which can be provided only in an in-patient facility;
> (ii) as a result of the mental disorder, the person is unable to fully understand and to make an informed decision regarding his need for treatment or care and supervision; and
> (iii) as a result of the mental disorder, the person is likely to cause harm to himself or to others or to suffer substantial mental or physical deterioration if he is not detained in an in-patient facility.

42 See, for example, from the Executive Summary of *Best Practices in Mental Health Reform* (Toronto: Clarke Institute of Psychiatry, University of Toronto, 1997):

> Among the core services and supports within a reformed system of care, case management and assertive community treatment (see Chapter 1, Literature Review, ANMH) have the most relevance to the creation of an integrated system of care. In these models of care delivery, accountability is clearly established at a local level, and continuity of care and access to comprehensive services are given priority. Assertive community treatment is the most comprehensive approach, combining in one team the elements of crisis intervention, treatment and individual support. It also has demonstrated economic effectiveness by reducing use of expensive inpatient hospitalization.

43 See Picard and Robertson, *supra* note 31, at 48.

44 The Saskatchewan Mental Health Services Act, supra note 4, makes no provision for the giving of consent to a CTO by a substitute decision-maker, appearing to leave the authority to impose a CTO in the hands of the attending physician. This may raise issues going to substituted consent and guardianship that go beyond the scope of this article.

45 Furthermore, the degree of competency necessary to understand the stipulation of the CCT (Compulsory Community Treatment) … is deemed different from the competency necessary to give informed consent—for if there is informed consent, there is no need for CCT. Nevertheless, it is highly unlikely one could consistently discern and standardize such a distinction between "levels of competency." One cannot underestimate the complexities involved in ascertaining that the uses of CCT will always be appropriate—even with an extremely refined set of criteria. See F. Boudreau and P. Lambert, "Compulsory Community Treatment? II. The Collision of Views and Complexities Involved: Is it 'The Best Possible Alternative?'" (1993) 12 *Can. J. of Community Mental Health* 79 at 87. See also the authors' immediately preceding article, "Compulsory Community Treatment? I. Ontario Stakeholders' Response to 'Helping Those Who Won't Help Themselves'" (1993) 12 *Can. J. of Community Mental Health* 57.

46 S.O. 1996, c. 2, Schedule A, s. 21(2)(a), *supra* note 33.

47 See in particular the article by Hinds, *supra* note 8.

48 Mental Health Services Act, S.S. 1984–85–86, as amended, s. 24.6, *supra* note 4.

49 The attending physician is relieved of liability for any "default or neglect" of other persons providing treatment under the plan (33.6(1)). By implication, the physician

appears not to be relieved of liability for default or neglect in his or her own responsibilities under the plan. Other health practitioners providing treatment under the plan "are responsible for implementing the plan to the extent indicated in it."

Saskatchewan's Mental Health Services Act, *supra* note 4 does not impose as many obligations of the physician issuing the CTO. Nevertheless, it likewise makes issuance conditional on the physician's believing the needed treatment services exist in the community, are available, and will be provided to the CTO subject. Further, section 24.7 states:

> Where a community treatment order has been validated pursuant to section 24.4, the attending physician shall endeavour, with all resources reasonably available in the community, to provide the person who is the subject of the order with services so that compulsory treatment or care and supervision of the person will no longer be required.

50 Torrey and Kaplan, *supra* note 9, at p. 783, quote the following statement by S.B. Silver in "Outpatient Commitment: Adapting Forensic Models to the Civil Context" (1991) 11 *Developments in Mental Health Law* 1 at 23: "Outpatient civil commitment may really affect provider behavior more significantly than patient behavior. We're not committing the patient, really, but rather the entire mental health community to be more accountable, to do the job well, to find somehow a treatment alliance with the patient."

51 See discussion by Kaiser, *supra* note 20 at 259–64.

52 It is worth noting that in the press release accompanying Bill 68, the Ontario government referred to continuing treatment orders as "legal agreements." Health and Long Term Care, press release, "Ontario introduces Brian's Law for better mental health treatment and safer communities" (25 April 2000).

53 *R. v. Oakes* (1986), 26 D.L.R. (4th) 200 (S.C.C.).

54 *Supra* note 20 at 238–40.

55 North Carolina, Washington and Hawaii are viewed as three such states, with possibly two others also having forms of preventive commitment. American commentators have noted that it is conceptually difficult to make community treatment available as an alternative to involuntary hospitalization when the latter is premised on committal criteria of dangerousness. In their excellent analysis of OPC provisions and the least restrictive alternative principle in the US, Schwartz and Costanzo use this to explain why the introduction of OPC laws tends to put pressure on legislators to lower criteria for civil commitment. *Supra* note 8.

56 Mental Health Act, *supra* note 2, ss. 20(1)(c) and 20.1(1.1).

57 Mental Health Act, R.S.B.C. 1996, c. 288, sections 37–9 (as amended by S.B.C. 1998, c. 35, s. 17), *supra* note 6.

58 *R. v. Big M Drug Mart* [1985] 1 S.C.R. 295 at 368, per Dickson C.J.: "[L]iberty does not mean mere freedom from physical restraint. In a free and democratic society, the individual must be left room for personal autonomy to live his or her own life and to make decisions that are of fundamental personal importance."

See also, *Godbout v. Longueuil (City)* [1997] 3 S.C.R. 844 at para. 66, per La Forest J.:

> The foregoing discussion serves simply to reiterate my general view that the right to liberty enshrined in s. 7 of the Charter protects within its ambit the right to an irreducible sphere of personal autonomy

wherein individuals may make inherently private choices free from state interference.

The foregoing passage was quoted with approval in *Blencoe v. British Columbia (Human Rights Commission)* [2000] S.C.J. 43 at para. 51, per Bastarache J.

59 *Law* v. *Canada, supra* note 28 at para. 53 (per Iacobucci, J.):

> Human dignity means that an individual or group feels self-respect and self-worth. It is concerned with physical and psychological integrity and empowerment. Human dignity is harmed by unfair treatment premised upon personal traits or circumstances which do not relate to individual needs, capacities or merits. ... Human dignity is harmed when individuals and groups are marginalized, ignored or devalued, and is enhanced when laws recognize the full place of all individuals and groups within Canadian society.

60 Since committal to a community treatment order is premised on the existence of chronic mental illness which requires ongoing therapeutic attention, the potential exists for an indefinite series of renewed orders. Section 24.7 of the Saskatchewan statute imposes an obligation on the attending physician to provide services "so that compulsory treatment or care or supervision of the order will no longer be required." There is no similar provision in the Ontario legislation.

61 Section 24(1) reads:

> Anyone whose rights or freedoms, as guaranteed by the Charter, have been infringed or denied may apply to a court of competent jurisdiction to obtain such remedy as the court considers appropriate and just in the circumstances.

62 In *Nova Scotia (Minister of Community Services)* v. *Moore*, [1995] N.S.J. No. 367, Daley, Fam. Ct. J., said (at para. 33) the following of the Minister's powers under that province's Adult Protection Act:

> Ms. Moore asked for an Order preventing or recommending against the use of needles to inject her medication. There is no authority under the APA to make such an Order nor does the Minister have the authority to order such injections. In fact, there is little authority that the Minister has over an adult in need of protection. ...That is a matter between the patient and her doctor. ...

Adult protection legislation, which exists in the four Atlantic provinces, and was recently introduced into the guardianship law in BC, is perhaps the next closest approximation of CTO legislation in Canada, after leave-of-absence provisions in mental health statutes. Under such legislation, public authorities are authorized to apply to court for an order permitting them to assess a vulnerable individual living in the community who is shown to be unable to protect him- or herself from neglect or abuse, and to provide social services to that person. The degree of compulsion which these statutes can authorize is one of several controversial issues surrounding these statutes. See discussion of adult protection legislation by Gordon and Verdun-Jones, *supra* note 32 at 2–1 to 2–59.

63 In *Granovsky* v. *Canada (Minister of Employment and Immigration)*, [2000] 1 S.C.R. 703, the Court described the identification of the comparator group as a "crucial" part of s. 15 analysis (at para. 45). In that case, the plaintiff alleged that the legislative scheme for Canadian Pension Plan disability benefits discriminated between able-bodied contributors to the Plan, and a person like himself who was *temporarily*

disabled during the contribution period. The Court rejected the claim in large part because it believed the appropriate comparison was with *permanently* disabled workers. Binnie J. later said that there could be "no stigma in being treated [by the Plan] as 'better off'" where in fact that is the reality of the appellant's medical history" (at para. 77).

7

HEALTH CARE REFORM
AND INTERNATIONAL TRADE

E. RICHARD GOLD

For most industrialized countries, and Canada in particular, health care goes far beyond the mere provision of health care services. Health care is a fundamental human right[1] and a right of citizenship.[2] As a society, we wish to ensure that health care services are provided to all Canadians without financial, geographic or other barriers and that health promotion and prevention are emphasized above treatment.[3] At the same time, in an age of financial restraint governments throughout the country are attempting to provide those services more efficiently.[4] Unfortunately, efficiency is hard to define, yet alone achieve, as the health care sector is renowned for market failure.[5]

If the forces of efficiency seem to be dominating other health care policies at the national level, these forces are even stronger at the international level. International trade agreements, which touch on health care in several ways, promote efficiency through reliance on open markets. The hope is that by promoting efficiency, we better promote other values. After all, if we are able to free up resources by using what we have more efficiently, we should be in a better position to address more concerns. Unfortunately, theory does not always turn into reality. This is because efficiency is not synonymous with the market, particularly in the health care sector.

In this chapter, I will examine the challenges faced by federal and provincial governments in reforming health care in light of international trade agreement obligations. In particular, I will focus on how these agreements affect Canada's ability to promote four critical, nonmarket-oriented goals of the Canadian health care system: universality, health promotion and prevention, removal of financial and geographic barriers to access health care services, and choice.[6] These are among the most important goals of the Canadian health care system and thus define the policy context for health care reform.

The nature of international trade agreements is to limit the choices of national governments. These agreements do so in order to ensure that governments do not choose policies that unduly shut non-nationals out of their economies. This means that these agreements limit the type of health care reform that the federal and provincial governments are free to implement. Because international trade agreements operate by limiting choice, they do not mandate a particular health policy; rather, they allow governments to make their own health policy choices provided that, at every stage, governments choose the same, or more market-orientated, approaches.

Later in this chapter I will examine how international trade arrangements, particularly the North American Free Trade Agreement[7] (NAFTA) and the World Trade Organization (WTO) agreements,[8] affect the choices available to Canadian health policy decision-makers. The situation is complicated by the fact that there are two levels of government involved in health care: the provinces provide health care services while the federal government provides some funding of those services. The situation is also unclear because the provisions of the international trade agreements that apply to health care were not drafted with health care specifically in mind, and have not been interpreted with sufficient clarity for us to understand how those provisions will, in fact, apply to this sector. Nevertheless, we can assess in general terms how these agreements may affect the formulation of health policy in Canada.

International trade agreements affect health care in three ways. First, health care services are governed by NAFTA and WTO rules applicable to all services. Essentially, these rules require that, to the extent that a government opens up health care services to market forces, the government may not return those services to the public sector without significant cost. Second, NAFTA and WTO rules provide for open markets in health care products, from pharmaceuticals to medical devices and medical equipment. Third, NAFTA and WTO agreements provide for a basic level of patent and other intellectual property rights that may affect the kind and amount of health care research conducted in Canada and elsewhere.

Health care reform may take different forms across Canada. We have already seen reform aimed at increasing private sector participation in health care. Alberta's Bill 11, which permits for-profit hospitals to perform certain surgical services, is an example of this type of reform.[9] While it is true that the Canadian health care system relies heavily on the private sector—after all, most doctors are in the private sector and there are many private clinics and laboratories—most serious medical procedures take place in public hospitals. Alberta has broken with this pattern, bringing about uncertain trade effects both on itself and, potentially, the federal government.

In the first part of this chapter I will summarize the ways in which NAFTA and WTO agreements apply to health services, health products and health research. I will follow this discussion in the second part with an examination of how these rules affect the formulation of Canadian health policy in the areas identified earlier—universality, emphasis on health promotion and prevention, and removal of barriers. My conclusion is that international trade agreements are unlikely to improve efficiency without undermining other values. At the same time, however, if governments are careful, the Canadian health care system need not be seriously affected. International trade agreements will, however, cause harm if governments move forward without sufficient planning and caution.

International Trade and Health Care

Both NAFTA and WTO agreements set out rules that affect health care services, products and research. In this part I will describe the general nature of these rules, discussing their implications on Canadian health care policy later. The reader must be careful when reading this section for two reasons. First, international trade agreements are, fundamentally, political compromises reached by countries with different political and social priorities and aspirations. Therefore, these agreements tend to be vague, both to cover over disagreements on policy and also to permit room for growth. This means that we are left to speculate on the meaning of vague terms and their application to health care. Second, neither NAFTA nor WTO agreements specifically address health care issues to any significant degree. The rules they set out in respect to the provision of services, distribution of products and conduct of research are general rules applying to many disparate fields. Because these rules are not tailored to health care, it is difficult to predict exactly how the rules will be applied to the health care sector. Thus the situation is one where not only are the rules vague, but their specific application to health care is quite uncertain.

Despite the uncertainties, we can confidently lay out the general schemes of NAFTA and WTO agreements and, less confidently, speculate on the application of these trade agreements to health care. I will start by describing the general layout of three international trade agreements: NAFTA, the General Agreement on Trade in Services[10] (GATS) and the agreement on Trade Related Aspects of Intellectual Property Rights[11] (TRIPs), the latter two made within the auspices of the WTO.

NAFTA

NAFTA is an international treaty between Canada, Mexico and the United States to create a free trade zone in goods and to open investment, intellectual property and services to market forces on a continent-wide basis. It does so by imposing certain rules on the type of legislation and regulation that the three countries can use in respect of the sale of goods and services, investments and intellectual property rights. These rules limit the choices available to the three countries in order to prevent them from adopting laws that prevent or undermine open trade. NAFTA follows on and effectively replaces the Canada-US Free Trade Agreement, although it carries forward many of the latter's provisions.

Because NAFTA is an international agreement signed by national governments, it only binds the federal governments of Mexico, the United States and Canada. It does not directly bind provinces or states. Nevertheless, since the idea behind NAFTA is to open trade in general, it contemplates that federal governments will pass down certain obligations to states and provinces.[12] An investor from the United States or Mexico who believes that a province may be violating these rules is entitled to seek damages from the Canadian federal government.[13]

The obligations of each province are independent from those of the other provinces. This means that the actions of one province cannot alter the nature of the obligations imposed on the remaining provinces. This will be important later, when I discuss some of the provisions of NAFTA.

1. NAFTA Obligations: Although NAFTA does not explicitly say that it applies to health services, it defines services so broadly as to encompass them.[14] Thus, both the federal and provincial governments must ensure that their health care laws and regulations conform to NAFTA.

The way that NAFTA sets out the rules that apply to health care at the federal and provincial levels is somewhat confusing. The general structure of the agreement separates out rules that apply to those who actually provide health services—the various health professionals—and rules that apply to those who invest in private clinics, hospitals, and other health-related enterprises. There are many similarities between these two sets of rules. In addition, NAFTA provides exemptions and reservations—ways for government to carve out law existing on the date that NAFTA came into force and laws relating to certain sectors—that permit governments to regulate in ways contrary to NAFTA rules. The outcome of these two disparate sets of rules is quite complicated.

To help sort through this morass of rules, I will divide NAFTA obligations differently than does the agreement. I will first discuss those obligations to which exemptions and/or reservations apply. After describing this first set of obligations and the nature of those exemptions and reservations, I will turn to those obligations that are absolute. These apply regardless of any exemption or reservation. As we will see, these latter obligations are likely to have a greater impact on health reform than the first group.

2. Rules Subject to Exemptions and/or Reservations: NAFTA establishes rules designed to ensure that Canadian law does not discriminate against nationals of Mexico or the United States. In certain circumstances, as I will discuss below, Canada is entitled to ignore these rules. Nevertheless, the baseline rule is that Canada must extend both national treatment and most-favoured-nation treatment to Mexican and American service providers and investors.[15] National treatment means that Canada must treat these service providers and investors (in terms of access to the Canadian market and the burden of regulations and obligations that governments impose on them) at least as well as service providers and investors from Canada. The most-favoured-nation obligation means that Canada must treat Mexican and American service providers and investors at least as well as those from any other country in the world. This means that, to the extent that a Canadian province opens its health care system to private Canadian companies, it must open its system to American and Mexican companies. This rule is supported by the obligation not to impose residency requirements on either service providers or those who run private clinics and hospitals in Canada.[16] Majority control restrictions do, however, apply. A province can also demand that a service provider meet provincial licensing requirements.[17]

3. NAFTA Exemptions and Reservations: As I stated earlier, the obligations to treat nationals of the United States and Mexico at least as well as Canadian and other nationals are not absolute. Canadian governments can rely on one exemption and two reservations to avoid these rules as they apply to health care. The difference between exemptions and reservations is subtle. An exemption provides a government with an absolute and continuous right to avoid particular NAFTA obligations. Therefore, to the extent that a government rule falls within the scope of a particular exemption, that rule is unimpeachable under NAFTA. On the other hand, reservations are more limited. They either have the effect of grandparenting existing government regulations—in which case any change to the regulation brings about a loss of the reservation—or they exclude the application of NAFTA from certain sectors of the economy on certain conditions.

The one exemption that may apply to health care states that NAFTA parties themselves need not follow the NAFTA obligations discussed above, with respect to their own procurement from investors.[18] Since only the federal government (and not the provincial governments) is a party to NAFTA, this exemption only applies to federal procurement. Since it is only the provincial governments (and not the federal government) that purchase the bulk of health care services in Canada, this exemption does little good. It may, however, assist the federal government in those very limited circumstances—for example, providing health care services to veterans—where it directly purchases health care services.

The two reservations may provide the provincial governments with some room to avoid the NAFTA rules set out above. As we will see, one of these ways is unlikely to succeed while the other is lost (for the government in question) as soon as a government takes a further step toward opening its health care market to the private sector.

The first set of reservations[19]—called Annex I reservations—permits provinces to exempt government measures that do not comply with the NAFTA rules set out earlier, as long as those measures were in place on the date that NAFTA took effect.[20] Essentially, this reservation freezes government regulation at the date that NAFTA came into effect. Any significant change to those regulations must either conform to NAFTA or at least not bring the regulations further out of line with NAFTA rules. That is, while particular government measures can be grandparented, they cannot be made worse from a trade liberalization point of view. Further, once a province modifies its regulations to make those regulations more consistent with NAFTA, the province cannot later return to the original measure. The reservation on the original measure is lost. This means that once a province opens the door to market forces it cannot later close that door.

Canada has a general reservation over all of its federal and provincial nonconforming measures, including those applicable to health care. Therefore, so long as the provinces do not modify the current rules regarding the roles of the public and private sectors in health care, the provinces are exempt from NAFTA obligations. As soon as a province opens this sector to greater participation by private enterprise, however, the NAFTA obligations on national treatment and most-favoured-nation treatment kick in.

The second set of reservations[21]—called Annex II reservations—exempts health services in Canada from the NAFTA rules discussed above, but only to the extent that those services are established or maintained for a public purpose.[22] Whether a province can shield its health care reform from NAFTA obligations depends on the meaning of "public purpose." Unfortunately, the meaning of this term is unclear.[23] Its use is a prime example of covering over political differences: Canada and the United States have radically different views on the meaning of this term. Canada argues that the meaning of "public purpose" is very broad, while the United States would restrict the meaning to exclude any services provided by the private sector.[24] Given rules of international treaty interpretation[25]—which favour giving effect to the overall

HEALTH CARE REFORM & THE LAW IN CANADA

intention of the treaty, here, opening of markets—the American position is arguably the better one.

At some point between Canada's current mixed health care system and a completely private health care system, we cross the line from health services maintained for a public purpose to those not maintained for this purpose. Where that line is still needs to be established. Nevertheless, given the uncertainty and the serious consequences of being wrong, provinces ought not to rely solely on this reservation as they move to increase private sector participation in health care.

The net effect of the above exemption and reservations is that as long as a province continues to provide health services through the current mixture of the public and private sectors, its activities are shielded from NAFTA rules which relate to most-favoured-nation treatment and national treatment. Once, however, a province opens a new area of health care services to private sector participation, that province will likely have to comply with all NAFTA obligations in respect of those services.

Generally, what one province does should not affect the others. This would not be true, however, if the federal government were to involve itself in increasing private sector participation. The federal government is bound directly by NAFTA obligations, including those that apply to health care. Like the provinces, the federal government can rely upon the reservations discussed above. While the federal government does not directly provide health services, it participates in health care funding through transfer payments. Thus, if the federal government were to use this funding to support private sector participation in health care, it too could be caught by NAFTA rules. If this were to occur the federal government would have to fund the private sector equally throughout Canada, even in those provinces that had not opened the health care sector to private enterprise. In addition, and as discussed earlier, the federal government is also entitled to rely on the purchasing exemption. However, this would only cover the direct purchase of health services by the federal government and would not, therefore, apply to the bulk of health services purchased in Canada.

4. Rules Not Subject to Exemption: Along with the rules outlined earlier that are subject to exemptions and reservations, other NAFTA rules are absolute. These rules apply to American and Mexican investors in private clinics, hospitals and other health-related enterprises. These rules establish minimum standards of treatment, prohibit restrictions on the transfer of investments and require the payment of compensation for substantial interference with the use of the investments. As I will discuss below, it is these provisions that make it more risky for governments to engage in health care reform.

In addition to the requirement that Canada treat investors from the United States and Mexico at least as well as it treats anyone else—whether Canadian or otherwise—the federal and provincial governments must ensure that they comply with international standards of fairness in dealing with these investors.[26] Government must further refrain from imposing performance requirements on investors. These performance requirements include obligations on the investor or the private clinic or hospital to purchase supplies locally, to export a certain amount of its services and to provide services on an exclusive basis to a specific region.[27] Further, neither the federal nor provincial governments may impede the free transfer by investors of private clinics or hospitals or any profits and fees arising from those clinics or hospitals.[28] Essentially, Canadian governments must assure that an investor in a private health care institution can freely sell that institution without delay.

The above rules limit the government's ability to select investors and to impose obligations on investors to run their businesses in accordance with government policy. The next rule goes beyond this. It prevents, for all practical purposes, governments from taking aspects of the health care system that they have opened to private enterprise back into the public sector.

NAFTA requires that government pay compensation for the nationalization or expropriation of an investment.[29] This provision is very broad in three respects. First, the word "expropriation" means much more than the taking over of an investment by or for the government; it means any regulation that substantially interferes with the use that the investor can make of the investment.[30] The effect of this broad meaning is that any government regulation that makes the use of a private health care institution substantially more difficult or costly would be considered an expropriation. Second, should a government expropriate an investment, it must pay the investor the fair market value of the loss. Fair market value means more than simply the value of the bricks and mortar of the investment; it also includes lost profit. This may amount to a very significant sum if the institution is or is likely to be profitable. Third, NAFTA provides investors from the United States and Mexico with a unique right to directly sue the Canadian government for compensation before an international arbitration tribunal.[31] This means that there is no political check on the use of this enforcement mechanism.

The net effect of the expropriation provision is that, for example, should a province let a national of the United States or Mexico operate a private clinic or hospital in the province—and it quite possibly must if it permits Canadian nationals to do so—the province would not be able to later close that clinic without paying the owner the fair market value (the present value of all future profits) of that clinic or hospital. These costs can easily amount to so much that a province could not afford to ever close the clinic or hospital, even if to do so were in the public interest. This is but one example of the risk that governments face in introducing health care reform on an experimental or limited basis.

B. GATS

When the World Trade Organization was created during the Uruguay Round of trade negotiations, a series of trade agreements were put into effect. Two of these are of interest in relation to their effect on health care. The first agreement, which I will discuss in this section, is GATS, dealing with trade rules applying to services, including health services. The second, which I discuss in the next section, is TRIPs, which establishes certain rules relating to patents and other intellectual property rights in, among other things, pharmaceuticals and medical devices.

All members of the WTO, including Canada, are members of GATS. Like NAFTA, GATS applies only directly to federal governments but, again like NAFTA, it requires these federal governments to pass down obligations to states and provinces.

GATS contemplates two types of obligations—general and specific. The general obligations are mandatory and apply to all sectors, including health care. The specific obligations apply only to the extent that a country has agreed to undertake those obligations.[32] Canada has chosen not to take on any specific obligations with respect to health services. This means that we need only concern ourselves with general GATS obligations, at least for the moment. GATS contemplates that countries will gradually open all sectors to market forces. Should Canada agree to do so in respect of health services, GATS may have more of an effect on Canadian health policy than at present.

There is only one general obligation that GATS imposes with which we need concern ourselves. This is the obligation—called most-favoured-nation treatment—to treat nationals of each member of GATS at least as well as nationals of any other country in the world (whether party to GATS or not).[33] This provision goes half as far as the NAFTA provisions dealing with equal treatment. Recall that, under NAFTA, Canada had to treat nationals of the United States and Mexico at least as well as the better of nationals of any other country or of Canada. This last part is missing from the general obligations under GATS (but appears under the specific obligations that do not apply to health care). This means that under GATS, but not under NAFTA, Canada can impose one set of rules for Canadians and another set of rules for foreigners.

While most-favoured-nation treatment does not seem to raise any concerns with respect to health care, it may when the effect of the GATS is combined with NAFTA. NAFTA, after all, requires that Canada treat nationals of the United States and Mexico the same as Canadians (subject to the reservations discussed earlier). Further, nationals of the United States and Mexico are entitled under NAFTA to compensation for expropriation. When these provisions are combined with most-favoured-nation treatment under GATS, it would appear that Canada must extend its treatment of Canadians to Americans and Mexicans under NAFTA and then to other WTO members under GATS' most-favoured-nation treatment.

GATS provides Canada, however, with a way out of this situation. GATS contemplates and encourages its members to enter into economic integration agreements.[34] Since NAFTA qualifies as such an agreement,[35] the benefits that Canada bestows on nationals of the United States and Mexico under NAFTA do not trigger most-favoured-nation treatment under GATS.

To the extent that Canada only permits its nationals and those of Mexico and the United States to enter into its health care market, GATS has no application. In addition, GATS exempts from its coverage services purchased by government for governmental purposes as long as these are not resold.[36] Therefore, GATS obligations would not kick in as long as provincial governments continue to purchase health care services for their residents, even if the service providers were in the private sector. Should a province provide, however, that residents purchase their health care services directly, this exemption would be lost. This means that if a province were to permit a national of a country other than the United States or Mexico to provide health services directly to its residents, it would have to permit nationals of all WTO member countries the same privilege.

C. TRIPs

The second WTO agreement of interest is TRIPs. It too applies to all WTO members at the federal level, including Canada. TRIPs attempts to standardize intellectual property rules (patents, copyright, trademarks) across member states. It does so in two ways. First, it binds all WTO members to other international agreements dealing with intellectual property rights. Since Canada was already a party to all major intellectual property agreements in one form or another, this does not raise any significant issues for health care. Second, TRIPs sets out minimal standards of protection for these rights. It is these latter standards that may very well affect health care in Canada. Since the federal government deals with intellectual property rights in Canada, there is no concern about the federal government passing down TRIPs obligations to the provinces.

While TRIPs deals with various forms of intellectual property rights, the ones of interest to us are patent rights. Patents cover inventions. These include new, not obvious, and useful pharmaceuticals, diagnostic procedures and medical devices. The person who holds a patent can prevent everyone else from using, making or selling the invention.

NAFTA itself contains provisions dealing with patent rights.[37] Since TRIPs mirrors most of those provisions in similar language, and since it applies to more countries, I will restrict my analysis in this chapter to TRIPs. However, the reader should be aware that Canada has taken on obligations with respect to patent rights under both international agreements.

The most important obligations that TRIPs imposes, in terms of health care, are the twenty-year minimum patent term;[38] the availability of patents over micro-organisms, genetic sequences and cells from living matter;[39] the equality of inventions;[40] and the restriction on the availability of compulsory licensing.[41] Because of a similar provision in NAFTA covering the twenty-year minimum term,[42] Canada had extended its patent term to twenty years previous to TRIPs. This meant that generic pharmaceutical manufacturers were prevented from entering the market with less expensive medications for a longer period. The second obligation requires that Canada must, subject to the exceptions that I will discuss below, continue its practice of granting patents over biological material. The obligation of equality means that Canada must treat biotechnological inventions in an equal manner to other inventions. This does not mean that Canada must treat biotechnological inventions exactly the same way as other inventions. There are, for example, separate rules on how to describe the inventions and the ability to deposit micro-organisms and cells instead of describing them in prose. But Canada must not treat biotech inventions in a substantively different manner from mousetraps or electronics.[43] The restriction on compulsory licensing means that Canada cannot, except in extraordinary circumstances, permit generic drug manufacturers to make or sell pharmaceutical products during the patent term. In anticipation of TRIPs and NAFTA, Canada ended its practice of compulsory licensing in 1993.[44]

TRIPs does allow some exceptions to patenting. For example, a country is not required to grant patents on medical therapies, diagnostic procedures and surgical procedures;[45] or on animals or plants[46] but, if it does so, it must follow the ordinary rules described above. So far, Canada does not permit patents on surgical procedures. The status of animal and plant patents in Canada will remain unclear until there is either a definitive judicial ruling or Parliamentary action.[47] Second, a country is entitled to withhold patents on a very limited class of inventions. These inventions, if sold, would disrupt public order or morality, or seriously endanger the environment.[48] Canada currently has no provision in its patent legislation to permit the withholding of patents for these reasons.

The overall effect of TRIPs is to increase the reach and force of patents in the health care sector. Patents cover more things for longer terms and are subject to fewer restrictions than before TRIPs (and NAFTA). In addition, the rule of equality means that Canada would have difficulty treating patents for biomedical inventions differently from other inventions in order to achieve its health policy goals.

Application of International Trade Agreements to the Formulation of Health Policy

Canadian health policy is founded on several premises. While there are many others, including comprehensiveness and public administration of the health care system, the values I wish to examine are universality, health promotion, access and freedom of choice. Universal health services are those offered to all Canadians regardless of income or location.[49] Health promotion involves the elimination or reduction of risk of contracting disease. This can occur both through individual action—for example, through general fitness and avoidance of smoking—and through community efforts to reduce environmental and occupational contributions to illness.[50] Access means that Canadians can practically access health services regardless of their location and ability to pay.[51] Freedom of choice means that the patient is entitled both to choose his or her health provider and method of treatment.[52]

In this part, I will examine how the international trade agreements just described affect Canadian health policymakers' freedom to achieve the values underlying the Canadian health care system. As I have described earlier, international trade agreements slowly push governments to open their economies, including the health care sector, to private actors. While these agreements do not dictate any particular action, once a country has (trade-) liberalized its health care sector, it is prevented from retreating from that liberalization. That is, once a government has permitted the private sector to enter into the provision of health care services, it cannot later change course. This factor, in addition to some of the specific rules set out in the various trade agreements, affects the four health policy goals that I have highlighted.

A. Universality

The concept of universality requires that all Canadians (or at least permanent residents) have an equal right to health care services. This is because we, as a society, accept that the costs of accidents and disease should not fall only on those stricken with illness. We accept these costs for two reasons. First, it is more expensive to deal with the social consequences of failing to help those in need of medical care than to treat them. Second, since we do not know which among us will be affected by disease, we believe that it is best to contribute to a common fund to pay the costs of those who happen to fall ill.[53]

Nothing in NAFTA, GATS or TRIPs specifically addresses the goal of universality. In fact, at first blush, they do not appear to even affect this goal. Nevertheless, when the functioning of NAFTA and TRIPs are examined. a different conclusion is reached.

1. NAFTA: NAFTA may limit a provincial government's ability to achieve universality, should the government wish to contract out certain health-related services to private actors. Consider, for example, a government decision to contract out all computer-assisted imaging services because of the high costs of keeping up with both technological change and demand. The government may contract all of these services out to a single actor, a group of private investors or some combination of private and public actors. In any case, in order to ensure that these imaging technologies are available to all residents of the province, the government would have to impose the obligation on all or some of these to provide services to all residents.

The first question that NAFTA raises is whether the province can restrict those with which it contracts to Canadians. The province is not entitled to the government purchasing exemption. The province would also not be able to rely on the Annex I reservation because the measure is less conforming to NAFTA—because it does not offer nationals of the United States and Mexico the same rights as Canadians—than the original rule. Thus, the only way that the province could avoid having to offer the contracts to investors in the United States and Mexico is if the province can rely on the Annex II reservation. This may be difficult since the health service is being provided for a profit. There is, therefore, a serious possibility that the province would have to make the computer-assisted imaging contract available to a company from Mexico or the United States.

Assuming, then, that either the province voluntarily offers imaging contracts to investors in the United States or Mexico or it is forced to do so by NAFTA, a provision requiring private actors to provide services to all residents could be challenged under the NAFTA expropriation and compensation provision. As discussed earlier, any substantial interference with the use of an investor's investment could be considered an expropriation. The imaging machines and related facilities would constitute the investment. The substantial interference is the requirement to use those machines to service all residents of the province. The investor could argue that, by imposing this requirement, the government is forcing it to invest more than makes sound business judgement, or at least making it incur more debt because it must buy more equipment. This interference can be substantial, even if imposed at the outset of the investment and thus could plausibly be considered to be an expropriation. This would trigger the investor's right to seek compensation directly from Canada through arbitration.

This challenge is highly speculative. Unfortunately, there is no clear, guiding decision on its merit. Nevertheless, given the language of NAFTA, its purpose and previous interpretations of trade agreements, a challenge along these lines is possible. A government formulating its health policy ought, therefore, to at least consider the risk that it could face a heavy financial penalty by proceeding along this route.

There is a second reason for government to take the risk of such a challenge seriously. This is because, if the challenge were successful, government would have no way out. For example, a provincial government would not be able to terminate the imaging contracts because of the enormous cost of doing so. After all, terminating the contracts would likely be considered an expropriation and thus itself trigger investors' rights to compensation. A government attempting to terminate these contracts would be liable, therefore, to pay the investor all lost profits that the investor would have made from continuing with the contract. This is likely to be prohibitively expensive.

2. TRIPs: If the concept of universality is understood to include the right of every person, regardless of type of illness, to similar assistance from the health care system, then it is worth looking at the incentives that TRIPs establishes for medical research. TRIPs was established to encourage industry to invent. It further relies on market forces to direct the selection of what to invent. Given the market failure in health care, this can lead to potentially troubling results.

TRIPs has the effect of encouraging research into common diseases at the expense of less common ones, and those most suffered by the wealthy and away from those most suffered by the poor. It does so by increasing our reliance on patent rights as the engine to encourage scientific development. Patents are expensive to attain and are only valuable to the extent that others would want to use the patented invention. This means that while patents may encourage companies to invest in finding therapies, diagnostics and medications for common disease, they will not do so for less common illnesses. Since TRIPs brings more basic research—genetic sequences, cell lines and, possibly, research animals—into the patent scheme, it has the effect of skewing research away from less common diseases and diseases which are disproportionately suffered by the poor.[54]

The effect of this skewing of research toward common diseases is subtle and long term. Over time, there will be ever greater numbers of products aimed at those suffering from common ailments. On the other hand, lacking the incentives provided by patents and facing competition from more lucrative areas of research, we expect fewer products aimed at those suffering from uncommon ailments. This means that, in the absence of other measures, health care may be technically universal—since it is available to all—but will be effectively less universal since the person suffering from the rare condition cannot expect the same level of services from the health care system as someone suffering from more common diseases.

TRIPs does not limit government ability to regulate health care, but it does present additional challenges to the formulation of health policy. Given the skewing in research, a government wishing to ensure substantive rather than simply formal universality will have to take corrective action. This may include establishing research funds for rare diseases, perhaps funded by taxes on those who benefit from patent incentives, or setting up other incentive schemes such as "orphan" drug protection (providing for research grants, tax incentives, approval assistance and market exclusivity) and for research into rare diseases.

B. Health Promotion

The prevention of disease is less costly than the cure. Therefore, one would think that the value of health promotion is well allied with efficiency. It is. But given market inefficiencies in health care, opening the market to health care providers and encouraging the use of patents on basic biomedical research actually provides an economic incentive to invest in treatment rather than prevention, with diagnosis lying in between. This does not mean that other interests will not profit from health promotion—health clubs, the weight control industry and even fad diet promoters all have their niche—but traditional health care providers and pharmaceutical companies profit more from illness than prevention, especially in a fee-for-service regime.

I. NAFTA: NAFTA aims to open sectors of the economy to market forces. In doing so, NAFTA creates the opportunity for private actors to develop new products that respond to the desires of the consumer. Often enough, the response is creative and unpredictable. Thus, if NAFTA was unleashed on the health care sector, novel approaches to health care, including health promotion, could be expected.

Caution should be used, however, before opening up the health care market. As I discussed earlier, the health care sector is fraught with market inefficiencies. The fiduciary nature of the physician-patient relationship, the intervention of insurance companies, the indirect effects of illness on families and communities, and the life and death nature of illness all lead to a situation in which the market is unlikely to achieve an efficient allocation of resources.

This market inefficiency means that government intervention is necessary. NAFTA may restrict government choice in establishing incentives because of its rules concerning the treatment of investors, particularly those prohibiting performance requirements. Nevertheless, NAFTA does not curtail all restrictions. Government can proceed as long as it does so cautiously.

With this caution in mind, however, opening the market to more players, particularly if government has established the right kind of incentives, can lead to more diversity in many areas, including the area of health promotion. To the extent, then, that NAFTA encourages this diversity, it helps promote some of the values behind our health care system.

2. TRIPs: Because of the skewing effect discussed earlier, TRIPs is likely to have a negative effect on increasing health promotion. TRIPs and the patent system encourage companies to invest in research that leads to identifiable and patentable products. In the biomedical field these are most often medications, other therapies and diagnostics.[55] While diagnostic procedures can contribute to health promotion, by encouraging individuals to take measures to reduce their risk of illness, the patent system generally encourages research aimed at treating disease. In addition, patent holders have the right to prevent others from using the invention. Thus, someone holding a patent over a gene sequence is entitled to prevent others from pursuing alternative research—even if aimed at health promotion.[56] By requiring WTO members to cover a broad range of biomedical innovation through patents, TRIPs amplifies the patent system's skewing effect.

As discussed earlier, the fact that TRIPs, through its reliance on patent law, skews research is not necessarily a problem, provided that governments respond with countervailing measures. But the government must respond; otherwise, we risk compromising one important value behind our health care system.

C. Access

It is not enough that Canadians have the right to health care services, especially health promotion services; they must be able to access those services without significant financial or geographic barriers. This means that we must design our health care systems to facilitate access. Governments can do this directly by providing services at no cost and in locations near to those in need. Alternatively, governments can outsource this function to the private sector. In doing the latter, governments must be aware of NAFTA's restrictions.

1. NAFTA: The hypothetical I raised earlier in my discussion of universality also raises the issue of accessibility. Recall that, in the hypothetical, the government wanted to ensure that imaging services would be available to all residents of the province. It is likely, however, that the government would want to go further than this. In particular, given the remoteness of many regions within each province, the government is likely to impose the obligation on its contractors to provide services to one or more of these regions on an exclusive basis, perhaps in return for the right to provide services in more lucrative locations.

This additional provision to provide services to remote locations raises more problems under NAFTA than did the original hypothetical. First, it strengthens the investor's claim that the obligation amounts to an expropriation and, second, it raises problems over the prohibition on performance requirements.

The claim to compensation for expropriation is made stronger because the investor can more easily make the claim that it is being forced to use its investment—machines and facilities—in an uneconomic manner. The investor could argue that it could more profitably operate its machines in a metropolitan centre. Because the government is forcing it to place these expensive machines in remote locations, it could claim compensation equal to the difference between the profits it would earn in a large city and its actual profits in the remote area.

In addition to the expropriation challenge, the investor could claim that the requirement to provide services to remote locations violates the rule against imposing performance requirements. This investor could argue that the province is requiring it "to act as the exclusive supplier of the ... services it provides to a specific region...."[57] That is, the requirement to provide imaging services on an exclusive basis to remote regions may not stand up under a NAFTA challenge.[58] This challenge can be brought directly against Canada by a Mexican or American investor without having to go through political channels. Canadian investors do not have these rights.

Consider an alternative to the imaging contracts. Instead of requiring investors to provide services in remote regions, a provincial government may offer a subsidy to those who do, in fact, provide imaging services in those remote regions. This subsidy would be premised on the fact that it would be more expensive and less profitable to operate imaging facilities in remote areas than in urban centres.

An investor from the United States or Mexico providing services in a major centre without this subsidy could try to challenge this subsidy, or at least try to lay claim to it. The investor's argument would be that, as a national of the United States or Mexico, he is entitled to the best treatment that the province provides to any similar service provider. Since the provincial government is offering some imaging service providers a subsidy, the investor should be entitled to the same subsidy. If the investor were successful, the government would have to pay the investor not only the regular fee for providing the imaging service, but would have to pay the subsidy as well.

There are certainly difficulties with this argument. Chief among them is that the investor is claiming that all imaging service providers must be treated the same. The province would presumably argue, however, that it is treating all imaging service providers in remote areas the same, regardless of national origin. The province would argue that the investor would be entitled to the subsidy if he provided services in the remote area. This is a strong, but not foolproof, argument. While chances are good that the province would win this argument, there are no guarantees, especially given that the dispute would be settled through private arbitration and not through political channels.

In summary, NAFTA poses certain difficulties for provinces attempting to further open their health care sectors to private competition, while maintaining the principle of accessibility. The threat of compensation awards should, at the very least, give provinces pause before enacting reforms.

D. Freedom of Choice

Health care in Canada is characterized by freedom of choice. Patients select their health practitioners and health practitioners, except in emergency situations, select their patients.[59] While the provincial governments pay directly for health services, control over the selection of service provider and service provided rests with the patient and physician.

There are different visions of health and health care that exist within Canada's heterogeneous population.[60] Different people, given the choice, would likely choose different types and modes of delivery of health care services. This is where NAFTA can bring us some benefit.

As I discussed earlier with respect to health promotion, NAFTA offers the possibility of opening up our markets to creative health services and creative modes of providing those services. This can be of great value, not only in terms of health promotion, but in extending Canadians' freedom of choice. At the same time, we must be aware that the health care sector is fraught with market failure. Thus, the government must carefully craft incentives in any open health care market to ensure that health policy goals are achieved. This not only requires careful thinking, but also necessitates an understanding of NAFTA and other trade agreements.

E. One-Way Street

Before concluding this discussion of how international trade agreements may affect provincial plans to implement health reform, it is worth reiterating one important fact about NAFTA—NAFTA makes experimentation potentially irreversible and, therefore, risky.

Once a government has opened up its health care sector to market forces, NAFTA makes it difficult to back up for two reasons. First, the government will lose its ability to rely on its old Annex I reservation, since the regulation of the health market will have changed. This means that the government cannot return to its old measures unless those old measures comply with NAFTA rules. Since the old measures almost always exclude private enterprise, they will not meet those rules. Thus, once the province has liberalized trade, it cannot reverse the process. This is unsurprising: it is, after all, the intention behind NAFTA. Second, the government will find it difficult to renationalize any service that it opens to the private sector because of the enormous cost of paying compensation. NAFTA forces governments that want to renationalize industry to pay full market compensation.

Given these effects, it would be foolhardy for any government to proceed with market-oriented reforms of the health care sector without taking adequate precautions. Before starting any experiment, the government must contemplate how it will reverse a failed experiment. Neglecting to do so will likely foreclose the possibility of correcting such mistakes.

One way for governments to employ caution is to open health care to the market slowly and, while doing so, linking the changes to clearly enunciated economic criteria. Therefore, instead of passing legislation that permits private sector participation in the health care sector, provinces should consider enacting legislation that contains limitations, tied to objective criteria, on the rights granted to the private sector. For example, instead of legislation that permits the government to contract out imaging services to the private sector, the legislation should provide that the government can provide limited rights to the private sector to engage in imaging services for so long as the total cost of those services to the province is less than the national average.

This form of legislation should stand up under NAFTA and not lead to compensation awards should it turn out that the imaging services cost more than the national average. There are two reasons for this. First, the requirement that the cost remain below the national average does not seem to violate the prohibition on performance requirements. This is because it does not impose any particular type of conduct on the investor. Second, because the government need not do anything to end private sector participation in the provision of imaging services, no compensation is payable. The private sector would simply and automatically lose the right to provide imaging service once the costs of those services exceed the national average.

Despite the logic of this approach, there are no guarantees that an arbitration panel will refrain from awarding compensation. This is because there are simply too many uncertainties concerning the meaning of NAFTA provisions. Nevertheless, governments ought to engage in some form of preventative action should they decide to open their health care sectors to market forces.

Conclusion

Canadian health care reform must take into account the effects that international trade agreements have both on legislative action and on the health care sector itself. The impact of these agreements on health care is unclear due to the vague language often used in these agreements, and the fact that no trade body has yet applied them in any substantive way to health care. Nevertheless, the trade agreements have two clear effects. First, to the extent that any province opens its health care sector to private enterprise, that opening is irreversible without the payment of substantial compensation. Second, Canada must abide by strict rules with respect to intellectual property protection over medical devices and pharmaceuticals, including limitations on compulsory licensing.

Outside of patents, neither NAFTA nor WTO agreements requires Canada to adopt a particular health care policy. The effect of these agreements is to slowly nudge the federal and provincial governments toward opening health care markets. The way in which this is done is up to the particular province. However, given the high cost of removing health care services from market forces, governments should proceed slowly and with caution. It would be unwise for a government to take trade liberalization action without, at the same time, limiting that action and defining a clear escape route. After all, even the most fervent supporter of the free market would have to agree that it is unlikely that all experiments in opening our health care sector to market forces will succeed. It would be irresponsible, therefore, not to contemplate in advance how we will deal with failed experiments. This should be done in a manner that will prevent exorbitant costs to government.

NOTES

1   International Covenant on Economic, Social and Cultural Rights, 16 December 1966, 993 U.N.T.S. 3, Can. T.S. 1976 No. 46, art. 12. See also B. von Tigerstrom, "Human Rights and Health Care Reform," *infra*.

2   Canada Health Act, R.S.C. 1990, c. C–6.

3   *Ibid.*, preamble.

4   Provincial governments have drastically reduced their health care spending. See, for example, D. Moulton, "Nova Scotia Slashes Health Care Spending" (2000) 162 *C.M.A.J.* 1722; L S. Williams, "The Good Ship Alberta Enters Uncharted Waters in Attempt to Make Huge Health Care Spending Cuts" (1994) 151 *C.M.A.J.* 1621. This reduction in spending takes place against a backdrop of rationalizing health care services. See "Intensive Care" (2000) 355:8164 *The Economist* 34; M.G. Brown, "Rationing Health Care in Canada" (1993) 2 *Annals of Health L.* 101.

5   E.R. Gold, "Reintegrating Basic Research, Health Policy, and Ethics into Patent Law" in T.A. Caulfield and B. Williams-Jones, eds., *The Commercialization of Genetic Research: Ethical, Legal, and Policy Issues* (New York: Kluwer Academic/Plenum Publishers, 1999) 63 at 68–9.

6   J.F. Kotalik, "Ontario's Bill 26 and Foundational Values of Canadian Health Care" (1996) *Health L. Rev.* 11.

7   North American Free Trade Agreement Between the Government of Canada, the Government of Mexico and the Government of the United States, 17 December 1992, Can. T.S. 1994 No.2, 32 I.L.M. 289 (entered into force 1 January 1994) [hereinafter NAFTA].

8   Agreement Establishing the World Trade Organization, 15 April 1994, 33 I.L.M. 1144 [hereinafter WTO Agreement].

9   Health Care Protection Act, S.A. 2000, c. H–3.3.[hereinafter Bill 11].

10 General Agreement on Trade in Services, 15 April 1994, 33 I.L.M. 1168 [hereinafter GATS].

11 Agreement on Trade Related Aspects of Intellectual Property Rights, 15 April 1994, 33 I.L.M. 1197 [hereinafter TRIPs].

12 NAFTA, *supra* note 7, art. 105.

13 NAFTA, *ibid.*, art. 1116 and 1135.

14 NAFTA does not define services; instead, it enumerates transactions related to services generally such as production, distribution, marketing, sale and delivery of a services. Given this broad coverage of services and given that international trade dispute panels have interpreted services broadly, it is fairly certain that health care services would be included within NAFTA. See "Certain Measures Affecting the Automotive Industry (Complaint by Japan and the European Communities)" (2000) WTO Doc. WT/DS139/AB/R, WT/DS142/AB/R (Appellate Body Report), online at http://www.wto.org/english/tratop_e/dispu_e/distab_e.htm (accessed on 28 July 2000). See also B. Appleton, "International agreements and National Health Plans: NAFTA" in D. Drache and T. Sullivan, eds., *Market Limits in Health Reform: Public Success, Private Failure* (New York: Routledge, 1999) 87 at 88–9.

15 NAFTA, *supra* note 7, art. 1102, 1202, 1103, and 1203.

16 NAFTA, *ibid.*, art. 1107 and 1205.

17 NAFTA, *ibid.*, art. 1210.

18 NAFTA, *ibid.*, art. 1108(7).

19 NAFTA, *ibid.*, art. 1108(1)(a)(2), Annex I.

20 1 January 1994.

21 NAFTA, *supra* note 7, art. 1108(1)(a)(1), Annex II.

22 NAFTA, *ibid.*, Annex II, Schedule of Canada at II–C–9.

23 Appleton, *supra* note 14 at 94–6.

24 Appleton, *ibid.* at 96.

25 See, generally, R. Jennings and A. Watts, eds, *Oppenheim's International Law* (Harlow, Essex: Longman, 1992) at 1242, 1272–5.

26 NAFTA, *supra* note 7, art. 1105.

27 NAFTA, *ibid.*, art. 1106(1).

28 NAFTA, *ibid.*, art. 1109.

29 NAFTA, *ibid.*, art. 1110.

30 Appleton, *supra* note 14 at 92–3.

31 NAFTA, *supra* note 7, art. 1135.

32 GATS, *supra* note 10, Part III.

33 GATS, *ibid.*, art. II.

34 GATS, *ibid.*, art. V.

35 Canada, Mexico and the United States notified the Council for Trade in Services on 1 March 1995 of their entrance into NAFTA and that NAFTA met the requirements of GATS art. V. WTO, Council for Trade in Services, "Joint Communication from Canada, Mexico and the United States," Doc. No. S/C/N/ 4 (1995).

36 GATS, *supra* note 10, art. XIII.

37 NAFTA, *supra* note 7, art. 1709.

38 TRIPs, *supra* note 11, art. 33.

39 TRIPs, *ibid.*, art. 27(3)(b). Some countries, such as Norway, have questioned whether article 27(3)(b) requires a country to grant patents over cells from plants and animals other than micro-organisms. See WTO, Communication from Norway to the Council for Trade-Related Aspects of Intellectual Property Rights, "Review of the Provisions of Article 27.3(b)," Doc. No. IP/C/W /167 (3 November 1999). This is not, however, the majority view.

40 TRIPs, *supra* note 11, art. 27(1).

41 TRIPs, *ibid.*, art. 31.

42 NAFTA, *supra* note 7, art. 1709(12).

43 "Canada—Patent Protection of Pharmaceutical Products" (complaint by the European Communities) (2000), WTO Doc. WT/DS114/R (Panel Report), online at http://www.wto.org/english/tratop_e/dispu_e/distab_e.htm (accessed 1 August 2000) para. 7.92.

44 Patent Act Amendment Act, 1992, S.C. 1993, c. 2.

45 TRIPs, *supra* note 11, art. 27(3)(a).

46 TRIPs, *ibid.*, art. 27(3)(b).

47 The Federal Court of Appeal held in *President and Fellows of Harvard College* v. *Canada (Commissioner of Patents)*, [2000] F.C.J. No. 1213 (QL), 3 August 2000, that higher life forms, such as nonhuman animals and plants were patentable in Canada. The Commissioner of Patents has, however, sought leave to appeal this decision to the Supreme Court of Canada. Thus, the patentability of plants and animals remains in doubt.

48 TRIPs, *supra* note 11, art. 27(2).

49 *Royal Commission on Health Services*, vol. I (Ottawa: Queen's Printer, 1964–65) at 11; Canada Health Act, *supra* note 2, preamble and s. 7(c).

50 Canada Health Act, *ibid.*, preamble.

51 Canada Health Act, *ibid.*, preamble and s. 7(e).

52 *Royal Commission on Health Services*, *supra* note 48 at 11; Kotalik, *supra* note 6 at 16.

53 *Royal Commission on Health Services*, *ibid.*, at 5.

54 Gold, *supra* note 5.

55 E.R. Gold, "Biomedical Patents and Ethics: A Canadian Solution" (2000) 45 *McGill L.J.* 413 at 429–30.

56 T.A. Caulfield and E.R. Gold, "Genetic Testing, Ethical Concerns, and the Role of Patent Law" (2000) 57 *Clinical Genetics* 370 at 372; T.A. Caulfield and E.R. Gold, "Whistling in the Wind" (2000) 15 *FORUM For Applied Research and Public Policy* 75 at 77.

57 NAFTA, *supra* note 7, art. 1106(1)(g).

58 The province may try to argue that it is permitted to impose this performance requirement under art. 1106(4) since it is providing an advantage—the right to provide services in a city—in exchange for the obligation to provide services to the remote region. Unfortunately for the province, the language of art. 1106(4) does not seem to support this. First, art. 1106(4) does not apply to a performance requirement prohibited by art. 1106(1)—in our case art. 1106(1)(g)—but only applies to requirements to provide the service "in its territory." The requirement here is not for the entire territory of the province, but a certain region. Thus, the province's argument is not likely to succeed.

59 *Royal Commission on Health Services*, *supra* note 48 at 11.

60 See, for example, D.M. Wilson and D.M. Kieser, "Values and Canadian Health Care: An Alberta Exploration" (1996) 3 *Nursing Ethics* 9 at 12.

Afterword

The Challenge
and the Future

Brent F. Windwick

Not since the birth of Medicare has health care been considered such a central national value. But the system so embraced by Canadians is changing dramatically. The current pace of change in medical science would have been difficult to fathom twenty years ago. The convergence of genetic knowledge and information technology promises a progressive increase in the speed and diversity of these developments.[1] Significant economic changes have parallelled scientific and technological changes. How can policy or law reasonably keep up?[2]

The answer, quite simply, is that they cannot keep up. Compared to the medical science/technology bounding hare, health policy, and particularly health law, always will be the plodding tortoises, and it is unrealistic to think that the future will hold any surprises in this respect.

However, no matter how rapidly and radically the technological/scientific/ medical universe unfolds, the use and distribution of the benefits of these developments will continue to be grounded upon some very practical issues: what services can we reasonably afford? How can we provide the same or more ambitious services with the same or less resources? Who should be permitted or asked to develop and deliver these services? Who will be the beneficiaries of these services? These are all questions which require, at the very least, some rules of engagement, which health law can and must supply.

This book has explored various private and public law concepts that can be brought to bear upon health reform. While each contributor has adopted a distinctive perspective and emphasis, at least five important factors have been identified which underpin the central challenge of health reform—how to manage health resources more efficiently, yet preserve and enhance the quality of individual care. This note attempts to identify the five factors and to offer some observations on how public and private law can help to achieve the objective.

1. Cost constraints are here to stay

Significant funding constraints have been a reality in Canadian health care for some time now. The recent restoration of some funding by provincial and federal governments has relieved, but not eliminated the pressures which those constraints have generated. Even if public surpluses persist, it is unrealistic to believe that, in the foreseeable future, funding of the Canadian system will ever sufficiently overtake public needs or, perhaps more importantly, public expectations so as to relieve these pressures.

2. Legal mechanisms will be stressed by existing and emerging forces within the Canadian health system

Two sets of forces within the current Canadian health system will exert the greatest pressure for health reform and health law reform in the next several years. One is already an old friend—cost containment. The other is a relatively new but assertive acquaintance—privately organized health care delivery.

Already, the consequences of these forces have begun to manifest themselves: actively, by the outsourcing of publicly supplied, acute care services to the private sector; and passively—by the "outsourcing" of patient care from regulated hospitals to unregulated community environments where the legal protection against restricted access and increased user cost is, at best, incomplete.

The next big step that is being urged by some is the integration of a broader range of privately owned and operated health care into the public system,[3] and possibly the introduction of for-profit facilities and programmes as an adjunct to the public system.

Sujit Choudhry has argued that Alberta's *Health Care Protection Act*, formerly known as Bill 11, may represent a turning point in the history of apathetic and confused federal responses to the perceived threat of private, for-profit health care. While there are good reasons to be sceptical about the level of political motivation to resolve this issue at a time when public health care funding is on the rise, there is no question that the public discussion around this legislation has sharpened the debate and may well give it some significant staying power. What is indisputable is that the debate about for-profit vs. non-profit health care must be extended and deepened beyond political rhetoric and simplistic labels.[4]

3. Advances in medical science and technology are as likely to increase as to decrease economic pressure on the health system

Medical/scientific and technological advances likely will be an additional source of pressure on the health system. As Colleen Flood has pointed out, technological and scientific advances are costly, and when patients expect to benefit from these advances, they also will expect these costs to be borne by the health system. If the health system cannot afford to incorporate such developments, these expectations will be frustrated and pressure for delivery alternatives will increase. The challenge will be to find an alternative that will not drive an increasingly large wedge of inaccessibility between citizens who are economically advantaged and those who are not. One manifestation of this trend is currently being observed, and hotly debated, at the international level in the context of medical research.[5]

4. Physicians will continue to drive the resource allocation bus and the destination is uncertain

For all of the talk about primary care reform,[6] it has to be questioned how successful these efforts have been to date. It is overly simplistic to blame the inefficiencies of the Canadian health system solely upon physician insensitivity to resource usage, or physician resistance to reforming fee-for-service medical care. There is little doubt that physicians have been handicapped by inadequate point-of-care information for making informed decisions about resource allocation, and this has had adverse impact upon both individual patients and the system as a whole. Rapid technological change in the near future has the potential to dramatically correct this information deficit.[7] However, it likely will be a slow process, not because its success depends on technological developments, but because it depends as much or more on the voluntary integration of that technology into physician practice, or the resolution of professional governance organizations to push implementation.

The related issue of how "moral hazard" can effectively be managed will remain difficult to resolve. Currently, neither standard compensation mechanisms nor liability risk considerations favour, much less encourage, efficient resource utilization by physicians. And unfortunately, there remains limited impetus for change in this area. For so long as public perception is that physician supply is inadequate, and international competition offers lucrative alternatives to Canadian medical practice, provincial governments will be deterred from significant reform of physician compensation. The widely publicized failures of managed care in the United States are likely to reinforce this reluctance.

5. Canadian health policy-makers and lawmakers will no longer have the luxury of thinking and acting locally in response to these pressures

The forces of globalization, international corporatism and commercialization are, and will continue to be facts of Canadian life. Health care is unlikely to be immune to their effects. As Barbara von Tigerstrom and Richard Gold have illustrated, principles and instruments of public international law could be employed to protect or to subvert individual rights to publicly funded health care in Canada. There is an inherent tension between international human rights law, on the one hand, and international trade law, on the other. The latter could well dominate the former, to the detriment of the Canadian health system unless, as Professor Gold counsels, great care and caution is undertaken.

How can health law reform assist health reform? Public law will be an important and powerful tool for achieving not only efficiency of resource allocation but also the protection of individual rights. However, both of these objectives will depend upon a more precise articulation of guiding principles and, most importantly, a mechanism that will enforce those principles in a fair and consistent manner. This in turn will depend upon three factors: greater legislative clarity, practical enforcement mechanisms, and the political will to activate those mechanisms. Changes in these three areas are equally relevant to the federal legislative arena (*Canada Health Act*) as in the provincial ones (for example, how *Brian's Law* in Ontario, or the *Health Protection Act* in Alberta—deconstructed in this book by Peter Carver and Sujit Choudhry, respectively—will work in the real world).

Private law will also be an important tool for protecting individual rights. Moe Litman and Timothy Caulfield have clearly stated the case for this position. However, private law also has the potential to impede health reform by discouraging, or at least impeding efficient resource management. Private law, and the courts that will apply its principles, must be sensitive to the risk to individual patients of an inadequately resourced health system, but also to the risk of discouraging the creativity and discipline that health providers will need in order to be truly effective agents of health reform.

Legal rules, and the negotiated resolution or adjudication of disputes based on those rules, are increasingly crucial to the stable functioning of systems where collective interests and individual rights are at odds. Health care exemplifies such a system. Scientific and technological advances may offer more choice to the individual patient, but increasingly at the expense of the health of the system as a whole. Will law reconcile this conflict of values or choose sides?

The process of health reform and health law reform will involve, fundamentally, a rebalancing of the interests and rights of individuals against those of the community. Much of Canadian social and political discourse these days revolves around "rights talk."[8] "Health reform talk" is no exception. Rights invariably conflict, and so, as Michael Ignatieff recently has argued, "rights never securely legitimize the status quo; they actually make grievance legitimate, and in so doing compel societies to continue their partial, inadequate and therefore unending process of reform...[rights talk] condemns modern societies to a permanent self-inquisition, a permanent self-questioning."[9]

How the necessary balance between these competing rights and interests will be effected in the health context is unclear at the moment. This is the challenge that health law reformers must now face. What is clear, however, is that both private and public law reform will need to happen. Neither alone will be sufficient.

NOTES

I acknowledge assistance provided by Carolyn Hutniak, Timothy Caulfield, and Barbara von Tigerstrom in preparing this article.

1   J. Rifkin, *The Biotech Century*, (New York: Jeremy P. Tarcher/Putnam, 1998). This book remains one of the most readable accounts of these developments.

2   Consider, for example, that between late September and early October 2000, a British court was asked to sanction the surgical euthanasia of one conjoined infant to preserve the life of another, and a Colorado family went public with their successful selective embryo screening and selection in order to give life to a baby boy who not only was healthy but whose genetic material could give health to his dying older sister. In relation to the former, see A (Children), Unreported, 22 September 2000 (C.A. Civil Division), online at http://www.courtservice.gov.uk (accessed 4 December 2000) and, for an example of commentary on the case, A. McCall Smith, "The Separating of Conjoined Twins" Brit. Med. J. (2000) 321 at 782. In relation to the latter, see, for example, A.N. Wente, "Brave New Baby" *The Globe and Mail* (12 October 2000), online at http://www.globeandmail.com (accessed 12 October 2000).

3   Perhaps as a trade-off against publicly funded expansion into pharmacare and home care? This interesting speculation was raised by Jeffrey Simpson on the eve of the 2000 federal election. See J. Simpson, "With Future Policies Expect the Unexpected" *The Globe and Mail* (27 November 2000, online at http://www.globeandmail.com (accessed 2 December 2000).

4   The federal election campaign of 2000 produced a flurry of such rhetoric: see, for example, "We Will Withdraw The Money" *Edmonton Journal* (14 November 2000) A1; R. Fife "I'll Punish Two-Tier Provinces: PM" *National Post* (14 November 2000) 1. C.F. Drohan, "Leaders' Health Care Debate Gave Everybody a Headache" *The Globe and Mail* (11 November 2000), online at http://www.globeandmail.com (accessed 14 November 2000).

5   See, for example, D.J. Rothman, The Shame of Medical Research, New York Review of Books, November 30, 2000, online at http://www.nybooks.com/ nyrev/WWWarchdisplay.cgi?20001130060F (accessed 1 December 2000).

6   As in, most recently, the Ontario government's "serious consideration" of a commission to "pick up the pace" of primary care reform. See I. Urquhart, "Tories ponder speeding up reform of primary care" The Toronto Star (18 November 2000), online at http://www.thestar.ca (accessed 5 December 2000).

7   Alberta's Wellnet, for example, currently is running a pilot project to bring sophisticated information technology to the bedside or examining room. For some anecdotal accounts from health care providers in other jurisdictions see, for example, S. Jauhar, "Residents Discover a Handy Helpmate" New York Times (25 October 2000), online: http://www.nytimes.com (accessed 25 October 2000).

8   For a recent exploration of this phenomenon (and characterisation of it as something distinctively Canadian), see M. Ignatieff, The Rights Revolution - 2000 Massey Lectures, (Toronto: Canadian Broadcasting Corporation/Anansi 2000).

9   Ibid. 32-33.

HEALTH CARE REFORM PROJECT BIBLIOGRAPHY

The following bibliography was compiled by the University of Alberta's Health Law Institute as part of its Health Reform Project. It consists of selected resources relating to law and health reform that are available at the University of Alberta's libraries, public libraries or on the Internet. The sources cited are primarily Canadian and American material published after 1985 and include journal articles, books and government publications. Earlier published material from other jurisdictions has been listed where appropriate.

The bibliography is divided into headings and subheadings; the main headings are in alphabetical order and the materials under each heading are in alphabetical order by author. Materials that are particularly relevant to more than one topic area have been cross-listed and included under more than one heading.

There is a large volume of published material on many of the topics covered by this bibliography. While the bibliography covers a broad range of subjects, it includes a selection of materials only and does not claim to be an exhaustive list of available resources on each topic. Furthermore, we have not included all of the materials cited by the authors of the chapters in this book, and thus the interested reader may also want to refer to footnotes of relevant chapters for additional sources. We hope this bibliography will be useful as a reference and as a starting point for research in the area of health care reform.

Vanessa Cosco and Barbara von Tigerstrom
Health Law Institute, University of Alberta

Accountability

Alberta Health, *Achieving Accountability in Alberta's Health System* (Edmonton: Alberta Health, 1998).

Alberta Health, *Achieving Accountability in Alberta's Health System: A Draft for Discussion* (Edmonton: Alberta Health, 1997).

Alberta Health, *Health and Health System Expectations and Measures: A Consultation Paper* (Edmonton: Alberta Health, 1998).

Alberta Health Planning Secretariat, *Starting Points: Recommendations for Creating a More Accountable and Affordable Health System* (Edmonton: Alberta Health Planning Secretariat, 1993).

M.L. Millenson, *Demanding Medical Excellence: Doctors and Accountability in the Information Age* (Chicago: Univ. of Chicago Press, 1997).

L. Priest, *Operating in the Dark: Accountability in our Health Care System: A Special Report* (Toronto: Atkinson Charitable Foundation, 1999).

Provincial Health Council of Alberta, *Citizen's Evaluation Criteria for a Reformed Health System: Discussion Paper* (Edmonton: Provincial Health Council of Alberta, 1997).

Provincial Health Council of Alberta, *The Evaluation Framework: The Provincial Health Council's Focus for Assessing the Progress of Health Reform* (Edmonton: Provincial Health Council of Alberta, 1997).

Provincial Health Council of Alberta, *Health Monitor: June 1996 Progress Report, Issue 1* (Edmonton: Provincial Health Council of Alberta, 1996).

Provincial Health Council of Alberta, *Initial Observations on What Results are Expected from a Reformed Health System* (Edmonton: Provincial Health Council of Alberta, 1996).

Provincial Health Council of Alberta, *Our Understanding of Health Reform* (Edmonton: Provincial Health Council of Alberta, 1996).

Provincial Health Council of Alberta, *Our Understanding of the Vision of the Alberta Health System* (Edmonton: Provincial Health Council of Alberta, 1996).

Provincial Health Council of Alberta, *Report Card on the Status of Health Reform in Alberta* (Edmonton: Provincial Health Council of Alberta, 1997).

Disputes/appeals

Provincial Health Council of Alberta, *Appeal Mechanisms Review Final Report* (Edmonton: Provincial Health Council of Alberta, 1996).

Alternative/Complementary Therapies

K.M. Boozang, "Is the Alternative Medicine? Managed Care Apparently Thinks So" (2000) 32 *Connecticut L. Rev.* 567.

M.H. Cohen, *Complementary and Alternative Medicine: Legal Boundaries and Regulatory Perspectives* (Baltimore: Johns Hopkins Univ. Press, 1998).

C. Feasby, "Determining Standard of Care in Alternative Contexts" (1997) 5 *Health L.J.* 45.

R.A. Haigh, "Reconstructing Paradise: Canada's Health Care System, Alternative Medicine and the Charter of Rights" (1999) 7 *Health L.J.* 141.

C. Johnston, "Health-care Consumers Redefining Primary Care," *Family Practice* (1 January 1996) 16.

A.A. Mickelson, *et al.*, "Managed Care Potpourri IV: Where Oh Where is Complementary/ Alternative Care?" (1997) 19 *Whittier L. Rev.* 119.

D. Young, *et al.*, "The Dilemma Posed by Minority Medical Traditions in Pluralistic Societies: the Case of China and Canada" (1995) 18 *Ethnic & Racial Studies* 494.

Canada Health Act

M. Begin, *The Future of Medicare: Recovering the Canada Health Act* (Ottawa: Canadian Centre for Policy Alternatives, 1999).

S. Choudhry, "The Enforcement of the Canada Health Act" (1996) 41 *McGill L.J.* 461.

D. Gibson, "The Canada Health Act and the Constitution" (1996) 4 *Health L.J.* 1.

M. Jackman, "The Regulation of Private Health Care Under the Canada Health Act and the Canadian Charter" (1995) 6 *Constitutional Forum* 54.

E. Nelson, "What's it all About?: The Canada Health Act" (1997) 21:3 *L. Now* 29.

S. Wharry, "The Canada Health Act Goes on Trial" (1999) 160 *CMAJ* 1751.

Charter

R.A. Haigh, "Reconstructing Paradise: Canada's Health Care System, Alternative Medicine and the Charter of Rights" (1999) 7 *Health L.J.* 141.

M. Jackman, "The Regulation of Private Health Care Under the Canada Health Act and the Canadian Charter" (1995) 6 *Constitutional Forum* 54.

M. Jackman, "The Right to Participate in Health Care and Health Resource Allocation Decisions under Section 7 of the Canadian Charter" (1995) 4:3 *Health L. Rev.* 3.

B. von Tigerstrom, P. Nugent and V. Cosco, "Alberta's Health Information Act and the *Charter*: A Discussion Paper" (May 2000) Health Law Institute, University of Alberta.

B.F. Windwick, "Health-care and section 7 of the Canadian Charter of Rights and Freedoms" (1994) 3:1 *Health L. Rev.* 20.

Cases

Auton (Guardian ad litem of) v. *British Columbia (Ministry of Health)* (2000) 78 B.C.L.R. (3d) 55 (B.C.S.C.).

Brown v. *British Columbia (Minister of Health)* (1990), 66 D.L.R. (4th) 444 (B.C.S.C.).

Cameron v. *Nova Scotia (Attorney General)*, [1999] N.S.J. No. 33, 172 N.S.R. (2d) 227 (N.S.S.C.); aff'd (1999), 177 D.L.R. (4th) 611 (N.S.C.A.).

Chaoulli c. Québec (Procureure générale) [2000] R.J.Q. 786 (Q.S.C.).

Eldridge v. *British Columbia (Attorney General)*, [1997] 151 D.L.R. (4th) 577 (S.C.C.).

Fernandes v. *Manitoba (Director of Social Services, Winnipeg Central)* [1992] 78 Man. R. (2d) 172 (Man. C.A.).

J.C. v. *Forensic Psychiatric Service Commissioner* (1992), 65 B.C.L.R. (2d) 386 (B.C.S.C.).

Ontario Nursing Home Association v. *Ontario* (1990), 74 O.R. (2d) 365 (Ont. H.C.J.).

Comparative

D. Chernichovsky, "Health System Reforms in Industrialized Democracies: An Emerging Paradigm" (1995) 73 *Milbank Q.* 339.

R.G. Evans, "The Canadian Health-Care Financing and Delivery System: Its Experience and Lessons for Other Nations" (1992) 10 *Yale L. & Policy Rev.* 362.

E.S. Gioiosa Dillabough, "An Ethical Approach to Health Care Reform in Canada: A Comparative Analysis" (1997) 25 *Man. L.J.* 153.

E.S. Gioiosa Dillabough, "An Ethical Approach to Health Care Reform in Canada: A Comparison of the Canadian and American Health Care Systems" (1998) 18:3 *Health L. in Can.* 75.

G. Gray, "Access to Medical Care under Strain: New Pressures in Canada and Australia" (1998) 23 *J. Health Politics, Policy & L.* 905.

J.K. Iglehart, "The United States Looks at Canadian Health Care" (1989) 321 *New Eng. J. Med.* 1767.

D.A. Redelmeier and V.R. Fuchs, "Hospital Expenditures in the United States and Canada" (1993) 328 *New Eng. J. Med.* 772.

M.A. Rodwin and A. Okamoto, "Physicians' Conflicts of Interest in Japan and the United States: Lessons for the United States" (2000) 25 *J. Health Politics, Policy & L.* 343.

S.A. Schroeder, "Rationing Medical Care: A Comparative Perspective" (1994) 331 *New Eng. J. Med.* 1089.

P. Vaillancourt Rosenau, "Impact of Political Structures and Informal Political Processes on Health Policy: Comparison of the United States and Canada" (1994) 13:3 *Policy Studies Rev.* 293.

Conflicts of interest

(*see also* managed care, conflict of interest)

American Medical Association, "E-8.032 Conflicts of Interest: Health Facility Ownership by a Physician," online at http://www.ama-assn.org/apps/pf_online/ pf_online?f_n=browse&doc= policyfiles/CEJA/E-8.032.HTM (accessed on 22 February 2000).

American Medical Association, "E-Addendum 1: Council on Ethical and Judicial Affairs Clarification of Self-Referral," online at http://www.ama-assn.org/apps/pf_online/ pf_online?f_n=browse&doc=policyfiles/CEJA/E- 001.00.HTM&&s_t=&st_p=&nth=1&nxt_pol=policyfiles/CEJA/E-000.01.HTM& (accessed on 7 February 2000).

M.G. Bloche, "Clinical Loyalties and the Social Purposes of Medicine" (1999) 281 *JAMA* 268.

L. Cohen, "Issue of Fraud Raised as MD Self-Referral Comes Under Spotlight in Ontario" (1996) 154 *CMAJ* 1744.

College of Physicians and Surgeons of Alberta, "Conflict of Interest Guidelines" (December 1994), online at http:www.cpsa.ab.ca/policyguidelines/conflict/html (accessed on 22 February 2000).

B.M. Dickens, "Conflict of Interest in Canadian Health Care Law" (1995) 21 *Amer. J.L. & Med.* 259

E.J. Emanuel and D. Steiner, "Institutional Conflict of Interest" (1995) 332 *New Eng. J. Med.* 262.

C.M. Flood, "Conflicts Between Professional Interests, the Public Interest, and Patient's Interests in an Era of Reform: Nova Scotia Registered Nurses" (1997) 5 *Health L.J.* 27.

T. Lemmens and P.A. Singer, "Bioethics for Clinicians: 17. Conflict of Interest in Research, Education and Patient Care" (1998) 159 *CMAJ* 960.

M.A. Rodwin and A.Z. Okamoto, "Physicians' Conflicts of Interest in Japan and the United States: Lessons for the United States" (2000) 25 *J. Health Politics, Policy & L.* 344.

S.M. Shortell, *et al.*, "Physicians as Double Agents: Maintaining Trust in an Era of Multiple Accountabilities" (1998) 280 *JAMA* 1102.

S. Tedrick, "Legal Issues in Physician Self-Referral and Other Health Care Business Relationships" (1992) 13 *J. Legal Med.* 521.

Cost-Containment

T.H. Boyd, "Cost Containment and the Physician's Fiduciary Duty to The Patient" (1989) 39 *DePaul L. Rev.* 131.

T.A. Caulfield and D.E. Ginn, "The High Price of Full Disclosure: Informed Consent and Cost Containment in Health Care" (1994) 22 *Man. L.J.* 328.

R.G. Elgie, "Health Care Cost Containment: United States and Canada Comparisons" (1994) 15 *Health L. in Can.* 3.

W.S. Feldman, "To Test or Not to Test: A Medicolegal Problem" (1996) 14:4 *Legal Aspects of Med. Practice* 6.

V.R. Fuchs, "No Pain, No Gain: Perspectives on Cost Containment" (1993) 269 *JAMA* 631.

B.R. Furrow, "The Ethics of Cost-Containment: Bureaucratic Medicine and the Doctor as Patient-Advocate" (1988) 3 *J.L. Ethics & Pub. Pol.* 187.

J.E. Gladieux, "Medicare+Choice Appeal Procedures: Reconciling Due Process Rights and Cost Containment" (1999) 25 *Am. J.L. & Med.* 61.

J.C. Irvine, "The Physician's Duty in the Age of Cost Containment" (1994) 22 *Man. L.J.* 345.

S. Lightstone, "Waiting-list Worries Cause Calgary MDs to Prepare Letter for Patients" (1999) 161 *CMAJ* 183.

E.H. Morreim, "Cost Containment and the Standard of Medical Care" (1987) 75 *Cal. L. Rev.* 1719.

P.A. Singer and F.H. Lowy, "Rationing, Patient Preferences, and Cost of Care at the End of Life" (1992) 152 *Arch. Intern. Med.* 478.

A.F. Walsh, "The Legal Attack on Cost Containment Mechanisms: The Expansion of Liability for Physicians and Managed Care Organizations" (1997) 31 *John Marshall L. Rev.* 207.

Cases

Canada

Law Estate v. *Simice*, [1994] B.C.J. No. 979 (B.C. S.C.), online: QL.; (1994), 21 C.C.L.T. (2d) 228 (B.C. S.C.).

J.C. Irvine, "Case Comment: *Law Estate* v. *Simice*" (1994) 21 C.C.L.T. (2d) 259.

United Kingdom

R. v. *Cambridge Health Authority, ex p B*, [1995] 2 All E.R. 129.

Fiduciary Duty

Alberta Association of Registered Nurses, *Position Statement on Client Advocacy* (Edmonton: Alberta Association of Registered Nurses, 1999).

P. Bartlett, "Doctors as Fiduciaries: Equitable Regulation of the Doctor-Patient Relationship" (1997) 1 *Medical L. Rev.* 193.

M.G. Bloche, "Clinical Loyalties and the Social Purposes of Medicine" (1999) 281 *JAMA* 268.

T.H. Boyd, "Cost Containment and the Physician's Fiduciary Duty to The Patient" (1989) 39 *DePaul L. Rev.* 131.

B.M. Dickens, "Medical Records: Patient's Right to Receive Copies—Physician's Fiduciary Duty of Disclosure: *McInerney* v. *MacDonald*" (1994) 73 *Can. Bar Rev.* 234.

McInerney v. *MacDonald* [1992] 2 S.C.R. 138

Norberg v. *Wynrib*, [1992] 2 S.C.R. 226.

W.M. Sage, "Physicians as Advocates" (1999) 35 *Houston L. Rev.* 1529.

World Medical Association, "World Medical Association Statement on Patient Advocacy and Confidentiality," online at http://www.wma.net/e/policy/17-oo_e.html (accessed on 16 September 1999).

Funding/Financing

D. Baxter and A. Ramlo, *Healthy Choices: Demographics and Health Spending in Canada, 1980–2035* (Vancouver: Urban Futures Institute, 1998).

Canadian Institute for Health Information, *National Health Expenditure Trends, 1975–1999* (Ottawa, 1999).

Canadian Medical Association, *Toward a New Consensus on health Care Financing in Canada* (Ottawa: Canadian Medical Association, 1993).

Health Canada, *National Health Expenditures in Canada*, (Ottawa: Health and Welfare Canada, 1973–).

"Health Cuts Hurt Everyone" (1997) 156 *CMAJ* 1523.

W. Kondro, "Canada: Ontario's Health Budget Cuts" (1993) 341 *Lancet* 1207.

O. Madore, *Established Programs Financing for Health Care* (Ottawa: Minister of Supply and Services Canada, 1991).

D. Moulton, "Nova Scotia Slashes Health Care Spending" (2000) 162 *CMAJ* 1722.

World Medical Association, "World Medical Association Resolution on Improved Investment in Health Care," online at http://www.wma.net/e/policy/20-1-96_e.html (accessed on 16 September 1999).

General Health Reform

J.D. Blum, "Balancing Regional Government Health Mandates with Federal Economic Imperatives: Perspectives from Nova Scotia and Illinois" (1997) 20 *Dal. L.J.* 359.

H. Brody, "The Place of Ethics in Health Care Reform: Framing the Health Reform Debate" (1994) 24:3 *Hastings Ctr. Rep.* 7.

M.G. Brown, "Rationing Health Care in Canada" (1993) 2 *Ann. Health L.* 101.

Canadian Medical Association, "In Search of Sustainability: Prospects for Canada's Health Care System" (13–16 August 2000), online at http://www.cma.ca/advocacy/medicare/Sustainability-2/index.htm (accessed on 18 August 2000).

R.A. Carr-Hill, "Efficiency and Equity Implications of the Health Care Reforms" (1994) 39 *Soc. Sci. Med.* 1189.

C. Chase, "A Values Framework for Health System Reform" (1992) 11:1 *Health Affairs* 84.

R. Grad, "Health Care Reform in Canada: Is There Room for Efficiency?" (1999) 20 *Health L. in Can.* 17.

R.B. Hackey, "Commentary: The Politics of Reform" (2000) 25 *J. Health Politics, Policy & L.* 211.

T.P. Hill, "Health Care: A Social Contract in Transition" (1996) 43 *Soc. Sci. Med.* 783.

J. Hurley, "When Tinkering is Not Enough: Provincial Reform to Manage Health Care Resources" (1994) 37 *Can. Pub. Adm.* 490.

J.K. Iglehart, "Canada's Health Care System" (1986) 315 *New Eng. J. Med.* 202.

M. Jérôme-Forget and C. Forget, *Who is the Master? A Blueprint for Canadian Health Care Reform* (Montreal: The Institute for Research on Public Policy, 1998).

J.F. Kotalik, "Ontario's Bill 26 and Foundational Values of Canadian Health Care" (1996) 5:2 *Health L. Rev.* 11.

M. Lamb and R.B. Deber, "Managed Care: What is it, and Can it be Applied to Canada" in R.B. Deber and G.G. Thompson, eds., *Restructuring Canada's Health Services System: How Do We Get There From Here?* [Canadian Conference on Health Economics, proceedings] (Toronto: Univ. of Toronto Press, 1992) 159.

National Forum on Health, *Canada Health Action: Building on the Legacy, Volume I: The Final Report of the National Forum on Health* (Ottawa: National Forum on Health, 1997).

National Forum on Health, *Canada Health Action: Building on the Legacy, Volume II: Synthesis Reports and Issues Papers* (Ottawa: National Forum on Health, 1997).

Nova Scotia Department of Health, *Good Medicine: Securing Doctors' Services for Nova Scotians* (Halifax: Nova Scotia Dept. of Health, 1997).

G. Sharpe and D.N. Weisstub, "Bill 26: Towards the Restructuring of Ontario's Health Care System" (1996) 17:2 *Health L. in Can.* 31.

J. Rafuse, "University Researchers Propose Major Reforms to Cut Health Care Costs" (1995) 152 *CMAJ* 410.

World Health Organization, *World Health Report 2000* (Geneva: WHO, 2000).

World Medical Association, "World Medical Association Twelve Principles of Provision of Health Care in any National Health Care System," online at http://www.wma.net/e/policy/10-90_e.html (accessed on 16 September 1999).

Alberta

Alberta Health, *Health Goals for Alberta: Progress Report* (Edmonton: Alberta Health, 1993).

Alberta Health, *Partners in Health: The Government of Alberta's Response to the Premier's Commission on Future Health Care for Albertans* (Edmonton: Alberta Health, 1991).

Alberta Health Planning Secretariat, *Starting Points: Recommendations for Creating a More Accountable and Affordable Health System* (Edmonton: Alberta Health Planning Secretariat, 1993).

Alberta Health and Wellness, *Policy Statement on the Delivery of Surgical Services: A discussion paper* (Edmonton: Alberta Health and Wellness, 1999).

Alberta Health and Wellness, *Policy Statement on the Delivery of Surgical Services: Questions and answers* (Edmonton: Alberta Health and Wellness, 2000).

R. Cairney, "Did Alberta Attempt to Cut Health Care Costs Too Quickly?" (1994) 150 *CMAJ* 1857.

T. McLaren, L. Oberg and GPC Government Policy Consultants, *Health Care in Transition: The Alberta Experience* (Edmonton: GPC, 1996).

D.J. Philippon and S.A. Wasylyshyn, "Health-Care Reform in Alberta" (1996) 39 *Can. Pub. Adm.* 70.

Provincial Health Council of Alberta, *The Evaluation Framework: The Provincial Health Council's Focus for Assessing the Progress of Health Reform* (January 1997)

Provincial Health Council of Alberta, *Health Monitor: June 1996 Progress Report, Issue 1* (Edmonton: Provincial Health Council of Alberta, 1996).

Provincial Health Council of Alberta, *Initial Observations on What Results are Expected from a Reformed Health System* (Edmonton: Provincial Health Council of Alberta, 1996).

Provincial Health Council of Alberta, *Our Understanding of Health Reform* (Edmonton: Provincial Health Council of Alberta, 1996).

Provincial Health Council of Alberta, *Our Understanding of the Vision of the Alberta Health System* (Edmonton: Provincial Health Council of Alberta, 1996).

Provincial Health Council of Alberta, *Report Card on the Status of Health Reform in Alberta* (Edmonton: Provincial Health Council of Alberta, 1997).

L.S. Williams, "Good Ship Alberta Enters Uncharted Waters in Attempt to Make Huge Health Care Spending Cuts" (1994) 151 *CMAJ* 1621.

D.M. Wilson and D.M. Kieser, "Values and Canadian Health Care: An Alberta Exploration" (1996) 3 *Nursing Ethics* 9.

Canada

Canadian College of Health Service Executives, *Health Reform Update: 1998–99* (Ottawa: Canadian College of Health Service Executives, 1999).

D. Gratzer, *Code Blue: Reviving Canada's health care system* (Toronto: ECW Press, 1999).

M. Rachlis, *Strong Medicine: How to Save Canada's Health Care System* (Toronto: HarperCollins Publishers, 1995).

Royal Commission on Health Services, *Report of the Royal Commission on Health Services, Vol. I & II* (Ottawa: Queen's Printer, 1964–1965).

Health Care Protection Act

Alberta, Legislative Assembly, "Canada Health Act and Alberta Bill 11" by J.C. Levy in *Sessional Papers* 482 (2000).

Alberta Medical Association, "President's Letter" [re. Bill 11] (18 April 2000), online at http://www.amda.ab.ca/general/private-surg/index.html (accessed on 4 July 2000).

Canadian Union of Public Employees, "CUPE Responds to Alberta Legal Opinion on Bill 11" (7 April 2000), online at http://www.cupe.ca/arvayvsalberta.html (accessed on 28 April 2000).

T.A. Caulfield, C.M. Flood and B. von Tigerstrom, "Comment: Bill 11, Health Care Protection Act" (2000) 9:11 *Health L. Rev.* 22.

Friends of Medicare, "Bill 11 [The Health Care Protection Act???]," online at http://www.friendsofmedicare.ab.ca/2000/bill11analysis.htm (accessed on 4 July 2000).

Health Care Protection Act, S.A. 2000, c. H–3.3.

Opinion Letter re. Bill 11-Health Care Protection Act and the NAFTA, Cruickshank Karvellas (23 March 2000), online at http://www.gov.ab.ca/acn/images/2000/400/8972.pdf (accessed on 22 August 2000).

Opinion Letter re. Canada Health Act and Alberta Bill 11, J.J. Arvay, Q.C. and T. Murray Rankin, Q.C. (8 March 2000), online at http://www.cupe.ca/arvay/1.asp (accessed on 22 August 2000).

Opinion Letter re. NAFTA Investment Chapter Implications of Alberta Bill–11, Appleton & Associates (10 April 2000), online at http://www.appletonlaw.com/cases/AltaGovtBll-Appleton.PDF (accessed on 22 August 2000).

L. Shanner, "Ethical Concerns about Bill 11" (University of Alberta, April 2000), online at http://www.friendsofmedicare.ab.ca/2000/bill11ethics.pdf (accessed on 4 July 2000).

S. Shrybman, "A Legal Opinion Concerning NAFTA Investment and Services Disciplines and Bill 11: Proposals by Alberta to Privatize the Delivery of Certain Insured Health Care Services," online at http://www.cupe.ca/Shrybman/ (accessed on 23 August 2000).

Health Information
Confidentiality and disclosure of health information
(*see also* managed care, confidentiality)

General

P.S. Appelbaum, "A 'Health Information Infrastructure' and the Threat to Confidentiality of Health Records" (1998) 49 *Psychiatric Services* 27.

B. Bennett, "Confidentiality" in *Law and Medicine* (Sydney: LBC Information Services, 1997) 11.

Canadian Medical Association, "The Medical Record: Confidentiality, Access and Disclosure (update 2000)," online on http://www.cma.ca/inside/policybase/2000/05-09.htm (accessed on 3 July 2000).

J.D. Cohen, "HIV/AIDS Confidentiality: Are Computerized Medical Records Making Confidentiality Impossible?" (1990) 4 *Software L.J.* 93.

College of Physicians and Surgeons, "CPSO Info: Patient Confidentiality," online at http://www.cpso.on.ca/faqanswer.asp?FAQNum=24 (accessed on 31 July 1998).

College of Physicians and Surgeons of Alberta, "A Physician's Guide to Confidentiality and the Release of Medical Information," online at http://www.cpsa.ab.ca/policyguidelines/confident.html (accessed on 31 July 1998).

College of Physicians and Surgeons of Alberta, "Physicians' Office Medical Records (Policy Issued December 1994)," online at http://www.cpsa.ab.ca/policyguidelines/medrecords.html (accessed on 31 July 1998).

College of Physicians and Surgeons of New Brunswick, "Guidelines: Confidentiality and Release of Information," online at http://www.cpsnb.org/english/Guidelines/guidelines-5.html (accessed on 31 July 1998).

E. Etchells, G. Sharpe, M.M. Burgess and P.A. Singer, "Bioethics for Clinicians: 2. Disclosure" (1996) 155 *CMAJ* 387.

B. Friedland, "Physician-Patient Confidentiality: Time to re-examine a venerable concept in light of contemporary society and advances in medicine" (1994) 15 *J. Legal Med.* 249.

J.H. Haydon, "Legal Aspects of Health Information" (1999) 20 *Health L. in Can.* 1.

B. Hoffman, "Disclosure of Medical Information Without Consent: The Patient's Right to Confidentiality" (1992) 13:2 *Health L. in Can.* 156.

I. Kleinman, F. Baylis, S. Rodgers and P. Singer, "Bioethics for Clinicians: 8. Confidentiality" (1997) 156 *CMAJ* 521.

R. MacMillan, "Confidentiality: A Physician/Bureaucrat's Perspective" (1992) 13:2 *Health L. in Can.* 150.

A.L. Mactavish, "Mandatory Reporting of Sexual Abuse Under the Regulated Health Professions Act" (1994) 14:4 *Health L. in Can.* 89.

F.H. Miller, "Health Care Information Technology and Informed Consent: Computers and the Doctor-Patient Relationship" (1998) 31 *Indiana L. Rev.* 1019.

J.J. Morris, "Health Records" in *Law for Canadian Health Care Administrators* (Toronto: Butterworths, 1996).

W. Renke, "The Confidentiality of Health Information in the Criminal Law" (1998) 6:3 *Health L. Rev.* 3.

G. Ringwood, "Confidentiality: A Health Record Department Perspective" (1992) 13:2 *Health L. in Can.* 162.

W.M. Sage, "Regulating Through Information: Disclosure Laws and American Health Care" (1999) 99 *Col. L. Rev.* 1701.

D. Timbrell, "Perspective on Confidentiality and Privacy" (1992) 13:2 *Health L. in Can.* 147.

University of Toronto Joint Centre for Bioethics Working Group, "Ethical and Legal Issues in Electronic Health Information Systems" (20 April 1998), online at http://www.utoronto.ca/jcb/health_information.htm (accessed on 31 July 1998).

Duty to warn

American Society of Human Genetics Social Issues Subcommittee on Familial Disclosure, "ASHG Statement: Professional Disclosure of Familial Genetic Information" (1998) 62 *Am. J. Hum. Genet.* 474.

W.W. Bera, "A Physician's Duty to Warn a Patient's Relatives of a Patient's Genetically Inheritable Disease" (1999) 36 *Houston L. Rev.* 559.

S.G. Coughlan, "Patients' Secrets and Threats to Third Parties: Where to Draw the Line" (1995) 15:4 *Health L. in Can.* 91

L.E. Ferris, "In the Public Interest: Disclosing Confidential Patient Information for the Health or Safety of Others" (1998) 18:4 *Health L. in Can.* 119.

F. Gelo, "Should We Protect Families from Patients: Commentary" (1998) 28:3 *Hastings Ctr. Rep.* 18.

B. O'Connor and W.Vaught, "Should We Protect Families from Patients: Commentary" (1998) 28:3 *Hastings Ctr. Rep.* 18.

Genetic information

American Society of Human Genetics Social Issues Subcommittee on Familial Disclosure, "ASHG Statement: Professional Disclosure of Familial Genetic Information" (1998) 62 *Am. J. Hum. Genet.* 474.

W.W. Bera, "A Physician's Duty to Warn a Patient's Relatives of a Patient's Genetically Inheritable Disease" (1999) 36 *Houston L. Rev.* 559.

P.L. Brockett and E.S.Tankersley, "The Genetics Revolution, Economics, Ethics and Insurance" (1997) 16 J. *Bus. Ethics* 1661.

B. Brown, "Genetic Testing, Access to Genetic Data, and Discrimination: Conceptual Legislative Models" (1993) 27 *Suffolk Univ. L. Rev.* 1573.

I.J. Brown and P. Gannon, "Confidentiality and the Human Genome Project: A Prophecy for Conflict?" in S.A.M. McLean ed., *Contemporary Issues in Law, Medicine and Ethics* (Aldershot: Dartmouth, 1996) 215.

J.W. Burnett, "A Physician's Duty to Warn a Patient's Relatives of a Patient's Genetically Inheritable Disease" (1999) 36 *Houston L. Rev.* 559.

L.O. Gostin, "Genetic Privacy" (1995) 23 J. *of L. Med. & Ethics* 320.

D. Halsey Lea, J.F. Jenkins and C.A. Francomano, *Genetics in Clinical Practice: New Directions for Nursing and Health Care* (Toronto: Jones and Bartlett, 1998).

P. Jensen, "Genetic Privacy: The Potential for Genetic Discrimination in Insurance" (1999) 29 *Victoria Univ. Wellington L. Rev.* 347.

J. Miller, "Physician-Patient Confidentiality and Familial Access to Genetic Information" (1994) 2 *Health L.J.* 141.

W.F. Mulholland, II and A.S. Jaeger, "Genetic Privacy and Discrimination: A Survey of State Legislation" (1999) 39 *Jurimetrics* 317.

J. Palca, "Keeping Genetic Information Under Wraps" (1997) 27:2 *Hastings Ctr. Rep.* 6.

Privacy Commissioner of Canada, *Genetic Testing and Privacy* (Ottawa: Minister of Supply and Services, 1992).

K.H. Rothenberg, "Genetic Information and Health Insurance: State Legislative Approaches" (1995) 23 *J.L. Med. & Ethics* 312.

M.A. Rothstein, "Genetic Privacy and Confidentiality: Why They are so Hard to Protect" (1998) 26 *J.L. Med. & Ethics* 198.

Government documents (reports, discussiosn papers etc.)

Advisory Council on Health Infostructure, *Canada Health Infoway: Paths to Better Health, Final Report* (Health Canada Reports, February 1999).

Advisory Council on Health Info-structure, *Connecting for Better Health: Strategic Issues, Interim Report* (Health Canada Publications, September 1998).

Alberta Health, *Striking the Right Balance: Access to Health Information, Protection of Privacy: A Discussion Paper* (Edmonton: Alberta Health, 1996).

Alberta Health, *Striking the Right Balance: Access to Health Information, Protection of Privacy: A Summary of Views* (Edmonton: Alberta Health, 1997).

Alberta Wellnet, *Telehealth Decision Document* (Edmonton: Alberta Wellnet, 1998).

Canadian Institute for Health Information, *Health Information Roadmap Beginning the Journey* (1999).

Canadian Institute for Health Information, *Health Information Roadmap Responding to Needs* (1999).

Manitoba Health, *Privacy Protection of Health Information: A Discussion Paper* (Winnipeg: Manitoba Health, 1996).

National Conference on Health Info-Structure, *Report of the National Conference on Health Info-Structure: Final Report (February 8–10, 1998)* (Health Canada Publications, 1998).

Nova Scotia Department of Health, *Health Information Systems Strategy: Summary Report* (Halifax: Nova Scotia Dept. of Health, 1995).

Saskatchewan Health, *Consultation Paper on Protection of Personal Health Information* (Regina: Saskatchewan Health, 1997).

Saskatchewan Health, *Report on the Public Consultations on the Protection of Personal Health Information* (Regina: Saskatchewan Health, 1998).

Health information privacy

A. Allison and A. Ewens, "Tensions in Sharing Client Confidences While Respecting Autonomy: Implications for Interprofessional Practice" (1998) 5 *Nursing Ethics* 441.

M. Azrael, "RX Privacy: Whose Right to Know?" (1999) 32 *Maryland Bar J.* 12.

L.C. Brown, W.C. Stanton and W. Paye, "Facing the Limits on Uses of Medical and Peer Review Information: Are High Technology and Confidentiality on a Collision Course?" (1997) 19 *Whittier L. Rev.* 97.

Canadian Institute for Health Information, *Canadian Health Information Framework: Working Document* (Ottawa: Canadian Institute for Health Information, 1995).

Canadian Institute for Health Information, *Privacy and Confidentiality of Health Information at CIHI: Principles and Policies for the Protection of Health Information, 2nd ed.* (Ottawa: Canadian Institute for Health Information, 1999).

Canadian Institute for Health Information, *Privacy and Confidentiality of Health Information: A Selected Annotated Bibliography* (Ottawa: Canadian Institute for Health Information, 1995).

Canadian Institute for Health Information, *Roadmap Initiative: Launching the Process* (Ottawa: Canadian Institute for Health Information, 2000).

Canadian Medical Association, "Health Information Privacy Code" (1998) 159 *CMAJ* 997.

P.I. Carter, "Health Information Privacy: Can Congress Protect Confidential Medical Information in the 'Information Age'?" (1999) 25 *William Mitchell L. Rev.* 223.

S.O. Cassidy and M.J. Sepulveda, "Health Information Privacy Reform" (1995) 37 *JOEM* 605.

A. Cavoukian, "Safeguarding Health Information" (1998) 18:4 *Health L. in Can.* 115.

R. Chamberlayne, *et al.*, "Creating a Population-Based Linked Health Database: A New Resource for Health Services Research" (1998) 89 *Can. J. Pub. Health* 270.

K. Corcoran and W.J. Winslade, "Eavesdropping on the 50-Minute Hour: Managed Mental Health Care and Confidentiality" (1994) 12 *Behavioral Sciences & the L.* 351.

J.R. Davidson and T. Davidson, "Confidentiality and Managed Care: Ethical and Legal Concerns" (1996) 21 *Health & Social Work* 208.

A. Etzioni, "Medical Records: Enhancing Privacy, Preserving the Common Good" (1999) 29:3 *Hastings Ctr. Rep.* 14.

D.H. Flaherty, "Privacy, Confidentiality, and the Use of Canadian Health Information for Research and Statistics" (1992) 35 *Can. Pub. Admin.* 75.

M.J. Glagola, "Access Control for Electronic Patient Records" (1998) 20 *Radiology Management* 44.

K.W. Goodman, *Ethics, Computing and Medicine: Informatics and the Transformation of Health Care* (New York: Cambridge University Press, 1998).

L.O. Gostin, "Health Information Privacy" (1995) 80 *Cornell L. Rev.* 451.

L.O. Gostin, "Personal Privacy in the Health Care System: Employer-Sponsored Insurance, Managed Care, and Integrated Delivery Systems" (1997) 7 *Kennedy Inst. Ethics J.* 361.

L.O. Gostin, "Privacy and Security of Health Information in the Emerging Health Care System" (1995) 5:1 *Health Matrix* 36.

L.O. Gostin, *et al.*, "Privacy and Security of Personal Information in a New Health Care System" (1993) 270 *JAMA* 2487.

L.O. Gostin, *et al.*, "The Public Health Information Infrastructure: A National Review of the Law on Health Information Privacy" (1996) 275 *JAMA* 1921.

Health Canada and Canadian Institute for Health Information, *Health Information Roadmap: Beginning the Journey* (Ottawa: Health Canada, 1999).

Health Canada and Canadian Institute for Health Informaiton, *Health Information Roadmap: Responding to Needs* (Ottawa: Health Canada, 1999).

M.A. Jagutis, "Insurer's Access to Genetic Information: The Call for Comprehensive Federal Legislation" (1999) 82 *Marquette L. Rev.* 429.

R.H. Jerry, "Health Insurer's Use of Genetic Information: A Missouri Perspective on a Changing Regulatory Landscape" (1999) 64 *Missouri L. Rev.* 759.

S. Kornetsky, "Employer Perspectives on Health Information Confidentiality Legislation" (1999) 25 *Employee Relations L.J.* 145.

R. MacMillan, "Health Information and Health Insurance" (1998) 18:4 *Health L. in Can.* 129.

C. Marwick, "Increasing Use of Computerized Recordkeeping Leads to Legislative Proposals for Medical Privacy" (1996) 276 *JAMA* 270.

J.F. Merz, B.J. Spina and P. Sankar, "Patient Consent for Release of Sensitive Information from their Medical Records: An Exploratory Study" (1999) 17 *Behav. Sci. L.* 445.

W.H. Minor, "Identity Cards and Databases in Health Care: The Need for Federal Privacy Protections" (1995) 28 *Colum. J.L. & Soc. Probs.* 253.

National Research Council, *For the Record: Protecting Electronic Health Information* (Washington: National Academy Press, 1997).

W.E. Parmet, "Panel Comment: Legislating Privacy: The HIV Experience" (1995) 23 *J. of L. Med. & Ethics* 371.

Privacy Commissioner of Canada, *Privacy and Health Information Networks: Can we have both?* (Notes of the Privacy Commissioner of Canada to the Canadian Medical Association's National Physician Workshop, Ottawa, Ontario) (3 April 1998), online at http://www.privcom.gc.ca/02_05_a_980403_e.html (accessed on 3 November 1999).

G. Ringwood, "Toward Secure Health Information and the Electronic Health Record" (1998) 18:4 *Health L. in Can.* 117.

B. Rock and E. Congress, "The New Confidentiality for the 21st Century in a Managed Care Environment" (1999) 44 *Social Work* 253.

H.G. Rubinstein, "If I Am Only for Myself, What Am I? A Communitarian Look at the Privacy Stalemate" (1999) 25 *Am. J.L. & Med.* 203.

Secretary of Health and Human Services, "Confidentiality of Individually-Identifiable Health Information: Recommendations pursuant to section 264 of the Health Insurance Portability and Accountability Act of 1996" (11 September 1997), online at Electronic Privacy

Information Centre http://www.epic.org/privacy/medical/
hhs_recommendations_1997.html (accessed on 24 October 1997).

D.C. Silverman, "The Electronic Medical Record System: Health Care Marvel or Morass?"
(1998) 24 *Physician Executive* 26.

P. Starr, "Health and the Right to Privacy" (1999) 25 *Am. J.L. & Med.* 193.

D.M. Studdert, "Direct Contracts, Data Sharing and Employee Risk Selection: New Stakes for
Patient Privacy in Tomorrow's Health Insurance Markets" (1999) 25 *Am. J.L. & Med.* 233.

P.K. Sutherland and G. Yarbrough, "High-Tech Gossip: Physician-Patient Confidentiality and
Computerized Managed Care" (1996) 32:11 *Trial* 58.

B. von Tigerstrom, "Protection of Health Information Privacy: The Challenges and Possibilities
of Technology" (1998) 4 *Appeal Rev. Current L. & L. Reform* 44.

A.A. Waller, "Health Care Information Issues in Health Care Reform" (1995) 16 *Whittier L. Rev.*
15.

D.J. Willison, "Health Services Research and Personal Health Information: Privacy Concerns,
New Legislation and Beyond" (1998) 159 *CMAJ* 1378.

Information systems

R. Chamberlayne, *et al.*, "Creating a Population-Based Linked Health Database: A New Resource
for Health Services Research" (1998) 89 *Can. J. Pub. Health* 270.

National Conference on Health Info-Structure, *Report of the National Conference on Health Info-
Structure: Final Report (February 8–10, 1998)* (Health Canada Publications, 1998).

University of Toronto Joint Centre for Bioethics Working Group, "Ethical and Legal Issues in
Electronic Health Information Systems" (20 April 1998), online at http://www.utoronto.ca/
jcb/health_information.htm (accessed on 31 July 1998).

Alberta Wellnet

Alberta Medical Association, "Alberta Wellnet: Physicians Integrating Care Across Alberta ,"
online at http://www.amda.ab.ca/general/communications/publications/add/1998/nov-
dec98/wellnet.html (accessed on 16 June 1999).

Alberta Wellnet, "About Wellnet," online at http://www.albertawellnet.org/about/html (accessed
on 22 February 2000).

Health Canada Infoway

Advisory Council on Health Infostructure, *Canada Health Infoway: Paths to Better Health, Final
Report* (Health Canada Reports, February 1999).

Saskatchewan Health Information Network

Saskatchewan Health Information Network, "About SHIN: SHIN Focuses on Privacy," online
at http://www.shin.sk.ca/SHIN/About/Privacy.htm (accessed on 10 November 1999).

Legislation, texts (legislation, bills, proposed drafts)

Alberta
Health Information Act S.A. 1999, c. H–4.8.

Canada
Personal Information Protection and Electronic Documents Act, R.S.C. 2000, c. 5.
Manitoba
The Personal Health Information Act, R.S.M. 1997, c. P33.5.
Ontario
Draft Personal Health Information Protection Act, 1997 (Queens Printer for Ontario, November
1997).

Draft Personal Health Information Protection Act, 1997, Overview (Queens Printer for Ontario,
November 1997).

Saskatchewan
The Health Information Protection Act, R.S.S. 1999, c. H–0.021.
New Zealand
Privacy Commissioner, "Health Information Privacy code, 1994 (amended to 12 February 1996)," online at http://www.privacy.org.nz/shealthf.html (accessed on 22 February 2000).

Legislation, commentary (relating to or commenting on actual or proposed legislation)

Alberta

Alberta Health, *Consultations on the Draft Health Information Protection Act: A Summary of Views* (Edmonton: Alberta Health, 1997).

Alberta Health and Provincial Steering Committee on the Health Information Protection Act, "Report and Recommendations" (30 June 1998), online at http://www.health.gov.ab.ca/public/document/hipa/index.htm (accessed on 8 June 1999).

Alberta Health and Wellness, *A Guide to Alberta's New Health Information Act* (Edmonton: Alberta Health and Wellness, 1999).

Alberta Health and Wellness, *A Summary of Alberta's New Health Information Act* (Edmonton: Alberta Health and Wellness, 1999).

Alberta Medical Association, "Alberta Medical Association Comments to Bill 30-Health Information Protection Act" (1997), online at http://www.amda.ab.ca/general/pc-info/bill30.htm (accessed on 2 December 1999).

Alberta Medical Association, "President's Letter" (re. Bill 40) (25 November 1999), online at http://www.amda.ab.ca/general/privacy/pres-let.html (accessed on 22 February 2000).

Information and Privacy Commissioner of Alberta, "Response to Bill 40: The Health Information Act" (22 November 1999), online at http://ipc.developersedge.com/other/bill40response.htm (accessed on 22 February 2000).

Office of the Information and Privacy Commissioner, *Response to Bill 30: Health Information Protection Act* (3 November 1997).

G.B. Robertson, "The Health Information Protection Act" (1997) 6:1 *Health L. Rev.* 8.

B. von Tigerstrom, "The Health Information Act: Controversial New Legislation for Alberta" (2000) 2:1 *Observations: Bulletin of the Telehealth Ethics Observatory*, online at Centre for Bioethics http://www.ircm.qc.ca/bioethique/english/telehealth/current_issue.html (accessed on 22 February 2000).

B. von Tigerstrom, P. Nugent and V. Cosco, "Alberta's Health Information Act and the Charter: A Discussion Paper" (May 2000) Health Law Institute, University of Alberta.

Canada

BC Public Interest Advocacy Centre, *Personal Health Information and the Right to Privacy: An Overview of Statutory, Common Law, Voluntary and Constitutional Privacy Protections* (Vancouver: BC Freedom of Information and Privacy Association, March 2000).

Canadian Institute for Health Information, *Legislation Protecting Personal Health Information in Canada and Overseas: A background paper prepared for the CIHI Advisory Group on Confidentiality, Privacy, and Health Data Sharing* (Ottawa: Canadian Institute for Health Information, 1995).

Canadian Medical Association, "'Putting Patients First': Comments on Bill C–6" (29 November 1999), online at http://www.cma.ca/advocacy/political/1999/11%2D29/index.htm (accessed on 22 August 2000).

Privacy Commissioner of Canada, "Remarks to the Senate Standing Committee on Social Affairs, Science and Technology: Bill C–6, the *Personal Information Protection and Electronic Documents Act*" (Ottawa: 1 December 1999), online at http://www.privcom.gc.ca/english/02_05_a_991201_e.html (accessed on 4 March 2000).

Task Force on Electronic Commerce, "Analysis of the Submission by the Ontario Ministry of Health to the Standing Committee on Industry" (16 July 1999), online at http://e-com.ic.gc.ca/english/privacy/632d296.html (accessed on 5 August 1999)

B. von Tigerstrom, "The 'Hidden Story of Bill C–54: The Personal Information Protection and Electronic Documents Act and Health Information" (1999) 8:2 *Health L. Rev.* 13.

Ontario

M. Bay, "A Tribunal's Perspective on Ontario's Proposed Health Information Law" (1998) 18:4 *Health L. in Can.* 131.

B.K. Brown, "The Personal Health Information Protection Act, 1997: The Police Perspective" (1998) 18:4 *Health L. in Can.* 126.

A. Carruthers, "A Health Information Statute for Ontario: A Consumer's Perspective" (1998) 18:4 *Health L. in Can.* 127.

A. Cavoukian, "The Application and Scope of the Proposed New Law" (1992) 13:2 *Health L. in Can.* 153.

Ontario, Ministry of Health, *A Legal Framework for Health Information: Consultation Paper* (Toronto: Ontario Ministry of Health, 1996).

United States

G.J. Annas, L.H. Glantz and P.A. Roche, "Drafting the Genetic Privacy Act: Science, Policy, and Practical Considerations" (1995) 23 *J.L. Med. & Ethics* 360.

S.E. Corsey, "The American Health Security Act and Privacy: What Does it Really Cost?" (1994) 12 *J. Computer & Information L.* 585.

"Model Health Information Disclosure Act" (1999) 25 *J. Corporation L.* 119.

P.R. Reilly, "Panel Comment: The Impact of the Genetic Privacy Act on Medicine" (1995) 23 *J.L. Med. & Ethics* 378.

Secretary of Health and Human Services, "Confidentiality of Individually-Identifiable Health Information: Recommendations pursuant to section 264 of the *Health Insurance Portability and Accountability Act* of 1996" (11 September 1997), online at http://www.epic.org/privacy/medical/hhs_recommendations_1997.html (accessed on 24 October 1997).

A.A. Waller, "Health Care Information Issues in Health Care Reform" (1995) 16 *Whittier L. Rev.* 15.

Patients' access to health information

S. Malcolmson, "Access by Patients to the Clinical Record" (1992) 13 *Health L. in Can.* 160.

P. Marck, "Access and Privacy Issues in Health Information: Views from the Nursing Profession" (1997) 6:1 *Health L. Rev.* 3.

McInerney v. *MacDonald* [1992] 2 S.C.R. 138

Personal identifiers

F.L. Komuves, "We've Got Your Number: An Overview of Legislation and Decisions to Control the Use of Social Security Numbers as Personal Identifiers" (1998) 16 *J. Computer & Information L.* 529.

Research

D.H. Flaherty, "Privacy, Confidentiality, and the Use of Canadian Health Information for Research and Statistics" (1992) 35 *Can. Pub. Admin.* 75.

H.T. Greely, "Breaking the Stalemate: A Prospective Regulatory Framework for Unforeseen Research Uses of Human Tissue Samples and Health Information" (1999) 34 *Wake Forest L. Rev.* 737.

D.E. Nease and D.J. Doukas, "Research Privacy or Freedom of Information?" (1999) 29:3 *Hastings Ctr. Rep.* 47.

D.J. Willison, "Health Services Research and Personal Health Information: Privacy Concerns, New Legislation and Beyond" (1998) 159 *CMAJ* 1378.

E. Wright Clayton, "Panel Comment: Why the Use of Anonymous Samples for Research Matters" (1995) *J.L. Med. & Ethics* 375.

Technology and privacy

D.D. Bradham, S. Morgan and M.E. Dailey, "The Information Superhighway and Telemedicine: Applications, Status, and Issues" (1995) 30 *Wake Forest L. Rev.* 145.

M. Campbell, "Advanced Technology in the Health Care Sector: Selected Legal Implications" (1992) 13:2 *Health L. in Can.* 164.

F. Gilbert, "Privacy of Medical Records? The Health Insurance Portability and Accountability Act of 1996 Creates a Framework for the Establishment of Security Standards and the Protection of Individually Identifiable Health Information" (1997) 73 *North Dakota L. Rev.* 93.

K.B. Keltner, "Networked Health Information: Assuring Quality Control on the Internet" (1998) 50 *Federal Communications L.J.* 417.

C. Marwick, "Increasing Use of Computerized Recordkeeping Leads to Legislative Proposals for Medical Privacy" (1996) 276 *JAMA* 270.

W.H. Minor, "Identity Cards and Databases in Health Care: The Need for Federal Privacy Protections" (1995) 28 *Colum. J.L. & Soc. Probs.* 253.

A. Naszlady and J. Naszlady, "Patient Health Record on a Smart Card" (1998) 48 *Int. J. Med. Informatics* 191.

R. Neame, "Smart Cards: The Key to Trustworthy Health Information Systems" (1997) 314 *BMJ* 573.

D.M. Robinson, "A Legal Examination of Computerized Health Information" (1993) 14:2 *Health L. in Can.* 40.

Health Professionals
(*see also* Managed Care)

G.J. Agich, "Rationing and Professional Autonomy" (1990) 18 *L. Med & Health Care* 77.

M.J. Astrue, "Health Care Reform and the Constitutional Limits on Private Accreditation as an Alternative to Direct Government Regulation" (1994) 57 *L. & Contemporary Problems* 75.

T. Bodenheimer, "The American Health Care System: Physicians and the Changing Medical Marketplace" (1999) 340 *New Eng. J. Med.* 584.

Canadian Nurses' Association, *The Future Supply of Registered Nurses in Canada: A Discussion Paper* (Ottawa: Canadian Nurses' Association, 1997).

E. Godley, "MDs Should Assume More Responsibility for Managing Health Care, Royal College Audience Told" (1994) 150 *CMAJ* 76.

J.K. Iglehart, "Addressing the Problem of Physician Supply" (1986) 315 *New Eng. J. Med.* 1623.

R.G. Lee and F.H. Miller, "The Doctor's Changing Role in Allocating US and British Medical Services" (1990) 18 *L. Med. & Health Care* 69.

J.J. Morris, M. Ferguson and M.J. Dykeman, *Canadian Nurses and the Law* (Markham, ON: Butterworths, 1999).

I.J. Norman and S. Cowley, eds., *The Changing Nature of Nursing in a Managerial Age* (Oxford: Blackwell Science, 1999).

J. Spetz and Public Policy Institute of California, *The Effects of Managed Care and Prospective Payment on the Demand for Hospital Nurses: Evidence from California* (San Francisco: Public Policy Institute of California, 1999).

W.M. Sullivan, "What Is Left of Professionalism after Managed Care?" (1999) 29:2 *Hastings Ctr. Rep.* 7.

Assistive personnel

P.G. Zimmermann, "Increased Use of Unlicensed Assistive Personnel: Pros and Cons" (1995) 21 *J. Emerg. Nursing* 541.

Compensation

Alberta Medical Association and Alberta Health and Wellness, "Look Again: Taking another look at alternative payment plans," online at http://www.amda.ab.ca/general/health-reform/index.html (accessed on 4 July 2000).

C.E. Bishop and S.S. Wallack, "National Health Expenditure Limits: The Case for a Global Budget Process" (1996) 74 *Milbank Q.* 361.

J. Hurley and R. Card, "Global Physician Budgets as Common-Property Resources: Some Implications for Physicians and Medical Associations" (1996) 154 *CMAJ* 1161.

Employment/labour

L. Duran-Arenas and M. Lopez-Cervantes, "Health Care Reform and the Labor Market" (1996) 43 *Soc. Sci. Med.* 791.

D.J. Hunter, "The Changing Roles of Health Care Personnel in Health and Health Care Management" (1996) 43 *Soc. Sci. Med.* 799.

P.B. Jurgeleit, "Physician's Employment Under Managed Care: Toward a Retaliatory Discharge Cause of Action for HMO-Affiliated Physicians" (1997) 73 *Indiana L.J.* 255.

E.L. Luepke, "White Coat, Blue Collar: Physician Unionization and Managed Care" (1999) 8 *Ann. Health L.* 275.

Nursing

The Working Group for Registered Nurses in Advanced Nursing Practice in Rural/Remote Communities, *Guidelines for Registered Nurses in Advanced Nursing Practice Providing Primary Health Care Services in Under-Serviced Communities in Alberta* (Edmonton: Alberta Health, 1994).

Practice guidelines

Canadian Medical Association, *Guidelines for Canadian Clinical Practice Guidelines* (Ottawa: Canadian Medical Association, 1994).

J.R. Matthews, "Practice Guidelines and Tort Reform: The Legal System Confronts the Technocratic Wish" (1999) 24 *J. Health Politics, Policy & L.* 275.

Professional regulation

Health Workforce Rebalancing Committee, *Discussion Paper II: A Report of the Health Workforce Rebalancing Committee* (Edmonton: Alberta Health Workforce Rebalancing Committee, 1995).

Health Workforce Rebalancing Committee, *New Directions for Legislation Regulating the Health Professions in Alberta: A Discussion Paper* (Edmonton: Alberta Health Workforce Rebalancing Committee, 1994).

Health Workforce Rebalancing Committee, *Principles and Recommendations for the Regulation of Health Professionals in Alberta: Final Report of the Health Workforce Rebalancing Committee* (Edmonton: Alberta Health Workforce Rebalancing Committee, 1995).

Manitoba Law Reform Commission, *Discussion Paper: The Future of Occupational Regulation in Manitoba* (Winnipeg: The Commission, 1993).

World Medical Association, "World Medical Association Statement on Health Promotion," online at http://www.wma.net/e/policy/10-75_e.html (accessed on 16 September 1999).

Supply/licensing

Alberta Medical Association, "Setting a Direction for Alberta's Physician Workforce" (15 February 2000), online at http://www.amda.ab.ca/general/health-reform/index.html (accessed on 4 July 2000).

M.L. Barer and G.L. Stoddart, *Improving Access to Needed Medical Services in Rural and Remote Canadian Communities: Recruitment and Retention Revisited* (Vancouver: Centre for Health Services Policy Research, Health Human Resources Unit, 1999).

S.G. Coughlan and D. Darling, "Constitutional Implications of Geographical Limits on Physician Deployment" (1993) 72 *Nova Scotia Medical J.* 79.

Physician Resource Planning Committee, *et al.*, *Setting a Direction for Alberta's Physician Workforce: February 2000 Report to the Minister of Alberta Health and Wellness and the Alberta Medical Association* (Edmonton: Physician Resource Planning Committee, 2000).

R.W. Pong and J.C. Hogenbirk, "Licensing Physicians for Telehealth Practice: Issues and Policy Options" (1999) 8:1 *Health L. Rev.* 3.

D.R. Wilson, S.C. Woodhead-Lyons and D.G. Moores, "Alberta's Rural Physician Action Plan: An integrated approach to education, recruitment and retention" (1998) 158 *CMAJ* 351.

Home Care

M. Anderson, K. Parent and S. Nishihama, *A Study Conducted by Queens Health Policy Research Unit for the Canadian Association for the Fifty-Plus* (Kingston, ON: Queen's Health Policy Research Unit, Queen's University, 1999).

T.A. Caulfield and D.E. Ginn, "The High Price of Full Disclosure: Informed Consent and Cost Containment in Health Care" (1994) 22 *Man. L.J.* 328.

P. Doty, J. Kasper and S. Litvak, "Consumer-Directed Models of Personal Care: Lessons from Medicaid" (1996) 74 *Milbank Q.* 377.

L. Forrow, "When Is Home Care Medically Necessary?" (1991) 21:4 *Hastings Ctr. Rep.* 36.

B. Havens, *Home Care Issues at the Approach of the 21st Century from a World Health Organization Perspective: A Literature Review* (Geneva: World Health Organization, 1999).

B. Havens, *Home Care Issues and Evidence* (Geneva: World Health Organization, 1999).

J.M. Keefe, *Final Report on Human Resource Issues in Home Care: Comparative Analysis of Employment Arrangements* (Halifax, NS: Dept of Gerontology, Mount Saint Vincent University, 1999).

M.A. MacAdam, *Human Resource Issues in Home Care in Canada: A Policy Perspective* (Ottawa: Home Care Development, 1999).

M.R. Morris, *et al.*, *The Changing Nature of Home Care and its Impact on Women's Vulnerability to Poverty* (Ottawa: Status of Women Canada, 1999).

National Conference on Home Care: Proceedings (Halifax, March 8–10, 1998) (Ottawa: Health Canada Publications, 1998).

National Roundtable on Home and Community Care, *Report on the National Roundtable on Home and Community Care* (Ottawa: Health Canada, Home Care Development, 1999).

A.M. Williams, "The Development of Ontario's Home Care Program: A Critical Geographical Analysis" (1996) 42 *Soc. Sci. Med.* 937.

Informed Consent
(*see also* Managed Care, Informed consent)

R. Gatter, "Informed Consent Law and the Forgotten Duty of Physician Inquiry" (2000) 31 *Loyola Univ. Chicago L.J.* 557.

M.A. Jones, "Informed Consent and other Fairy Stories" (1999) 7 *Medical L. Rev.* 103.

J.H. Krause, "Reconceptualizing Informed Consent in an Era of Health Care Cost Containment" (1999) 85 *Iowa L. Rev.* 261.

F.H. Miller, "Health Care Information Technology and Informed Consent: Computers and the Doctor-Patient Relationship" (1998) 31 *Indiana L. Rev.* 1019.

A.J. Rosoff, "Informed Consent in the Electronic Age" (1999) 25 *Am. J.L. & Med.* 367.

J. Sugarman, *et al.*, "Empirical Research on Informed Consent: An Annotated Bibliography" (1999) 29:1 *Hastings Ctr. Rep.* S1.

Insurance

A.E. Cantor, "Insurance: Policies Can Be Held Discriminatory Under the ADA" (1999) *J.L. Med. & Ethics* 102.

O. Carrasquillo, "A Reappraisal of Private Employers' Role in Providing Health Insurance" (1999) 340 *New Eng. J. Med.* 109.

D. Cook, "Genetics and the British Insurance Industry" (1999) 25 *J. Med. Ethics* 157.

A. English, "The New Children's Health Insurance Program: Early Implementation and Issues for Special Populations" (1999) 32:9–10 *Clearinghouse Rev.* 429.

R.B. Hackey, "Commentary: The Politics of Reform" (2000) 25 *J. Health Politics, Policy & L.* 211.

J.J. Hasman and W.A. Chittenden III, "Recent Developments in Health Insurance, Life Insurance, and Disability Insurance Case Law" (2000) 35 *Tort & Insurance L.J.* 369.

J.K. Iglehart, "The American Health Care System—Medicaid" (1999) 340 *New Eng. J. Med.* 403.

J.K. Iglehart, "The American Health Care System—Medicare" (1999) 340 *New Eng. J. Med.* 327.

J.M. Jendusa, "Pandora's Box Exposed: Untangling the Web of the Double Helix in Light of Insurance and Managed Care" (1999) 49 *DePaul L. Rev.* 161.

C.N. Kahn, "Patients' Rights Proposals: The Insurers' Perspective" (1999) 281 *JAMA* 858.

J.M. Kelly, "HIV and Insurance" in D.C. Jayasuriya, ed., *HIV Law, Ethics and Human Rights: Text and Materials* (New Delhi: UNDP Regional Project on HIV and Development, 1995).

R. Kuttner, "The American Health Care System: Employer-Sponsored Health Coverage" (1999) 340 *New Eng. J. Med.* 248.

R. Kuttner, "The American Health Care System: Health Insurance Coverage" (1999) 340 *New Eng. J. Med.* 163.

D.W. Light, "Good Managed Care Needs Universal Health Insurance" (1999) 130 *Ann. Intern. Med.* 686.

R. MacMillan, "Health Information and Health Insurance" (1998) 18:4 *Health L. in Can.* 129.

S.H. Miles, "Gender and Health Insurance" (1997) 23 *William Mitchell L. Rev.* 313.

T.R. Oliver, "Commentary: Dynamics without Change: The New Generation" (2000) 25 *J. Health Politics, Policy & L.* 225.

J.E. Sabin and N. Daniels, "Making Insurance Coverage for New Technologies Reasonable and Accountable" (1998) 279 *JAMA* 703.

D.M. Studdert, "Direct Contracts, Data Sharing and Employee Risk Selection: New Stakes for Patient Privacy in Tomorrow's Health Insurance Markets" (1999) 25 *Am. J.L. & Med.* 33.

J.P. Vistnes, et al., *Health Insurance Status of the Civilian Noninstitutionalized Population* (Rockville, MD: US Dept. of Health and Human Services, Public Health Service, Agency for Health Care Policy and Research, 1999).

Managed Care

Capitation

F.H. Miller, "Capitation and Physician Autonomy: Master of the Universe or Just Another Prisoner's Dilemma?" (1996) 6:1 *Health Matrix* 89.

S.D. Pearson, J.E. Sabin and E.J. Emanuel, "Ethical Guidelines for Physician Compensation Based on Capitation" (1998) 339 *New Eng. J. Med.* 689.

S.K. Reed, "Serious Mental Illness and Capitation Financing" (1994) 12 *Behavioral Sciences & the L.* 379.

D.C. Wyld, "The Capitation Revolution in Health Care: Implications for the Field of Nursing" (1996) 20 *Nurs. Admin. Q.* 1.

Cases

Andrews-Clarke v. *Travelers Ins. Co.*, 984 F.Supp. 49 (D.Mass. 1997).

Corcoran v. *United Healthcare, Inc.*, 965 F.2d 1321 (5th Cir. 1992).

Danca v. *Emerson Hospital*, 9 F.Supp.2d 27 (D.Mass. 1998).
Davies v. *Genesis Medical Center*, 994 F.Supp. 1078 (S.D.Iowa 1998).
Moscovitch v. *Danbury Hospital*, 25 F.Supp.2d 74 (D.Conn. 1998).
Pegram v. *Herdrich*, 120 S. Ct. 2143 (2000), rev'g 154 F. 3d 362 (7th Cir. 1998).
Shea v. *Emmanuel College*, 682 N.E.2d 1348 (Mass. 1997).
Weiss v. *Cigna Healthcare, Inc.*, 972 F.Supp. 748 (S.D.N.Y. 1997).
Wickline v. *State of California*, 228 Cal.Rptr. 661 (Cal.App. 2 Dist. 1986).
Wilson v. *Blue Cross of Southern California*, 271 Cal.Rptr. 876 (Cal.App. 2 Dist. 1990).

Confidentiality
(*see also* Health Information,
Confidentiality and disclosure)

E. Brooks, *et al.*, "Confidentiality and Right to Privacy Issues in Mental Health Managed Care" (1997) 19 *Whittier L. Rev.* 39.

K. Corcoran and W.J. Winslade, "Eavesdropping on the 50-Minute Hour: Managed Mental Health Care and Confidentiality" (1994) 12 *Behavioral Sciences & the L.* 351.

J.R. Davidson and T. Davidson, "Confidentiality and Managed Care: Ethical and Legal Concerns" (1996) 21 *Health & Social Work* 208.

L.O. Gostin, "Personal Privacy in the Health Care System: Employer-Sponsored Insurance, Managed Care, and Integrated Delivery Systems" (1997) 7 *Kennedy Inst. Ethics J.* 361.

B. Rock and E. Congress, "The New Confidentiality for the 21st Century in a Managed Care Environment" (1999) 44 *Social Work* 253.

P.K. Sutherland and G. Yarbrough, "High-Tech Gossip: Physician-Patient Confidentiality and Computerized Managed Care" (1996) 32:11 *Trial* 58.

Conflicts of interest (*see also* conflicts of interest)

K.T. Christensen, "Commentary: A Physician's Perspective on Conflicts of Interest" (1997) 25 *J.L. Med. & Ethics* 199.

B.J. Culliton, "Managed Care and Conflict of Interest" (1996) 2 *Nature Medicine* 489.

B.M. Dickens, "Conflicts of Interest in Canadian Health Care Law" (1995) 21 *Am. J.L. & Med.* 259.

E.J. Emanuel and L. Goldman, "Protecting Patient Welfare in Managed Care: Six Safeguards" (1998) 23 *J. Health Politics, Policy & L.* 635.

S. Gordon and C.M. Fagin, "Preserving the Moral High Ground" (1996) 96 *AJN* 31.

H.T. Greely, "Direct Financial Incentives in Managed Care: Unanswered Questions" (1996) 6:1 *Health Matrix* 53.

M. Gunderson, "Eliminating Conflicts of Interest in Managed Care Organizations Through Disclosure and Consent" (1997) 25 *J.L. Med. & Ethics* 192.

M.R. Haack, "Payment Incentives and Conflicts of Interest Within a Managed Care Environment" (1997) 23 *J. Gerontological Nursing* 22.

T.S. Hall, "Third-Party Payor Conflicts of Interest in Managed Care: A Proposal for Regulation Based on the Model Rules of Professional Conduct" (1998) 29 *Seton Hall L. Rev.* 95.

M.A. Hall and R.A. Berenson, "Ethical Practice in Managed Care: A Dose of Realism" (1998) 128 *Ann. Intern. Med.* 395.

R.S. Johnson, "ERISA Doctor in the House? The Duty to Disclose Physician Incentives to Limit Health Care" (1998) 82 *Minnesota L. Rev.* 1631.

G.P. Lenehan, "On the Dark Side of 'Corporate Care': Conflicts of Interest and the Growing Need for Regulation" [editorial] (1996) 22 *J. Emerg. Nurs.* 95.

D.C. McGraw, "Financial Incentives to Limit Services: Should Physicians be Required to Disclose these to Patients" (1995) 83 *Georgetown L.J.* 1821.

J.P. Merritt, [letter] (1997) 12 *Am. J. Medical Quality* 135.

C. Michna, "The Patient Has Not Been Informed: A Proposal for a Physician Conflict of Interest Disclosure Law" (1992) 27 *Valparaiso Univ. L. Rev.* 495.

T.E. Miller and W.M. Sage, "Disclosing Physician Financial Incentives" (1999) 281 *JAMA* 1424.

E.H. Morreim, "Revenue Streams and Clinical Discretion" (1998) 46 *JAGS* 331.

M.A. Rodwin, "Conflicts of Interest and Accountability in Managed Care: The Aging of Medical Ethics" (1998) 46 *JAGS* 338.

D.F. Thompson, "Understanding Financial Conflicts of Interest" (1993) 329 *New Eng. J. Med.* 573.

M. Waldman, "Conflict of Interest, Physicians and Physiotherapy" (1996) 154 *CMAJ* 1737.

Disputes/appeals

M. Anderlik, "The Rising Number of Complaints Against HMOs, and What to Make of It" (15 October 1998), online at http://www.law.uh.edu/healthlawperspectives/Managed/981015Complaints.html (accessed on 22 February 2000)

H. Bailit, "When the Benefit is in Doubt, Who Decides?" (1998) 46 *JAGS* 342.

A.E. Bierman, "A Modest Proposal: Model Arbitration Provisions in the Age of Managed Care" (1999) 45 *Wayne L. Rev.* 173.

G. Bonnyman and M.M. Johnson, "Unseen Peril: Inadequate Enrollee Grievance Protections in Public Managed Care Programs" (1998) 65 *Tennessee L. Rev.* 359.

J.J. Fins, "A Medical Trust Fund for Managed Care: The Legacy of *Hughley* vs *Rocky Mountain Health Care Maintenance Organization*" (1998) 46 *JAGS* 365.

J.E. Gladieux, "Medicare+Choice Appeal Procedures: Reconciling Due Process Rights and Cost Containment" (1999) 25 *Am. J.L. & Med.* 61.

E.D. Kinney, "Resolving Consumer Grievances in a Managed Care Environment" (1996) 6:1 *Health Matrix* 147.

R.B. Mathews, "The Role of the ADR in Managed Care Disputes" (1999) 54 *Dispute Resolution J.* 8.

T.E. Miller, "Center Stage on the Patient Protection Agenda: Grievance and Appeal Rights" (1998) 26 *J.L. Med. & Ethics* 89.

N. Neveloff Dubler, "Mediation and Managed Care" (1998) 46 *JAGS* 359.

Drug benefits

D.A. Balto, "A Whole New World?: Pharmaceutical Responses to the Managed Care Revolution" (1997) 52 *Food & Drug L.J.* 83.

J.J. Fins, "Drug Benefits in Managed Care: Seeking Ethical Guidance from the Formulary?" (1998) 46 *JAGS* 346.

Education

R. Michels, "Medical Education and Managed Care" (1999) 340 *New Eng. J. Med.* 959.

S. Moriber Katz, " Medical Education and Managed Care: Keeping Pace" (1998) 46 *JAGS* 381.

Empirical studies (*see also* Studies)

M.R. Anderlik, "The Impact of Physician Financial Incentives" (31 December 1998), online at http://www.law.uh.edu/healthlawperspectives/Managed/981231Financial.html (accessed on 22 February 2000).

L.C. Baker, "Association of Managed Care Market Share and Health Expenditures for Fee-for-Service Medicare Patients" (1999) 281 *JAMA* 432.

D.S. Feldman, D.H. Novack and E. Gracely, "Effects of Managed Care on Physician-Patient Relationships, Quality of Care, and the Ethical Practice of Medicine" (1998) 158 *Arch. Intern. Med.* 1626.

J.F. Griffin, *et al.*, "The Effect of a Medicaid Managed Care Program on the Adequacy of Prenatal Care Utilization in Rhode Island" (1999) 89 *Am. J. Pub. Health* 497.

K. Grumbach, *et al.*, "Primary Care Physicians' Experience of Financial Incentives in Managed-Care Systems" (1998) 339 *New Eng. J. Med.* 1516.

K. Grumbach, *et al.*, "Resolving the Gatekeeper Conundrum" (1999) 282 *JAMA* 261.

J.M. Hutchinson, "Method of Physician Remuneration and Rates of Antibiotic Prescription" (1999) 160 *CMAJ* 1013.

N.S. Jecker and A.R. Jonsen, "Managed Care: A House of Mirrors" (1997) 8 *J. Clinical Ethics 230*.

A.C. Kao, D.C. Green, A.M. Zaslavsky, J.P. Koplan and P.D. Cleary, "The Relationship Between Method of Physician Payment and Patient Trust" (1998) 280 *JAMA* 1708.

H. Kattlove, A. Liberati, E. Keeler and R.H. Brook, "Benefits and Costs of Screening and Treatment for Early Breast Cancer: Development of a Basic Benefit Package" (1995) 273 *JAMA* 142.

V. Mooney, "The Impact of Managed Care on Musculoskeletal Physical Treatment" (1995) 18 *Orthopedics* 1063.

L. Patrick-Cooper, "Race, Gender, and Partnership in the Patient-Physician Relationship" (1999) 282 *JAMA* 583.

R.L. Scott, "Relationship of Physician and Insurer in Determining Access to Health Care" (11 March 1998), online at Health Law Perspectives, University of Houston Law Center http://www.law.uh.edu/healthlawperspectives/Managed/980311Relation.html (accessed on 22 February 2000).

S.R. Simon, *et al.*, "Views of Managed Care: A Survey of Students, Residents, Faculty, and Deans at Medical Schools in the United States" (1999) 340 *New Eng. J. Med.* 928.

J.E. Ware, M.S. Bayliss, W.H. Rogers, M. Kosinski and A.R. Tarlov, "Difference in 4-Year Health Outcomes for Elderly and Poor, Chronically Ill Patients Treated in HMO and Fee-for-Service Systems" (1996) 276 *JAMA* 1039.

ERISA

M. Anderlik, "A New Weapon Against Managed Care Organizations: ERISA" (28 September 1998), online at http://www.law.uh.edu/healthlawperspectives/Managed/980928NewWeapon.html (accessed on 22 February 2000).

K.S. Bartholomew, "ERISA Preemption of Medical Malpractice Claims in Managed Care: Asserting a New Statutory Interpretation" (1999) 52 *Vanderbilt L. Rev.* 1131.

S. Carter, "Health Care and ERISA" (1999) 36 *Harvard J. on Leg.* 561.

M.G. Farrell, "ERISA Preemption and Regulation of Managed Health Care: The Case for Managed Federalism" (1997) 23 *Am. J.L. & Med.* 251.

P.D. Jacobson and S.D. Pomfret, "ERISA Litigation and Physician Autonomy" (2000) 283 *JAMA* 921.

R.S. Johnson, "ERISA Doctor in the House? The Duty to Disclose Physician Incentives to Limit Health Care" (1998) 82 *Minnesota L. Rev.* 1631.

W.J. Kilberg, "The Impending Collision Between HMOs and ERISA: Can Either Emerge Unscathed?" (2000) 25 *Employee Relations L.J.* 1.

A.S. Korte, "The Model Health Care Accountability and Information Act: Managed Care and Medical Malpractice Liability under an Amended ERISA" (1999) 55 *Washington Univ. J. Urban & Contemporary L.* 161.

P. Laufer, "Managed Care: ERISA Held Not to Preempt State Tax on Health Care Facilities" (1998) 26 *J.L. Med. & Ethics* 78.

R.L. Scott, "Court Upholds Right to Sue MCOs, but Independent Review Process Limited" (22 September 1998), online at http://www.law.uh.edu/healthlawperspectives/Managed/980922Court.html (accessed on 22 February 2000).

H. Shapiro and R. Rachal, "The Duty to Inform and Fiduciary Breaches: The "New Frontier" in ERISA Litigation" (1999) 14 *Labor Lawyer* 503.

T.F. Theodos, "The Patients' Bill of Rights: Women's Rights Under Managed Care and ERISA Preemption" (2000) 26 *Am. J.L. & Med.* 89.

Ethics

E. Alexander and H. Brody, "Ethics by the Numbers: Monitoring Physicians' Integrity in Managed Care" (1998) 9 *J. Clinical Ethics* 297.

British Medical Association Medical Ethics Department, "Duty of Candour? Truth Telling and Rationing of Resources," online at http://www.bma.org.uk/public/ethics/candour.htm (accessed on 31 July 2000).

A. Buchanan, "Managed Care: Rationing without Justice, But Not Unjustly" (1998) 23 *J. Health Politics, Policy & L.* 617.

D. Callahan, "Managed Care and the Goals of Medicine" (1998) 46 *JAGS* 385.

J.A. Carrese and S.M. Wright, "Time to Teach about Ethical Issues Encountered in Managed Care" (1998) 73 *Academic Med.* 1128.

J.F. Childress, "Conscience and Conscientious Actions in the Context of MCOs" (1997) 7 *Kennedy Inst. Ethics J.* 403.

L.R. Churchill, "'Damaged Humanity': The Call for a Patient-Centered Medical Ethic in the Managed Care Era" (1997) 18 *Theoretical Med.* 113.

Council on Ethical and Judicial Affairs, American Medical Association, "Ethical Issues in Managed Care" (1995) 273 *JAMA* 330.

N. Daniels and J.E. Sabin, "Last Chance Therapies and Managed Care: Pluralism, Fair Procedures, and Legitimacy" (1998) 28:2 *Hastings Ctr. Rep.* 27.

E. Elhauge, "Allocating Health Care Morally" (1994) 82 *Cal. L. Rev.* 1449.

J.A. Erlen and M.P. Mellors, "Managed Care and the Nurse's Ethical Obligations to Patients" (1995) 14 *Orthopaedic Nursing* 42.

R.G. Evans, "Ethical Ambiguities and Economic Consequences in the Allocation of Health Care" in B. Dickens and M. Ouellette, eds., *Health Care, Ethics and Law* (Montreal: Éditions Thémis, 1993) 47.

J.J. Fins, E. Blacksher, "The Ethics of Managed Care: Report on a Congress of Clinical Societies" (1998) 46 *JAGS* 309.

B.R. Furrow, "The Ethics of Cost-Containment: Bureaucratic Medicine and the Doctor as Patient-Advocate" (1988) 3 *J.L. Ethics & Public Policy* 187.

K.G. Gervais, *Ethical Challenges in Managed Care: A Casebook* (Washington: Georgetown Univ. Press, 1999).

M.A. Hall, "Ethical Practice in Managed Care: A Dose of Realism" (1998) 128 *Ann. Intern. Med.* 395.

W.L. Holleman, M.C. Holleman and J.G. Moy, "Are Ethics and Managed Care Strange Bedfellows or a Marriage Made in Heaven?" (1997) 349 *Lancet* 350.

J.P. Kassirer, "Managing Care: Should We Adopt a New Ethic" (1998) 339 *New Eng. J. Med.* 397.

P. Menzel, *et al.*, "Towards a Broader View of Values in Cost-Effectiveness Analysis of Health" (1999) 29:3 *Hastings Ctr. Rep.* 7.

D.M. Mirvis, "Managed Care, Managing Ethics" (1998) 46 *JAGS* 389.

P.A.F. Morrin, "Ethical Implications of Resource Allocation: Part II" (1995) *Ont. Med. Rev.* 80.

S.D. Pearson, J.E. Sabin and E.J. Emanuel, "Ethical Guidelines for Physician Compensation Based on Capitation" (1998) 339 *New Eng. J. Med.* 689.

E.D. Pellegrino, "Managed Care at the Bedside: How Do We Look in the Moral Mirror?" (1997) 7 *Kennedy Inst. Ethics* 321.

D.F. Phillips, "Erecting an Ethical Framework for Managed Care" (1998) 280 JAMA 2060.

T. Reay, "Allocating Scarce Resources in a Publicly Funded Health System: Ethical Considerations of a Canadian Managed Care Proposal" (1999) 6 *Nursing Ethics* 240.

J.E. Sabin, "Caring About Patients and Caring About Money: The American Psychiatric Association Code of Ethics Meets Managed Care" (1994) 12 *Behavioral Sciences & the L.* 317.

B.J. Spielman, "Managed Care Regulation and the Physician-Advocate" (1999) 47 *Drake L. Rev.* 713.

D.C. Thomasma, "The Ethics of Managed Care: Challenges to the Principles of Relationship-Centered Care" (1996) 25 *J. Allied Health* 233.

A. Williams, "Cost-effectiveness Analysis: Is it Ethical?" (1992) 18 *J. Medical Ethics* 7.

Gag clauses

B.A. Liang, "The Practical Utility of Gag Clause Legislation" (1998) 13 *J. General Intern. Med.* 419.

P.M. Maloney, "Gagging Physicians: Is That What the Legislature Intended?" (1998) 35 *San Diego L. Rev.* 547.

J.A. Martin and L.K. Bjerknes, "The Legal and Ethical Implications of Gag Clauses in Physician Contracts" (1996) 22 *Am. J.L. & Med.* 433.

B.J. Spielman, "Managed Care Regulation and the Physician-Advocate" (1999) 47 *Drake L. Rev.* 713.

General

G.J. Annas, *Some Choice: Law, Medicine, and the Market* (New York, NY: Oxford University Press, 1998).

S.J. Balla, "Markets, Governments, and HMO Development in the 1990s" (1999) 24 *J. Health Politics, Policy & L.* 215.

A.J. Barsky and J.F. Borus, "Somatization and Medicalization in the Era of Managed Care" (1995) 274 *JAMA* 1931.

R. Bowser and L.O. Gostin, "Managed Care and the Health of a Nation" (1999) 72 *Southern Cal. L. Rev.* 1209.

V.Y. Brown and B.R. Hartung, "Managed Care at the Crossroads: Can Managed Care Organizations Survive Government Regulation?" (1998) 7 *Ann. Health L.* 25.

F. Davidoff, "Medicine and Commerce: Is Managed Care a 'Monstrous Hybrid'?" (1998) 128 *Ann. Intern. Med.* 496.

D.M. Fox, "Managed Care: The Third Reorganization of Health Care" (1998) 46 *JAGS* 314.

E. Ginzberg, "The Uncertain Future of Managed Care" (1999) 340 *New Eng. J. Med.* 144.

A. Hampton, "Resurrection of the Prohibition on the Corporate Practice of Medicine: Teaching Old Dogma New Tricks" (1998) 66 *Univ. Cincinnati L. Rev.* 489.

C.C. Havighurst, "Foreword: Managed Care—Work in Progress or Stalled Experiment?" (1999) 35 *Houston L. Rev.* 1385.

C.C. Havighurst, "Managed Care—Work in Progress or Stalled Experiment" (1999) 35 *Houston L. Rev.* 1385.

S.M. Keigher, "Managed Care's Silent Seduction of America and the New Politics of Choice" (1995) 20 *Health & Social Work* 146.

R. Kuttner, "Must Good HMOs Go Bad? The Commercialization of PrePaid Group Health Care" (1998) 338 *New Eng. J. Med.* 1558.

R. Kuttner, "Must Good HMOs Go Bad? The Search for Checks and Balances" (1998) 338 *New Eng. J. Med.* 1635.

S.R. Latham, "Regulation of Managed Care Incentive Payments to Physicians" (1996) 22 *Am. J.L. & Med.* 399.

Managed Care Phase Two—Structural Changes and Equity Issues (1997) 23 *Am. J.L. & Med.* 187.

D. Orentlicher, "Paying Physicians More to do Less: Financial Incentives to Limit Care" (1996) 30 *Univ. Richmond L. Rev.* 155.

M. Powers, "Managed Care: How Economic Incentive Reforms Went Wrong" (1997) 7 *Kennedy Inst. Ethics J.* 353.

E.C. Price, "The Evolution of Health Care Decision Making: The Political Paradigm and Beyond" (1998) 65 *Tennessee L. Rev.* 619.

R.E. Rosenblatt, "Medicaid Primary Care Case Management, The Doctor-Patient Relationship, and the Politics of Privatization" (1986) 36 *Case West. Reserve L. Rev.* 915.

P.C. Sorum, "Striking Against Managed Care: The Last Gasp of?" (1998) 280 *JAMA* 659.

J.D. Stobo, "Who Should Manage Care? The Case for Providers" (1997) 7 *Kennedy Inst. Ethics J.* 387.

R.M. Veatch, "Who Should Manage Care? The Case for Patients" (1997) 7 *Kennedy Inst. Ethics J.* 391.

Informed consent

M.G. Bloche, "Managed Care, Medical Privacy, and the Paradigm of Consent" (1997) 7 *Kennedy Inst. Ethics J.* 381.

T. Chambers, "Letting the Patient Backstage: Informed Consent for HMO Enrollees" (1998) 46 *JAGS* 355.

R.R. Faden, "Managed Care and Informed Consent" (1997) 7 *Kennedy Inst. Ethics J.* 377.

V. Khanna, H. Silverman and J. Schwartz, "Disclosure of Operating Practices by Managed-Care Organizations to Consumers of Healthcare: Obligations of Informed Consent" (1998) 9 *J. Clinical Ethics* 291.

F.H. Miller, "Denial of Health Care and Informed Consent in English and American Law" (1992) 18 *Am. J.L. & Med.* 37.

S.M. Wolf, "Toward a Systematic Theory of Informed Consent" (1999) 35 *Houston L. Rev.* 1631.

Liability (*see also* Tort Law/Liability)

J. Alderman, "Managed Care: HMOs Liable for Bad Faith, Cost-Motivated Refusal to Authorize Care" (1998) 26 *J.L. Med. & Ethics* 78.

S.J. Arkin, "A Litigator's Perspective on HMO Liability: The View from the Plaintiff's Side" (1998) 22 *Am. J. Trial Advocacy* 131.

J. Bartimus and C.A. Wright, "HMO Liability: From Corporate Negligence Claims for Negligent Credentialing and Utilization Review to Bad Faith" (1998) 66 *UMKC L. Rev.* 763.

C.E. Brasel, "Managed Care Liability: State Legislation May Arm Angry Members with Legal Ammo to Fire at their MCOs for Cost Containment Tactics—But Could it Backfire?" (1999) 27 *Capital Univ. L. Rev.* 449.

J.B. Buckhalter, "ERISA Preemption of Medical Malpractice Claims: Can Managed Care Organizations Avoid Vicarious Liability?" (1999) 22 *Seattle Univ. L. Rev.* 1165.

H. Burghardt, "Fraud and Abuse: RICO Cause of Action Against MCOs—*Humana Inc.* v. *Forsyth*" (1999) 25 *Am. J.L. & Med.* 178.

D.C. DiCicco, "HMO Liability for the Medical Negligence of Member Physicians" (1998) 43 *Villanova L. Rev.* 499.

S.M. Glenn, "Tort Liability of Integrated Health Care Delivery Systems: Beyond Enterprise Liability" (1994) 29 *Wake Forest L. Rev.* 305.

L.S. Goldsmith, "New Health Care Liabilities in the New Millennium" (2000) 23:1 *Trial Lawyer* 21.

J.L. Gonzalez, "A Managed Care Organization's Medical Malpractice Liability for Denial of Care: The Lost World" (1998) 35 *Houston L. Rev.* 715.

R.J. Herrington, "*Herdrich* v. *Pegram*: ERISA Fiduciary Liability and Physician Incentives to Deny Care" (2000) 71 *Univ. Colorado L. Rev.* 715.

D.W. Larios, "Barbarians at the Gate? An Essay on Payor Liability in an Era of Managed Care" (1998) 65 *Tennessee L. Rev.* 445.

J.K. Locke, "The ERISA Amendment: A Prescription to Sue MCOs for Wrongful Treatment Decisions" (1999) 83 *Minnesota L. Rev.* 1027.

E.H. Morreim, "Confusion in the Courts: Managed Care Financial Structures and their Impact on Medical Care" (2000) 35 *Tort & Insurance L.J.* 699.

E.H. Moskowitz, "Clinical Responsibility and Legal Liability in Managed Care" (1998) 46 *JAGS* 373.

C.P. Parver and K.A. Martinez, "Holding Decision Makers Liable: Assessing Liability Under a Managed Health Care System" (1999) 51 *Admin. L. Rev.* 199.

D.G. Savage, "Cost-Cutting Consequences" (2000) 86 *ABA J.* 30.

J.P. Smith, "Managed Care: California Jury Awards $121 Mil. in Denial of Benefits Case against Aetna" (1999) 27 *J.L. Med. & Ethics* 104.

C. Stewart, "Tragic Choices and the Role of Administrative Law" (2000) 321 *BMJ* 105.

P.R. Sugarman, "Admissibility of Managed Care Financial Incentives in Medical Malpractice Cases" (1999) 34 *Tort & Insurance L.J.* 735.

D.L. Trueman, "As Managed Care Plans Increase, How Can Patients Hold HMOs Liable for Their Actions?" (1999) 71 *NY State Bar J.* 6.

D.L. Trueman, "Physicians' Liability Under Managed Care" (1999) 222 *NY L.J.* 1.

A.F. Walsh, "The Legal Attack on Cost Containment Mechanisms: The Expansion of Liability for Physicians and Managed Care Organizations" (1997) 31 *John Marshall L. Rev.* 207.

J.L. Wood, "Expanding Liability for Managed Care Entities" (1999) 32 *Maryland Bar J.* 30.

Mental health

M.L. Durham, "Healthcare's Greatest Challenge: Providing Services for People with Severe Mental Illness in Managed Care" (1994) 12 *Behavioral Sciences & the L.* 331.

J.A. Goldner, "Managed Care and Mental Health: Clinical Perspectives and Legal Realities" (1999) 35 *Houston L. Rev.* 1437.

C. McDaniel and J. Erlen, "Ethics and Mental Health Service Delivery Under Managed Care" (1996) 17 *Issues in Mental Health Nursing* 11.

S.K. Reed, "Serious Mental Illness and Capitation Financing" (1994) 12 *Behavioral Sciences & the L.* 379.

R.N. Swidler, "Special Needs Plans: Adapting Medicaid Managed Care for Persons with Serious Mental Illness or HIV/AIDS" (1998) 61 *Albany L. Rev.* 1113.

Physicians' duties

E.J. Cassell, "The Future of the Doctor-Payer-Patient Relationship" (1998) 46 *JAGS* 318.

F.A. Chervenak, "Responding to the Ethical Challenges Posed by the Business Tools of Managed Care in the Practice of Obstetrics and Gynecology" (1996) 175 *Am J. Obstet. Gynecol.* 523.

E.J. Emanuel and N. Neveloff Dubler, "Preserving the Physician-Patient Relationship in the Era of Managed Care" (1995) 273 *JAMA* 323.

B. Friedland, "Managed Care and the Expanding Scope of Primary Care Physicians' Duties: A Proposal to Redefine Explicitly the Standard of Care" (1998) 26 *J.L. Med. & Ethics* 100.

S.D. Goold, "Money and Trust: Relationships between Patients, Physicians, and Health Plans" (1998) 23 *J. Health Politics, Policy & L.* 687.

G.B. Hickson, "Don't Let Primary Care Physicians off the Hook so Easily" (1998) 26 *J.L. Med. & Ethics* 113.

A.J. Lairson, "Reexamining the Physician's Duty of Care in Response to Medicare's Prospective Payment System" (1987) 62 *Wash. L. Rev.* 791.

G. Martin, "Resource Allocation in the Health-Care Reform Era: implications for the doctor-patient relationship" (1994) *Ont. Med. Rev.* 52.

D. Mechanic, "The Functions and Limitations of Trust in the Provision of Medical Care" (1998) 23 *J. Health Politics, Policy & L.* 661.

Physician/Patient Relationships Ad Hoc Committee to Defend Health Care, [Physicians' Call to Action] "For Our Patients, Not for Profits: A Call to Action" (1997) 278 *JAMA* 1733.

M.A. Rodwin, "Strains in the Fiduciary Metaphor: Divided Physician Loyalties and Obligations in a Changing Health Care System" (1995) 21 *Am. J.L. & Med.* 241.

R.E. Rosenblatt, "Medicaid Primary Care Case Management, The Doctor-Patient Relationship, and the Politics of Privatization" (1986) 36 *Case West. Reserve L. Rev.* 915.

H. Shapiro and R. Rachal, "The Duty to Inform and Fiduciary Breaches: The "New Frontier" in ERISA Litigation" (1999) 14 *Labor Lawyer* 503.

L. Snyder and J. Tooker, "Obligations and Opportunities: The Role of Clinical Societies in the Ethics of Managed Care" (1998) 46 *JAGS* 378.

Practice guidelines

I. Durand-Zaleski, C. Colin and C. Blum-Boisgard, "An Attempt to Save Money by Using Mandatory Practice Guidelines in France" (1997) 315 *BMJ* 943.

B.R. Furrow, "Broadcasting Clinical Guidelines on the Internet: Will Physicians Tune In?" (1999) 25 *Am. J.L. & Med.* 403.

O.F. Norheim, "Healthcare Rationing: Are Additional Criteria Needed for Assessing Evidence Based Clinical Practice Guidelines?" (1999) 319 *BMJ* 1426.

D. Orentlicher, "Practice Guidelines: A Limited Role in Resolving Rationing Decisions" (1998) 46 *JAGS* 369.

R. Porter, "Doctors May Not Follow Practice Guidelines, Study Finds" (2000) 36:2 *Trial* 99.

Professional relationships

A.S. Brett, "Relationships Between Primary Care Physicians and Consultants in Managed Care" (1997) 8 *J. Clinical Ethics* 60.

G.J. Povar, "The Quality of Primary Care/Consultant Relationships in Managed Care: Have We Gone Forward or Backward?" (1997) 8 *J. Clinical Ethics* 66.

Regulation

M.R. Anderlik, "Efforts to Regulate Physician Financial Incentives" (20 January 1999), online at http://www.law.uh.edu/healthlawperspectives/Managed/990120Efforts.html (accessed on 7 February 2000).

V.Y. Brown and B.R. Hartung, "Managed Care at the Crossroads: Can Managed Care Organizations Survive Government Regulation?" (1998) 7 *Ann. Health L.* 25.

J.F. Doherty Jr., "Managed Care in the Cross Hairs: Regulating a Moving Target" (1999) 32 *Maryland Bar J.* 18.

D.M. Frankford, "Regulating Managed Care: Pulling the Tails to Wag the Dogs" (1999) 24 *J. Health Politics, Policy & L.* 1191.

T.E. Miller, "Managed Care Regulation in the Laboratory of the States" (1997) 278 *JAMA* 1102.

A.A. Noble and T.A. Brennan, "The Stages of Managed Care Regulation: Developing Better Rules" (1999) 24 *J. Health Politics, Policy & L.* 1275

L.I. Sederer, "Judicial and Legislative Responses to Cost Containment" (1992) 149 *Am. J. Psychiatry* 1157.

J. Schwartz, "State Regulation of Managed Care: Fragments of Reform" (1997) 7 *Kennedy Inst. Ethics J.* 345.

Risk selection (cream skimming)

W.W. Bera, "Preventing 'Patient Dumping': The Supreme Court Turns Away the Sixth Circuit's Interpretation of EMTALA" (1999) 36 *Houston L. Rev.* 615.

J.M. Jendusa, "Pandora's Box Exposed: Untangling the Web of the Double Helix in Light of Insurance and Managed Care" (1999) 49 *DePaul L. Rev.* 161.

M.A. Rothstein and S. Hoffman, "Genetic Testing, Genetic Medicine, and Managed Care" (1999) 34 *Wake Forest L. Rev.* 849.

E.M. van Barneveld, R.C.J.A. van Vliet and W.P.M.M. van de Ven, "Mandatory High-Risk Pooling: An Approach to Reducing Incentives for Cream Skimming" (1996) 33 *Inquiry* 133.

Mental Health

J. Arboleda-Flórez and M. Copithorne, *Mental Health Law and Practice: A Guide to the Alberta Mental Health Act and Related Canadian Legislation* (Calgary: Carswell, 1994).

G.A.H. Benjamin, *Law and Mental Health Professionals* (Washington, DC: American Psychological Association, 1995).

J.E. Gray, M.A. Shone and P.F. Liddle, *Canadian Mental Health Law and Policy* (Markham, ON: Butterworths, 2000).

Health Systems Research Unit, Clarke Institute of Psychiatry, *Best Practices in Mental Health Reform: Discussion Paper* (Ottawa: Health Canada, 1997).

B.M. Hogett, *Mental Health Law* (London: Sweet and Maxwell, 1996).

K. Johns and R.C. Dillehay, *Law and Mental Health Professionals* (Washington, DC: American Psychological Association, 1998).

J.E. Sabin and N. Daniels, "Determining 'Medical Necessity' in Mental Health Practice" (1994) 24:6 *Hastings Ctr. Rep.* 5.

Other Jurisdictions

Australia

B. Gaze, "Resource Allocation—The Legal Implications" (1993) 9 *J. Contemporary Health L. & Policy* 91.

K. Wheelwright, "Commonwealth and State Powers in Health—A Constitutional Diagnosis" (1995) 21 *Monash Univ. L. Rev.* 53.

Netherlands

S.M. MacLeod and J. Bienenstock, "Evidence-Based Rationing: Dutch Pragmatism or Government Insensitivity?" (1998) 158 *CMAJ* 213.

New Zealand

C.M. Flood, "Prospects for New Zealand's Reformed Health System" (1996) 4 *Health L.J.* 87.

United Kingdom

M. Elsenaar, "Law, Accountability and the Private Finance Initiative in the National Health Service" *Pub. L.* (Spring 1999) 35.

R.G. Lee and F.H. Miller, "The Doctor's Changing Role in Allocating US and British Medical Services" (1990) 18 *L. Med. & Health Care* 69.

G.L. Maddox, "General Practice Fundholding in the British National Health Service Reform, 1991–1997: GP Accounts of the Dynamics of Change" (1999) 24 *J. Health Politics, Policy & L.* 815.

A. Maynard, "Distributing Health Care: Rationing and the Role of the Physician in the United Kingdom National Health Service" (1994) 4:2 *Health Matrix* 259.

C. Newdick, "Resource Allocation in the National Health Service" (1997) 23 *Am. J.L. & Med.* 291.

C. Newdick, "Rights to NHS Resources After the 1990 Act" (1993) 1 *Med. L. Rev.* 53.

C. Newdick, *Who Should We Treat?: Law, Patients and Resources in the NHS* (New York, NY: Oxford Univ. Press, 1995).

J.H. Tingle, "The Allocation of Healthcare Resources in the National Health Service in England: Professional and Legal Issues" (1993) 2 *Ann. Health L.* 195.

United States (*see also* managed care)

J.R. Antos and L. Bilheimer, "Medicare Reform: Obstacles and Options" (1999) 89 *Am. Ec. Rev.* 217.

R. Bayer and D. Callahan, "Medicare Reform: Social and Ethical Perspectives" (1985) 10 *J. Health Politics, Policy & L.* 533.

J.F. Blumstein and F.A. Sloan, "Health Care Reform Through Medicaid Managed Care: Tennessee (TennCare) as a Case Study and a Paradigm" (2000) 53 *Vanderbilt L. Rev.* 123.

L.D. Brown, "The Politics of Medicare and Health Reform, Then and Now" (1996) 18 *Health Care Financing Rev.* 163.

D.H. Caldwell, Jr., *US Health Law and Policy* (Chicago: American Hospital Publishing, 1998).

N. Daniels and J.E. Sabin, "The Yin and Yang of Health Care System Reform: Professional and Political Strategies for Setting Limits" (1995) 4 *Arch. Fam. Med.* 67.

R.G. Lee and F.H. Miller, "The Doctor's Changing Role in Allocating US and British Medical Services" (1990) 18 *L. Med. & Health Care* 69

M. Moon, "Medicare and Health Care Reform" (1994) 6 *J. Aging & Soc. Policy* 27.

P.A. Paul-Shaheen, "The States and Health Care Reform: The Road Traveled and Lessons Learned from Seven That Took the Lead" (1998) 23 *J. Health Politics, Policy & L.*319.

L.Z. Rubenstein, *et al.*, "Medicare: Challenges and Future Directions in a Changing Health Care Environment" (1994) 34 *Gerontologist* 620.

A Symposium on Health Care Reform—Perspectives in the 1990s (1994) 46 *Wash. Univ. J. Urban & Contemporary L.* 1.

Patients' Rights

R. Baker, "American Independence and the Right to Emergency Care" (1999) 281 *JAMA* 859.

D.A. Hyman, "Regulating Managed Care: What's Wrong with a Patient Bill of Rights" (2000) 73 *Southern Cal. L. Rev.* 221.

C.N. Kahn, "Patients' Rights Proposals: The Insurers' Perspective" (1999) 281 *JAMA* 858.

W.K. Mariner, "Going Hollywood with Patient Rights in Managed Care" (1999) 281 *JAMA* 861.

W.K. Mariner, "Patients' Rights after Health Care Reform: Who Decides What Is Medically Necessary?" (1994) 84 *Am. J. Public Health* 1515.

D.E. Shalala, "A Patients' Bill of Rights: The Medical Student's Role" (1999) 281 *JAMA* 857.

R. Sorian and J. Feder, "Why We Need a Patients' Bill of Rights" (1999) 24 *J. Health Politics, Policy & L.* 1137.

T.F. Theodos, "The Patients' Bill of Rights: Women's Rights Under Managed Care and ERISA Preemption" (2000) 26 *Am. J.L. & Med.* 89.

S.C. Weiss, "Defining a 'Patients' Bill of Rights' for the Next Century" (1999) 281 *JAMA* 856.

M.H. Wilson Silver, "Patients' Rights in England and the United States of America: The Patient's Charter and the New Jersey Patient Bill of Rights: A Comparison" (1997) 23 *J. Med. Ethics* 213.

World Medical Association, "World Medical Association Declaration on the Rights of the Patient," online at http://www.wma.net/e/policy/17-h_e.html (accessed on 16 September 1999).

Pharmaceuticals

A.F. Holmer, "Direct-to-Consumer Prescription Drug Advertising Builds Bridges Between Patients and Physicians" (1999) 281 *JAMA* 380.

National Forum on Health, "Directions for a Pharmaceutical Policy in Canada" in *National Forum on Health, Canada Health Action: Building on the Legacy, Volume II: Synthesis Reports and Issues Papers* (Ottawa: National Forum on Health, 1997).

R. Porter, "Internet Pharmacies: Who's Minding the Store" (2000) 36:5 *Trial* 12.

A. Robinson, "After Years of Steady Growth, Winds of Restraint Blowing on Prescription-Drug Industry" (1995) 153 *CMAJ* 85.

Primary Care

L.S. Bohnen, "Primary Care in Ontario: Legal Issues" (1998) 19:1 *Health L. in Can.* 24.

B. Friedland, "Managed Care and the Expanding Scope of Primary Care Physicians' Duties: A Proposal to Redefine Explicitly the Standard of Care" (1998) 26 *J.L. Med. & Ethics* 100.

K. Grumbach, *et al.*, "Resolving the Gatekeeper Conundrum: What Patients Value in Primary Care and Referrals to Specialists" (1999) 282 *JAMA* 261.

G.B. Hickson, "Don't Let Primary Care Physicians off the Hook so Easily" (1998) 26 *J.L. Med. & Ethics* 113.

C. Johnston, "Health-care Consumers Redefining Primary Care" (1 January 1996) *Family Practice* 16.

Ontario College of Family Physicians, *Family Medicine in the 21st Century: A Prescription for Excellent Healthcare* (Toronto: Ontario College of Family Physicians, 1999).

B. Sibbald, "Is fee-for-service on the way out for Ontario FPs?" (1999) 161 *CMAJ* 861.

J.L. Reichert, "Many Doctors Pressured to Wear too Many Hats, Study Says" (2000) 36:3 *Trial* 110.

Privatization

Alberta Health and Wellness, *Policy Statement on the Delivery of Surgical Services: A discussion paper* (Edmonton: Alberta Health and Wellness, 1999).

Alberta Health and Wellness, *Policy Statement on the Delivery of Surgical Services: Questions and Answers* (Edmonton: Alberta Health and Wellness, 2000).

Alberta Medical Association, "AMA Position Statement: RHA Contracting with Private Surgical Facilities" (Approved 10 March 2000), online at http://www.amda.ab.ca/general/private-surg/index.html (accessed on 4 July 2000).

S. Alvi, *Health Costs and Private Sector Competitiveness* (Conference Board of Canada, Human Resources Research Group, 1995).

S.S. Bachman, "Why Do States Privatize Mental Health Services? Six State Experiences" (1996) 21 *J. Health Politics, Policy & L.* 807.

H.P. Bartlett and D.R. Phillips, "Policy Issues in the Private Health Sector: Examples from Long-Term Care in the UK" (1996) 43 *Soc. Sci. Med.* 731.

Bill 37 Review Panel, *Report of the Bill 37 Review Panel* (Edmonton: The Review Panel, 1999).

A. Brotman, "Privatization of Mental Health Services: The Massachusetts Experiment" (1992) 17 *J. Health Politics, Policy & L.* 541.

A. Buchanan, "Privatization and Just Healthcare" (1995) 9 *Bioethics* 220.

C. Carruthers, "Saying Goodbye to Canada's Single-Payer System" (1995) 152 *CMAJ* 731

A.C. Enthoven, "On the Ideal Market Structure for Third-Party Purchasing of Health Care" (1994) 39 *Soc. Sci. Med.* 1413.

K.P. Feehan, "Access to Service: Threats and Opportunities—The Role of the Private Sector in Alberta's New Health System" (1995) 16:1 *Health L. in Can.* 17.

C.M. Flood, "Contracting for Health Care Services in the Public Sector" (1999) 31 *Can. Bus. L.J.* 175.

D.M. Frankford, "Privatizing Health Care: Economic Magic to Cure Legal Medicine" (1992) 66 *Southern Cal. L. Rev.* 1.

Friends of Medicare, "The Case Against Private For-Profit Hospitals" (September 1998), online at http://www.friendsofmedicare.ab.ca/briefs/0998full.htm (accessed on 21 January 2000).

M. Gordon, J. Mintz and D. Chen, "Funding Canada's Health Care System: a Tax-Based Alternative to Privatization" (1998) 159 *CMAJ* 493.

M. Jackman, "The Regulation of Private Health Care Under the Canada Health Act and the Canadian Charter" (1995) 6 *Constitutional Forum* 54.

G.D. Marriott, "The Regional Health Authorities Act and the Privatization of Health Care in Alberta" (1994) 3:3 *Health L. Rev.* 35.

A. Maynard, "Can Competition Enhance Efficiency in Health Care? Lessons from the Reform of the U.K. National Health Service" (1994) 39 *Soc. Sci. Med.* 1433.

National Advisory Council on Aging, *The NACA Position on the Privatization of Health Care* (Ottawa: Minister of Public Works and Government Services, 1997).

National Forum on Health, *The Public and Private Financing of Canada's Health System—A Discussion Paper* (Ottawa: National Forum on Health, 1995).

K. Patterson, "PFI in the Health Sector" (1996) 41 *J. of the Law Society of Scotland* 344.

R. Plain, *The Privatization and the Commercialization of Public Hospital Based Medical Services within the Province of Alberta: An Economic Overview from a Public Interest Perspective* (Edmonton: University of Alberta, Medicare Economics Group, 2000).

J.J. Polder, J. Hoogland, H. Jochemsen and S. Strijbos, "Profession, Practice and Profits: Competition in the Core of Health Care System" (1997) 14 *Syst. Res. Behav. Sci.* 409.

J. Rafuse, "Private-Sector Share of Health Spending Hits Record Level" (1996) 155 *CMAJ* 749.

S. Rathgeb Smith and M. Lipsky, "Privatization in Health and Human Services: A Critique" (1992) 17 *J. Health Politics, Policy & L.* 233.

R.E. Rosenblatt, "Medicaid Primary Care Case Management, The Doctor-Patient Relationship, and the Politics of Privatization" (1986) 36 *Case West. Reserve L. Rev.* 915.

J.L. Scarpaci, "HMO Promotion and the Privatization of Health Care in Chile" (1987) 12 *J. Health Politics, Policy & L.* 551.

T. Schrecker, "Private Health Care for Canada: North of the Border, an Idea Whose Time Shouldn't Come?" (1998) 26 *J. L. Med. & Ethics* 138.

K. Taft and G. Steward, *Clear Answers: The Economics and Politics of For-Profit Medicine* (Edmonton: Duval House Publishing, 2000).

K. Taft and G. Steward, *Private Profit or the Public Good: The Economics and Politics of the Privatization of Health Care in Alberta* (Edmonton: Parkland Institute, University of Alberta, 2000).

V.I. Tarman, *Privatization and Health Care: The Case of Ontario Nursing Homes* (Toronto: Garamond Press, 1990).

United Nations Division for Public Economics and Public Administration, *et al.*, *Privatization of Public Sector Activities: With a Special Focus on Telecommunications, Energy, Health and Community Services* (New York, NY: United Nations, 1999).

J. von der Schulenburg, "Forming and Reforming the Market for Third-Party Purchasing of Health Care: A German Perspective" (1994) 39 *Soc. Sci. Med.* 1473.

D.G. Whiteis, "Unhealthy Cities: Corporate Medicine, Community Economic Underdevelopment, and Public Health" (1997) 27 *Inter. J. Health Services* 227.

D. Wilson, "Legislative Protections in a Privatized Health System: The Antitrust Solution?" (1998/99) 7:3 *Health L. Rev.* 23.

R.L. Wisor, "Community Care, Competition and Coercion: A Legal Perspective on Privatized Mental Health Care" (1993) 19 *Am. J.L. & Med.* 145.

S. Woolhandler and D.Y. Himmelstein, "When Money is the Mission—The High Costs of Investor-Owned Care" (1999) 341 *New Eng. J. Med.* 444.

Public Health

S. Burris, "Law as a Structural Factor in the Spread of Communicable Disease" (1999) 36 *Houston L. Rev.* 1755.

Canadian Public Health Association, "Focus on Health: Public Health in Health Services Restructuring," online at http://www.cpha.ca/cpha.docs/Focus.eng.html (accessed on 28 January 2000).

Canadian Public Health Association, "Public Health Infrastructure in Canada: Summary Document" (December 1997), online at http://www.cpha.ca/cpha.docs/PHIC/Main.html (accessed on 28 January 2000).

L.O. Gostin, S. Burris and Z. Lazzarini, "The Law and the Public's Health: A Study of Infectious Disease Law in the United States" (1999) 99 *Colum. L. Rev.* 59.

B.F. Neidl, "The Lesser of Two Evils: New York's New HIV/AIDS Partner Notification Law and Why the Right of Privacy Must Yield to Public Health" (1999) 73 *St. John's L. Rev.* 1191.

Regionalization

Canadian Medical Association, "Regionalization (update 1998)" (19 June 1998), online at http://www.cma.ca/inside/policybase/1998/06-19e.htm (accessed on 20 February 2000).

J.L. Dorland and S. Mathwin, *How Many Roads? Queen's-CMA Conference on Regionalization and Decentralization in Health Care* (Kingston, ON: Teaching Health Unit, Queen's Health Policy, School of Policy Studies, Queen's University, 1996).

Health Plan Coordination Project, *Getting Started II: Health Business Plan Guidebook* (Calgary, Health Plan Coordination Project, 1994).

G.D. Marriott, "The Regional Health Authorities Act and the Privatization of Health Care in Alberta" (1994) 3:3 *Health L. Rev.* 35.

L. McNamara-Paetz, "Can Regionalization Live Up to its Economic Reputation?" (1999) 4:3 *Health L. Rev.* 2.

Regional Health Authorities Health Plan Coordination Project, *Getting Started: An Orientation for RHAs* (Calgary: Health Plan Coordination Project, 1994).

Resource Allocation

G.J. Agich, "Rationing and Professional Autonomy" (1990) 18 *L. Med & Health Care* 77.

American Medical Association, "E–2.03 Allocation of Limited Medical Resources," online at http://www.ama-assn.org/apps/pf_online/pf_online?f_n=browse&doc=policyfiles/CEJA/E-2.03.HTM&&s_t=&st_p=&nth=1&prev_pol=policyfiles/CEJA/E-1.02.HTM&nxt_pol=policyfiles/CEJA/E-2.01.HTM& (accessed on 22 February 2000).

R. Baker, "Rationing, Rhetoric, and Rationality: A review of the health care rationing debate in American and Europe" in J.M. Humber and R.F. Almeder, eds., *Biomedical Ethics Reviews* (Totowa, NJ: Humana Press, 1995) 55.

R.H. Blank, "Rationing Medicine: A Comparative Analysis" (1993) 21 *Western State Univ. L. Rev.* 11.

R.H. Blank, "Regulatory Rationing: A Solution to Health Care Resource Allocation" (1992) 140 *Univ. Penn. L. Rev.* 1573.

M.G. Brown, "Rationing Health Care in Canada" (1993) 2 *Ann. Health L.* 101.

Canadian Medical Association, "CMA Policy Summary: Core and Comprehensive Health Care Services" (1995)152 *CMAJ* 740A.

Canadian Medical Association, *Core and Comprehensive Health Care Services: A Framework for Decision-Making* (Ottawa: Canadian Medical Association, 1994).

Canadian Psychiatric Association, "Access to New Medications," online at http://cpa.medical.org/pubs/papers/access.html (accessed on 27 October 1999).

Catholic Health Association of Canada, *Resource Allocation in the Healthcare Sector: An Aid for Ethical Decision-Making* (Ottawa: Catholic Health Association of Canada, 1996).

N. Daniels, "Technology and Resource Allocation: Old Problems in New Clothes" (1991) 65 *Southern Cal. L. Rev.* 225.

M. Feldstein, "Prefunding Medicare" (1999) 89 *Am. Ec. Rev.* 222.

E. Friedman, "Freedom, Fault and Default" (1992) 14 *Health Management Q.* 10.

B. Gaze, "Resource Allocation—the Legal Implications" (1993) 9 *J. Contemporary Health L. & Policy* 91.

M. Jackman, "The Right to Participate in Health Care and Health Resource Allocation Decisions under Section 7 of the Canadian Charter" (1995) 4:3 *Health L. Rev.* 3.

L. Jacobs, T. Marmor and J. Oberlander, "The Oregon Health Plan and the Political Paradox of Rationing: What Advocates and Critics have Claimed and what Oregon Did" (1999) 24 *J. Health Politics, Policy & L.* 161.

N.S. Jecker, "Futility and Rationing" (1992) 92 *Am. J. Med.* 189.

C. Johnson Redden, "Rationing Care in the Community: Engaging Citizens in Health Care Decision Making" (1999) 24 *J. Health Politics, Policy & L.* 1363.

M.B. Kapp, "*De Facto* Health-Care Rationing by Age," (1998) 19 *J. Legal Med.* 323.

J.F. Kilner, "Age as a Basis for Allocating Lifesaving Medical Resources: An Ethical Analysis" (1988) 13 *J. Health Politics, Policy & L.* 405.

P.W. Kryworuk, B.T. Butler and A.L. Otten, "Liability in the Allocation of Scarce Health Care Resources" (1996) 16:3 *Health L. in Can.* 65.

P.W. Kryworuk, B.T. Butler and A.L. Otten, "Potential Legal Liability in the Allocation of Scarce Health Care Resources" (1994) 14:4 *Health L. in Can.* 95.

R.G. Lee and F.H. Miller, "The Doctor's Changing Role in Allocating US and British Medical Services" (1990) 18 *L. Med. & Health Care* 69.

H.M. Leichter, "Oregon's Bold Experiment: Whatever Happened to Rationing?" (1999) 24 *J. Health Politics, Policy & L.* 147.

L. Lemieux-Charles, *et al.*, "Ethical Issues Faced by Clinician/Managers in Resource-Allocation Decisions" 38:2 *Hosp. & Health Services Admin.* 267.

F.H. Lowy, "Restructuring Health Care: Rationing and Compromise" (1992) 8 *Humane Med.* 263.

S.M. MacLeod and J. Bienenstock, "Evidence-Based Rationing: Dutch Pragmatism or Government Insensitivity?" (1998) 158 *CMAJ* 213.

A. Maynard, "Distributing Health Care: Rationing and the Role of the Physician in the United Kingdom National Health Service" (1994) 4:2 *Health Matrix* 259.

S. Mhatre and R. Deber, "From Equal Access to Health Care to Equitable Access to Health: A Review of Canadian Provincial Health Commissions and Reports" (1992) 22 *Inter. J. Health Services* 645.

D. Naylor and A.L. Linton, "Allocation of Health Care Resources: A Challenge for the Medical Profession" (1986) 134 *CMAJ* 333.

C. Newdick, "Resource Allocation in the National Health Service" (1997) 23 *Am. J.L. & Med.* 291.

C. Newdick, "Rights to NHS Resources After the 1990 Act" (1993) 1 *Med. L. Rev.* 53.

O.F. Norheim, "Healthcare Rationing: Are Additional Criteria Needed for Assessing Evidence Based Clinical Practice Guidelines?" (1999) 319 *BMJ* 1426.

C. Perry, "When Medical Need Exceeds Medical Resources and When Medical Want Exceeds Medical Need" (1993) 21 *Western State Univ. L. Rev.* 39.

A.K. Rai, "Reflective Choice in Health Care: Using Information Technology to Present Allocation Options" (1999) 25 *Am. J.L. & Med.* 387.

M. Rivet, "Allocation and Rationing of Health Care Resources: Patients' Challenges to Decision-Making" in B. Dickens and M. Ouellette, eds., *Health Care, Ethics and Law* (Montreal: Éditions Thémis, 1993) 17.

D. Sawyer and J. Williams, "Core and Comprehensive Health Care Services: 3. Ethical Issues" (1995) 152 *CMAJ* 1409.

S.A. Schroeder, "Rationing Medical Care—A comparative perspective" (1994) 331 *New Eng. J. Med.* 1089.

H.A. Shenkin, *Current Dilemmas in Medical-Care Rationing: A Pragmatic Approach* (Lanham, MD: Univ. Press of Am., 1996).

G.P. Smith II, "Death be not Proud: Medical, Ethical and Legal Dilemmas in Resource Allocation" (1987) 3 *J. Contemporary Health L. & Policy* 47.

T. Stoltzfus Jost, "Health Care Rationing in the Courts: A Comparative Study" (1998) 21 *Hastings Int'l & Comp. L. Rev.* 639.

R.A. Stradiotto and J.I. Boudreau, "Resource Allocation and Accountability in Health Care" (2000) 20:3 *Health L. in Can.* 40.

"Symposium: Health Care Reform and Rationing" (1993) 21 *Western State Univ. L. Rev.* 1.

J.H. Tingle, "The Allocation of Healthcare Resources in the National Health Service in England: Professional and Legal Issues" (1993) 2 *Ann. Health L.* 195.

P.A. Ubel, R.M. Arnold and A.L. Caplan, "Rationing Failure: The Ethical Lessons of the Retransplantation of Scarce Vital Organs" (1993) 270 *JAMA* 2469.

R.M. Wachter, "Rationing Health Care: Preparing for New Era" (1995) 88 *Southern Medical J.* 25.

L.W. White and M.E. Waithe, "The Ethics of Health Care Rationing as a Strategy of Cost Containment" in J.M. Humber and R.F. Almeder, eds., *Biomedical Ethics Reviews* (Totowa, NJ: Humana Press, 1995) 21.

A.M.F. Wong, "The Inhumanity of Fairness: Rationing Resources for Reconstructive Breast Surgery" (1995) 152 *CMAJ* 577.

G. Yamey, "Health Secretary Admits that NHS Rationing is Government Policy" (2000) 320 *BMJ* 10.

Access

R.J. Anderson, "Seeking Social Justice" (1992) 14 *Health Management Q.* 18.

S. Birch and J. Abelson, "Is Reasonable Access What We Want? Implications of, and Challenges to, Current Canadian Policy on Equity in Health Care" (1993) 23 *Inter. J. Health Services* 629.

British Medical Association, "Access to Health Care for Asylum Seekers Following the Implementation of the Asylum and Immigration Act 1996," online at http://web.bma.org.uk/public/ethics.nsf/39f32339ff78cd6b802566a6003f3311/c2f6a9b8982c05c9802566a6003d5dd6?OpenDocument (accessed on 22 February 2000).

R. Chernomas, "Comments on Birch and Abelson's 'Is Reasonable Access What We Want?'" "Ensuring (E)qual(ity) Health Care for Poor Americans: Symposium" (1994) 60 *Brooklyn L. Rev.* 1–490.

M.A. Hall, "Rationing Health Care at the Bedside" (1994) 69 *NY Univ. L. Rev.* 693.

Health Law and Policy Institute, University of Houston Law Center, "Nonfinancial Barriers to Health Care: Executive Summary," online at http://www.law.uh.edu/healthlaw/nfbstudy.html (accessed on 22 February 2000).

"Institutionalised Racism in Health Care" (1999) 353 *Lancet* 765.

G.L. Larkin, J.E. Weber and A.R. Derse, "Universal Emergency Access under Managed Care: Universal Doubt or Mission Impossible?" (1999) 8 *Cambridge Q. Healthcare Ethics* 213.

M. Lowe, I.H. Kerridge and K.R. Mitchell, "'These sorts of people don't do very well': Race and Allocation of Health Care Resources" (1995) 21 *J. Medical Ethics* 356.

M. Powell, "Ensuring Access to Abortion in an Era of Cutbacks" (1997) 156 *CMAJ* 1545.

T. Reay, "Allocating Scarce Resources in a Publicly Funded Health System: Ethical Considerations of a Canadian Managed Care Proposal" (1999) 6 *Nursing Ethics* 240.

W.M. Sage, "Funding Fairness: Public Investment, Proprietary Rights and Access to Health Care Technology" (1996) 82 *Virginia L. Rev.* 1737.

B. Starfield, "Access—Perceived or Real, and to What?" (1995) 274 *JAMA* 346.

S.D. Watson, "Minority Access and Health Reform: A Civil Right to Health Care" (1994) 22 *J.L. Med. & Ethics* 127.

K.A. White, "Crisis of Conscience: Reconciling Religious Health Care Providers' Beliefs and Patients' Rights" (1999) 51 *Stanford L. Rev.* 1703.

World Medical Association, "World Medical Association Statement on Access to Health Care," online at http://www.wma.net/e/policy/10-70_e.html (accessed on 16 September 1999).

Medically necessary/core health services

T.P. Blanchard, "Medicare Medical Necessity Determinations Revisited: Abuse of Discretion and Abuse of Process in the War Against Medicare Fraud and Abuse" (1999) 43 *Saint Louis Univ. L.J.* 91.

J.T. Boese, "When Angry Patients Become Angry Prosecutors: Medical Necessity Determinations, Quality of Care and the Qui Tam Law" (1999) 43 *Saint Louis Univ. L.J.* 53.

A.V. Campbell, "Defining Core Health Services: The New Zealand Experience" (1995) 9 *Bioethics* 252.

T.A. Caulfield, "Wishful Thinking: Defining 'Medically Necessary' in Canada" (1996) 4 *Health L.J.* 63.

C. Charles, J. Lomas and M. Giacomini, "Medical Necessity in Canadian Health Policy: Four Meanings and a Funeral?" (1997) 75 *Milbank Q.* 365.

L. Forrow, "When Is Home Care Medically Necessary?" (1991) 21:4 *Hastings Ctr. Rep.* 36; discussions 36–8.

E.B. Hirshfeld, "Medical Necessity Determinations: The Need for a New Legal Structure" (1996) 6:1 *Health Matrix* 50.

W.K. Mariner, "Patients' Rights after Health Care Reform: Who Decides What Is Medically Necessary?" (1994) 84 *Am. J. Public Health* 1515.

J. Menikoff, "Demanded Medical Care" (1998) 30 *Ariz. St. L.J.* 1091.

M.M. Rachlis, "Defining Basic Services and De-Insuring the Rest: The Wrong Diagnosis and the Wrong Prescription" (1995) 152 *CMAJ* 1401.

S. Rosenbaum, D.M. Frankford, and B. Moore, "Who Should Determine When Health Care Is Medically Necessary" (1999) 340 *New Eng. J. of Med.* 229.

J.E. Sabin and N. Daniels, "Determining 'Medical Necessity' in Mental Health Practice" (1994) 24:6 *Hastings Ctr. Rep.* 5.

T. Stoltzfus Jost, "The American Difference in Health Care Costs: Is There a Problem? Is Medical Necessity the Solution?" (1999) 43 *Saint Louis Univ. L.J.* 1.

[sh 3] Cases

Auton (Guardian ad litem of) v. *British Columbia (Ministry of Health)* (2000) 78 B.C.L.R. (3d) 55 (B.C.S.C.).

Cameron v. *Nova Scotia (Attorney General)*, [1999] N.S.J. No. 33, 172 N.S.R. (2d) 227 (N.S. S.C.); aff'd (1999), 177 D.L.R. (4th) 6171 (N.S.C.A.).

Right to Health

Brown v. British Columbia (Minister of Health) (1990), 66 D.L.R. (4th) 444.

A. den Exter and H. Hermans, *The Right to Health Care in Several European Countries* (Cambridge, MA: Kluwer Law International, 1999).

S.D. Watson, "Minority Access and Health Reform: A Civil Right to Health Care" (1994) 22 *J.L. Med. & Ethics* 127.

World Medical Association, "World Medical Association Declaration of Ottawa on the Rights of the Child to Health Care," online at http://www.wma.net/e/policy/17-170_e.html (accessed on 16 September 1999).

Specific Populations

A. English, "The New Children's Health Insurance Program: Early Implementation and Issues for Special Populations" (1999) 32:9–10 *Clearinghouse Rev.* 429.

F.M. McClellan, "Is Managed Care Good for What Ails You? Ruminations on Race, Age and Class" (1999) 44 *Villanova L. Rev.* 227.

Chronic populations

J.S. Hacker, "Medicare HMOs: Making Them Work for the Chronically Ill" (1999) 24 *J. Health Politics, Policy & L.* 1230.

J.V. Jacobi, "Canaries in the Coal Mine: the Chronically Ill in Managed Care" (1999) 9:1 *Health Matrix* 79.

S.A. Somers, K. Brodsky and V. Harr, "The Coverage of Chronic Populations Under Medicaid Managed Care: An Essay on Emerging Challenges" (1998) 65 *Tennessee L. Rev.* 649.

Disability

A. Abbe, "'Meaningful Access' to Health Care and the Remedies Available to Medicaid Managed Care Recipients under the ADA and the Rehabilitation Act" (1999) 147 *Univ. Penn. L. Rev.* 1161.

M. Crossley, "Medicaid Managed Care and Disability Discrimination Issues" (1998) 65 *Tennessee L. Rev.* 419.

Elderly

Alberta Medical Association, "Alberta Medical Association Response to *Healthy Aging: New Directions for Care*: Long Term Care Review Final Report of the Policy Advisory Committee," online at http://www.amda.ca/general/health-reform/index.html (accessed on 4 July 2000).

R.H. Binstock, "Older People and Health Care Reform" (1993) 36 *Am. Behavioral Scientist* 823.

R.N. Butler, F.T. Sherman, E. Rhinehart, S. Klein, J.C. Rother, "Managed Care: What to Expect as Medicare-HMO Enrollment Grows" (1996) 51 *Geriatrics* 35.

M.B. Gerety, "Healthcare Reform: Benefits or Hazards for the Frail and Their Doctors" (1995) 43 *JAGS* 718.

M.B. Gerety, "Health Care Reform from the View of a Geriatrician" (1994) 34 *Gerontologist* 590.

R.L. Kane and R.A. Kane, "Effects of the Clinton Health Reform on Older Persons and Their Families: A Health Care Systems Perspective" (1994) 34 *Gerontologist* 598.

M.B. Kapp, "*De Facto* Health-Care Rationing by Age," (1998) 19 *J. Legal Med.* 323.

M.B. Kapp, "Health Care Delivery and the Elderly: Teaching Old Patients New Tricks" (1987) 17 *Cumberland L. Rev.* 437.

J.L. O'Sullivan, "Managed Care and the Elderly" (1998) 31 *Maryland Bar J.* 18.

D.C. Rasinski-Gregory and M. Piven Cotler, "The Elderly and Health Care Reform: Needs, Concerns, Responsibilities and Obligations" (1993) 21 *Western State Univ. L. Rev.* 65.

G.P. Smith, *Legal and Healthcare Ethics for the Elderly* (Washington, DC: Taylor & Francis, 1996).

E.H. Wagner, "The Promise and Performance of HMOs in Improving Outcomes in Older Adults" (1996) 44 *JAGS* 1251.

Ethnicity/race

L. Patrick-Cooper, "Race, Gender, and Partnership in the Patient-Physician Relationship" (1999) 282 *JAMA* 583.

Gender

Association féminine d'éducation et d'action sociale, *et al.*, *Who Will Be Responsible for Providing Care? The Impact of the Shift to Ambulatory Care and of Social Economy Policies on Quebec Women* (March 1998).

C.M.T. Gijsbers Van Wijk, K.P. Van Vliet and A.M. Kolk, "Gender Perspectives and Quality of Care: Towards Appropriate and Adequate Health Care for Women" (1996) 43 *Soc. Sci. Med.* 707.

M. Harrington Meyer and E.K. Pavalko, "Family, Work, and Access to Health Insurance Among Mature Women" (1996) 37 *J. Health & Social Behavior* 311.

Ministry of Health and Ministry Responsible for Seniors, Women's Health Bureau, *Women's Health in the Context of Restructuring: summary report* (Victoria, BC: Ministry of Health and Ministry Responsible for Seniors, Women's Health Bureau, 1998).

K.L. Moss, ed., *Man-Made Medicine: Women's Health, Public Policy, and Reform* (Durham: Duke Univ. Press, 1996).

National Forum on Health, "An Overview of Women's Health" in National Forum on Health, *Canada Health Action: Building on the Legacy, Volume II: Synthesis Reports and Issues Papers* (Ottawa: National Forum on Health, 1997).

M. Oberman and M. Schaps, "Women's Health and Managed Care" (1998) 65 *Tennessee L. Rev.* 555.

L. Patrick-Cooper, "Race, Gender, and Partnership in the Patient-Physician Relationship" (1999) 282 *JAMA* 583.

T.F. Theodos, "The Patients' Bill of Rights: Women's Rights Under Managed Care and ERISA Preemption" (2000) 26 *Am. J.L. & Med.* 89.

C. Ungerson, "Gender, Cash and Informal Care: European Perspectives and Dilemmas" (1995) 24 *J. Soc. Pol.* 31.

United Nations World Health Organization and United Nations Population Fund, *Women and Health: Mainstreaming the Gender Perspective into the Health Sector* (Report of the Expert Group Meeting 28 September–2 October 1998, Tunis (United Nations, 1999).

Studies
(*see also* managed care, empirical studies)

A.B. Bindman, K. Grumbach, D. Osmond, M. Komaromy, K. Vranizan, N. Lurie, J. Billings and A. Stewart, "Preventable Hospitalizations and Access to Health Care" (1995) 274 *JAMA* 305.

R.J. Blendon, *et al.*, "Physicians' Perspectives on Caring for Patients in the United States, Canada, and West Germany" (1993) 328 *New Eng. J. Med.* 1011.

M. Demers, "Frequent Users of Ambulatory Health Care in Quebec: The Case of Doctor-Shoppers" (1995) 153 *CMAJ* 37.

T.M. Gill and A.R. Feinstein, "A Critical Appraisal of the Quality of Quality-of-Life Measurements" (1994) 272 *JAMA* 619.

M. Goldszmidt, C. Levitt, E. Duarte-Franco and J. Kaczorowski, "Complementary Health Care Services: A Survey of General Practitioners' Views" (1995) 153 *CMAJ* 29.

H. Kattlove, A. Liberati, E. Keeler and R.H. Brook, "Benefits and Costs of Screening and Treatment for Early Breast Cancer: Development of a Basic Benefit Package" (1995) 273 *JAMA* 142.

S.J. Katz and T.P. Hofer, "Socioeconomic Disparities in Preventive Care Persist Despite Universal Coverage: Breast and Cervical Cancer Screening in Ontario and the United States" (1994) 272 *JAMA* 530.

G.R. Langley, A.M. MacLellan, H.J. Sutherland and J.E. Till, "Effect of Nonmedical Factors on Family Physicians' Decisions About Referral for Consultation" (1992) 147 *CMAJ* 659.

J.L. Reichert, "Many Doctors Pressured to Wear too Many Hats, Study Says" (2000) 36:3 *Trial* 110.

R. Sturm and K.B. Wells, "How Can Care for Depression Become More Cost-Effective?" (1995) 273 *JAMA* 51.

P.A. Ubel, R.M. Arnold and A.L. Caplan, "Rationing Failure: The Ethical Lessons of the Retransplantation of Scarce Vital Organs" (1993) 270 *JAMA* 2469.

P.F.M.M. van Bergen, J.J.C. Jonker, B.A. van Hout, R.T. van Domburg, J.W. Deckers, A.J. Azar and A. Hofman, "Costs and Effects of Long-term Oral Anticoagulant Treatment After Myocardial Infarction" (1995) 273 *JAMA* 925.

C. Vincent, M. Young and A. Phillips, "Why Do People Sue Doctors? A Study of Patients and Relatives Taking Legal Action" (1994) 343 *Lancet* 1609.

R.M. Wachter, J.M. Luce, S. Safrin, D.C. Berrios, E. Charlebois and A.A. Scitovsky, "Cost and Outcome of Intensive Care for Patients With AIDS, *Pneumocystis carinii* Pneumonia, and Severe Respiratory Failure" (1995) 273 *JAMA* 230.

Telehealth

J.D. Blum, "Telemedicine Poses New Challenges for the Law" (1999) 20:1 *Health L. in Canada* 115.

D.D. Bradham, S. Morgan and M.E. Dailey, "The Information Superhighway: A Critical Discussion of its Possibilities and Legal Implications" (1995) 30 *Wake Forest L. Rev.* 145.

C. Chase, "How Will the Internet Change our Health System?" (2000) 19:1 *Health Affairs* 148.

E.R. Cohen, "The Brave New World of Internet Telemedicine" (1999) 158 *New Jersey L.J.* 33.

J.F. Daar and S. Koerner, "Telemedicine: Legal and Practical Implications" (1997) 19 *Whittier L. Rev.* 3.

A.P. Frank, *et al.*, "Anonymous HIV Testing Using Home Collection and Telemedicine Counseling" (1997) 157 *Arch. Intern. Med.* 309.

L.S. Goldsmith, "New Health Care Liabilities in the New Millennium" (2000) 23:1 *Trial Lawyer* 21.

J. Grigsby and J.H. Sanders, "Telemedicine: Where It Is and Where It's Going" (1998) 129 *Ann. Intern. Med.* 123.

C. Guttman-McCabe, "Telemedicine's Imperiled Future? Funding, Reimbursement, Licensing and Privacy Hurdles Face a Developing Technology" (1997) 14 *J. Contemporary Health L. & Policy* 161.

P.C. Kuszler, "Telemedicine and Integrated Health Care Delivery: Compounding Malpractice Liability" (1999) 25 *Am. J.L. & Med.* 297.

D.A.B. Lindberg and B.L. Humphreys, "Medical Informatics" (1997) 277 *JAMA* 1870.

K.D. Mandl, I.S. Kohane and A.M. Brandt "Electronic Patient-Physician Communication: Problems and Promise" (1998) 129 *Ann. Intern. Med.* 495.

D.F. Meek, "Telemedicine: How an Apple (or Another Computer) May Bring Your Doctor Closer" (1998) 29 *Cumberland L. Rev.* 173.

R.W. Pong and J.C. Hogenbirk, "Licensing Physicians for Telehealth Practice: Issues and Policy Options" (1999) 8:1 *Health L. Rev.* 3.

R.W. Pong and J.C. Hogenbirk, "Reimbursing Physicians for Telehealth Practice: Issues and Policy Options" (2000) 9:1 *Health L. Rev.* 3.

R. Porter, "Internet Pharmacies: Who's Minding the Store" (2000) 36:5 *Trial* 12.

C.M. Rackett, "Telemedicine Today and Tomorrow: Why 'Virtual' Privacy is Not Enough" (1997) 25 *Fordham Urban L.J.* 167.

J.B. Rosenblum, "A Telemedicine Primer" (1999) 45:3 *The Practical Lawyer* 23.

A.J. Rosoff, "Informed Consent in the Electronic Age" (1999) 25 *Am. J.L. & Med.* 367.

S. Savkar and R.J. Waters, "Telemedicine: Implications for Patient Confidentiality and Privacy" (1995), online at http://www.arentfox.com/quickguide/businesslines/e-health/e-health_telemed/e-healthnewsalerts/licenseimplic/licenseimplic.html (accessed on 22 February 2000).

F.J. Serbaroli, "Telemedicine and the Internet" (1999) 222 *NY L.J.* 3.

A.R. Spielberg, "Online Without a Net: Physician-Patient Communications by Electronic Mail" (1999) 25 *Am. J.L. & Med.* 267.

A.M. Sulentic, "Crossing Borders: The Licensure of Interstate Telemedicine Practitioners" (1999) 25 *J. Legislation* 1.

N.P. Terry, "Cyber-Malpractice: Legal Exposure for Cybermedicine" (1999) 25 *Am. J.L. & Med.* 327.

United States Department of Commerce, "Telemedicine Report to Congress" (31 January 1997), online at http://www.ntia.doc.gov/reports/telemed/cover.htm (accessed on 27 July 1999).

R.V. Wiesemann, "On-Line or On-Call? Legal and Ethical Challenges Emerging in Cybermedicine" (1999) 43 *St. Louis Univ. L.J.* 1119.

World Medical Association, "World Medical Association Statement on Home Medical Monitoring, 'Tele-Medicine' and Medical Ethics," online at http://www.wma.net/e/policy/17-35_e.html (accessed on 16 September 1999).

C.J. Young, "Telemedicine: Patient Privacy Rights of Electronic Medical Records" (1998) 66 *UMKC L. Rev.* 921.

Tort Law/Liability
(*see also* Managed Care, Liability)

K. Barker, "NHS Contracting: Shadows in the Law of Tort?" (1995) 3 *Med. L. Rev.* 161.

B. Chapman, "Controlling the Costs of Medical Malpractice: An Argument for Strict Hospital Liability" (1990) 28 *Osgoode Hall L.J.* 523.

P.M. Danzon, "The Swedish Patient Compensation System" (1994) 15 *J. Legal Med.* 199.

R.G. Elgie, T.A. Caulfield and M.I. Christie, "Medical Injuries and Malpractice: Is it Time for 'No Fault?'" (1993) 1 *Health L.J.* 97.

C. Feasby, "Determining Standard of Care in Alternative Contexts" (1997) 5 *Health L.J.* 45.

L.S. Goldsmith, "New Health Care Liabilities in the New Millennium" (2000) 23:1 *Trial Lawyer* 21.

G. Javitt and E. Lu, "Capping the Crisis: Medical Malpractice and Tort Reform" (1992) *L. Med. & Health Care* 258.

P.W. Kryworuk, B.T. Butler and A.L. Otten, "Liability in the Allocation of Scarce Health Care Resources" (1996) 16:3 *Health L. in Can.* 65.

P.W. Kryworuk, B.T. Butler and A.L. Otten, "Potential Legal Liability in the Allocation of Scarce Health Care Resources" (1994) 14:4 *Health L. in Can.* 95.

P.C. Kuszler, "Telemedicine and Integrated Health Care Delivery: Compounding Malpractice Liability" (1999) 25 *Am. J.L. & Med.* 297.

J.R. Matthews, "Practice Guidelines and Tort Reform: The Legal System Confronts the Technocratic Wish" (1999) 24 *J. Health Politics, Policy & L.* 275.

E.H. Morreim, "Cost Containment and the Standard of Medical Care" (1987) 75 *Cal. L. Rev.* 1719.

E.H. Morreim, "Stratified Scarcity: Redefining the Standard of Care" (1989) 17 *L. Med. & Health Care* 356.

E.H. Morreim, "Whodunit? Causal Responsibility of Utilization Review for Physicians' Decisions, Patients' Outcomes" (1992) 20 *L. Med. & Health Care* 40.

N. Priday, "The Effect of the Nature of the Health Care System on Malpractice Jurisprudence in Canada and the United States" (1994) 15 *Health L. in Can.* 10.

G.B. Robertson, "The Efficacy of the Medical Malpractice System: A Canadian Perspective" (1994) 3 *Ann. Health L.* 167.

C.E. Schneider, "Regulating Doctors" (1999) 29:4 *Hastings Ctr. Rep.* 21.

N.J. Squillante, "Expanding the Potential Tort Liability of Physicians: A Legal Portrait of 'Nontraditional Patients' and Proposals for Change" (1993) 40 *UCLA L. Rev.* 1617.

N.P. Terry, "Cyber-Malpractice: Legal Exposure for Cybermedicine" (1999) 25 *Am. J.L. & Med.* 327.

P.C. Weiler, J.P. Newhouse and H.H. Hiatt, "Proposal for Medical Liability Reform" (1992) 267 *JAMA* 2355.

R.B. Whitehead, "The Effect of Malpractice Legislation on the Doctor-Patient Relationship" (1993) 40 *Medical Trial Technique Q.* 170.

Trade Agreements

Friends of Medicare, "#6 Canadian Medicare and the International Trade Agreements" (January 2000), online at http://www.friendsofmedicare.ab.ca/1999/kleinagenda/agenda6.htm (accessed on 21 January 2000).

P. Goldman, "The Legal Effect of Trade Agreements on Domestic Health and Environmental Regulation" (1992) 7 *J. Environmental L. & Litigation* 11.

Gottlieb and Pearson, "International trade standards and the regulatory powers of governments at the end of the 20th century, with special emphasis on public health standards and the Canadian public health system," online at http://www.healthcoalition.ca/gottlieb.html.

E-H.W. Kluge, "Competition and Function: The Canada-US Free Trade Agreement and the Philosophy of Health Care" (1991) 10 *Business & Professional Ethics J.* 29.

Opinion Letter re. Bill 11-Health Care Protection Act and the NAFTA, Cruickshank Karvellas (23 March 2000), online at http://www.gov.ab.ca/acn/images/2000/400/8972.pdf (accessed on 22 August 2000).

Opinion Letter re. NAFTA Investment Chapter Implications of Alberta Bill-11, Appleton & Associates (10 April 2000), online at http://www.appletonlaw.com/cases/AltaGovtBll-Appleton.PDF (accessed on 22 August 2000).

B. Schwartz, "How Possible Increases in the Scope of the Agreement on Internal Trade Would Affect the Health and Social Services Sectors" (1998) 7:2 *Health L. Rev.* 3.

B. Schwartz, "NAFTA Reservations in the Areas of Health Care" (1997) 5 *Health L. J.* 99.

S. Shrybman, "A Legal Opinion Concerning NAFTA Investment and Services Disciplines and Bill 11: Proposals by Alberta to Privatize the Delivery of Certain Insured Health Care Services," online at http://www.cupe.ca/Shrybman/ (accessed on 23 August 2000).

Waiting Lists

D.A. Alter, *et al.*, "Fairness in the coronary angiography queue" (1999) 161 *CMAJ* 813.

British Columbia Medical Association, "Wait List Report," online at http://www.bcma.org/concerns/waitlist.asp (accessed on 19 June 2000).

Canadian Medical Association, "Operational Principles for the Measurement and Management of Waiting Lists," online at http://www.cma.ca/inside/policybase/1999/11-27.htm (accessed on 30 June 2000).

D.C. Hadorn, "What Can Comparisons of Mortality Rates Tell Us About Waiting Lists?" (2000) 21 *CMAJ* 794.

H. Kent, "Waiting-list Web site 'inaccurate' and 'misleading,' BC doctors complain" (1999) 161 *CMAJ* 181.

E. LeBourdais, "Preferential treatment for WCB patients angers some MDs" (1999) 161 CMAJ 859.

S. Lewis, *et al.*, "Ending Waiting-List Mismanagement: Principles and Practice" (2000) 162 *CMAJ* 1297.

C.D. Naylor, J.P. Szalai and M. Katic, "Benchmarking the Vital Risk of Waiting for Coronary Artery Bypass Surgery in Ontario" (2000) 162 *CMAJ* 775.

"New Cures For the Queue: Lining up to Treat Health Care's Long Waits" (Spring 2000) 3:1 *Health Policy Forum* 24.

S.E.D. Shortt, "Waiting for medical care: Is it who you know that counts?" (1999) 161 *CMAJ* 823.

D. Spurgeon, "Patients with Cancer Asked to Sign Waivers on Dangers of Delays" (2000) 320 *BMJ* 203.